Test Question Logic

(TQLogic™) for Beginning Nursing Students

FOURTH REVISED EDITION

PATRICIA A. HOEFLER, M.S.N., R.N.
AUTHOR

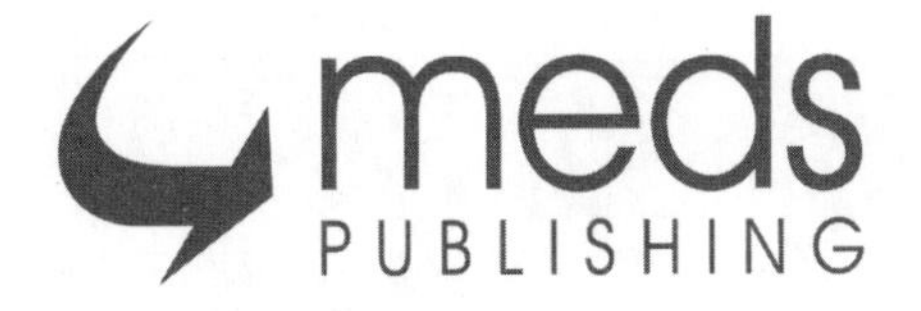

MEDICAL EDUCATION DEVELOPMENT SERVICES
7901 Sandy Spring Road, Suite 203
Laurel, MD 20707
www.medspub.com

Editor: Mark Williams-Abrams

FOURTH REVISED EDITION 2005

The author and the publisher have prepared this work for student nurses. Care has been taken to confirm the accuracy of the information presented and to describe generally-accepted practices. Nevertheless, it is difficult to ensure that all the information presented is entirely accurate for all circumstances, and the authors and the publisher cannot accept any responsibility for any errors or omissions. The authors and the publisher make no warranty, express or implied, with respect to this work, and disclaim any liability, loss, or damage as a consequence, directly or indirectly, of the use and application of any of the contents of this work.

Copies of this book may be obtained from:
MEDICAL EDUCATION DEVELOPMENT SERVICES
7901 Sandy Spring Road, Suite 203
Laurel, Maryland 20707
www.medspub.com

ISBN: 1-56533-506-6
Printed in the United States of America.

Table of Contents

Introduction

Why a Book on Problem-Solving and Test-Taking for Nursing Students?

The purpose of this book is to help you to become a successful and confident professional nurse. To do this, you need to succeed in your nursing courses and exams—and, when you graduate, on the NCLEX exam for licensure.

To succeed as a nursing student and as a professional nurse, you need to develop your ability to apply the *nursing process.* The nursing process is the method that professional nurses use *to solve clinical problems and apply nursing knowledge.* Learning to use the nursing process is a central focus of this book.

This book will show you how to identify clinical problems and compare solutions. It will also teach you the special test-taking, time management and study skills that you need to succeed in your nursing education program. Time management is a critical issue for so many of today's nursing students who have jobs and families in addition to their nursing studies.

The study and review techniques in this book will actually save you time and help you get the most out of your nursing program.

In the past, problem-solving and test-taking were not taught in most nursing programs. There just didn't seem to be a place for them in the curriculum. Today, though, they are recognized by nurse educators as *essential professional skills* that nurses will need throughout their careers.

Why Are Nursing Exams So Hard?

Nursing students from all backgrounds tell us that nursing exams are very difficult. And it's true!

Nursing exams are different, and more difficult, because *nursing requires constant problem solving.* Nurses must constantly make decisions and set priorities.

On nursing exams, you have to identify clinical problems and choose the best solution. So just remembering nursing information isn't enough. You also need top-notch problem-solving skills. Nursing exams test your *nursing judgment.* You need special skills to demonstrate your nursing judgment on a multiple choice exam.

Nursing instructors frequently hear beginning nursing students say:

- "I do very well clinically. However, when it come to the nursing exams, I do poorly."
- "Sometimes the amount of material covered on an exam is overwhelming! I study very hard, but my nursing grades do not show it."
- "I get excellent grades clinically, but the results on my nursing exams decrease my overall grade in nursing."

Does this sound like you? Well, you are not alone—and this book has the help you need to succeed in your nursing courses and on your exams.

If you would like to become more skilled—and more confident—at taking nursing exams, this book is just what you need.

Are There Special Test-Taking Skills for Nursing Exams?

No one likes taking exams, and nursing students are no exception.

Nursing students find their multiple choice examinations to be anxiety-provoking. The questions ask you to solve urgent or complex problems. Sometimes it is hard to understand what the question is asking. It is often hard to choose between the options. And what can you do when you just don't know the answer?

Do you become confused when a question presents a clinical scenario and asks you to "identify the manifestation that should receive the nurse's immediate attention"? What about questions that ask you to "select the highest (or lowest) priority nursing intervention" in a clinical scenario?

Sometimes a question gives you so much information that it's hard to tell which facts are most important. And sometimes you find a question that seems to have two, three, or even four correct answers!

Students often think these questions are "trick questions." But the questions on nursing exams actually use a special kind of "test-taking logic." For example, in a clinical situation, many actions might be *appropriate;* however, on an exam only one action can be the *best* or *priority* action. This is how the exam tests your *nursing judgment* as well as your nursing knowledge. It is very important to know how to go about answering judgment questions!

The good news is that there are special test-taking skills to help you answer these difficult questions. These skills will give you a new way to approach a nursing test question. With these skills, you can focus on answering the question, and not become distracted or confused. Using these skills, you will be able to *make the most of your nursing knowledge* on an exam.

Are There Special Study Skills for Nursing Exams, Too?

Absolutely!

Preparing for an exam that goes beyond just recalling facts requires a special approach.

To solve a problem presented in a nursing exam question, you use the nursing process. If you use the nursing process when *reviewing* nursing content, you will be well prepared for the exam. This book will show you how to do this. This book will also give you tips on time-saving ways to prepare for class and how to take good class notes.

Can Everyone Learn To Be A Good Test Taker?

Yes! The good news is that becoming a test-wise nursing student or NCLEX candidate is a skill you can learn!

Learning how to do well on nursing exams is a skill like learning a musical instrument or a sport. Becoming a musician or an athlete involves learning skills that must be developed over time with skilled instruction. You can learn to become a good test-taker with the right tips and enough practice. Think of this book as a coaching session by an expert who will "teach you the ropes" and offer tips and suggestions to help you do your best.

As with any other skill, "practice makes perfect"—so we have provided drill questions and a "Final Exam" to help you practice your new skills. As you use these practice questions, you will see how the techniques work, and you will increase your confidence as a test-taker.

What is the NCLEX Examination?

Issued by the National Council of State Boards of Nursing, the NCLEX is designed to test competence: knowledge, skills, and abilities essential to the safe and effective practice of nursing at the entry level for both RN and PN candidates.

NCLEX exam results are an important component used by boards of nursing to make decisions about licensure. Only state boards of nursing can release NCLEX exam results to candidates.

The NCLEX examination is administered in the United States, American Samoa, Guam, the Northern Mariana Islands, Puerto Rico, and the Virgin Islands. The use of the same exam by all jurisdictions facilitates licensure by endorsement from one board of nursing to another.

The National Council posts a bulletin on its website, www.ncsbn.org, to address the many questions candidates have about the NCLEX. Online test plans explain the manner in which cognitive ability, integrated concepts and processes are tested. They provide a valuable break-down of NCLEX content distribution. The site also reports on any upcoming pilot studies, anticipated policy or exam changes.

Computerized Adaptive Testing and the NCLEX

Pencil and paper are out for those taking the NCLEX exam. Computerized Adaptive Testing (CAT) is in!

The National Council's position is that CAT provides a more accurate measure of a candidate's competency determined by the *difficulty* of questions answered correctly, *not* by *how many* questions are answered correctly.

NCLEX questions are all multiple choice, designed to assess the candidates problem solving skills and cognitive abilities. There are some 3,000 items in the NCLEX pool. Test items include making client assignments, prioritizing care and analyzing complex client data to determine the appropriate nursing response.

With CAT, each candidate's test is unique: it is assembled interactively as the individual is tested.

As the candidate answers each question, the computer calculates a competence estimate based on all earlier answers. The exam is constructed to recognize that each candidate will have strengths and weaknesses in particular subject areas. A question determined to measure the candidate's ability most precisely in the appropriate test plan area is selected. The process is repeated for each question, creating an examination tailored to the individual's knowledge and skills while fulfilling all NCLEX test plan requirements. The examination continues in this way until a pass or fail decision is made.

An RN candidate must answer a minimum of 75 questions (from a total of 265); A PN candidate must answer a minimum 85 questions (from a total of 205). The maximum testing time is five hours.

Prep and Practice with MEDS

Clearly, it is advantageous for you to prepare for the computerized NCLEX with simulation NCLEX-style exams like those published by meds (see product index). As future nurses you must leave your technology fears behind, get on the computer, pop in the meds companion exam disk and practice, practice, practice!

Now, let's resume preparation and get on with *Test Question Logic for Beginning Nursing Students.*

Can This Book Really Help Me Pass the NCLEX exam?

Yes, it can! Thousands of nursing students across the United States and Canada have increased their test scores using the techniques in this book.

Research has shown that *the test-wise candidate will score higher, on average, than the less skilled test-taker* every time. This is also true for nursing exams. If you know how to prepare for an exam and have good test-taking skills, you will be able to *make the most of your nursing knowledge* when you take an exam.

Nursing exams are difficult—but they are only multiple choice exams! If you have the ability to do well clinically, you have the ability to do well on exams. By becoming a skilled problem solver and test-taker and learning how to prepare for an exam, you can decrease your test-taking anxiety and increase your test scores.

What Are the Main Skills Needed to Answer Nursing Exam Questions?

The questions on nursing exams go beyond testing your ability to *recall* nursing information. They are designed to test your *comprehension* and your ability to *apply* your nursing knowledge. In fact, they are designed to test your *competency to practice nursing safely.* For this reason, nursing exams have their own distinctive characteristics and use several *different types of questions* when testing a given clinical area.

On nursing exams, you will find the questions you probably expect—questions about body mechanics, ambulating and transferring clients, safety and infection control, in addition to questions about pathophysiology, medications, nursing interventions and their rationales, and how to provide pre- and post-operative care.

However, an exam in any clinical area may also include communication questions as well as questions about client teaching, privacy and client rights, and special aspects of providing care to infants and children, pregnant clients and new mothers, elderly clients, clients with sensory impairments, confused clients, or clients with other special needs. In fact, you may need to apply your knowledge of everything from growth and development to special diets!

You will need special study skills to *prepare* for this kind of an exam, in addition to special test-taking techniques. We will show you how to organize your study and review of your course materials, and we will teach you the skills you need to answer the test questions. The key to answering complex nursing exam questions is *knowing how to identify what they are really about*! In this book, you will learn a quick method for correctly interpreting a test questions. You will also learn special guidelines for answering communication questions and questions that select priorities. And we will focus on *using the nursing process to identify and solve the different types of nursing problems* described in these questions. With good test-taking skills and careful preparation, you can "ace" your nursing exams!

What Will I Get Out Of This Book?

This book will show you how to prepare for class, take good lecture notes, and review nursing content. It will show you how to use the nursing process to become a good problem solver. And it will give you the test-taking techniques you need to succeed!

Test Question Logic for Beginning Nursing Students teaches the specialized three-step method developed by MEDS Publishing for correctly interpreting test questions. We developed this method over more than a decade of grass-roots experience. It has been perfected in our NCLEX review courses and test-taking workshops. Using this method, thousands of nursing students have increased their exam scores and passed the NCLEX on their first try.

As a skilled test-taker, you will not become confused or distracted when answering complex questions. You will know how to use pacing strategy to make the most of the time allowed for an exam. Mastering these skills will also increase your confidence and decrease your anxiety when taking an exam.

Test Question Logic for Beginning Nursing Students unlocks the mysteries of the unique "test-taking logic" of nursing exams. With MEDS Publishing's unique strategies, you will be able to decode even the most difficult questions and decide between possible options.

As you will see, all of the skills and techniques presented in this book respect the nursing profession and use the nursing process. The nursing educators at MEDS Publishing hope that this book will be interesting as well as helpful for nursing students from all backgrounds. We hope you will enjoy *Test Question Logic for Beginning Nursing Students*—and we wish you much success and fulfillment in your nursing career.

Sincerely,

Patricia A. Hoefler, M.S.N., R.N.
President
MEDS Publishing

Chapter 1

HOW TO USE THIS BOOK

Learning Objectives

Test Question Logic for Beginning Nursing Students will teach you the specialized skills you need to increase your scores on nursing course exams. It will also help improve your professional problem-solving skills and become a better and more confident professional nurse!

This book will show you how to:

- ✓ "Study smarter" for your nursing courses.
- ✓ Plan your review of nursing content at exam time.
- ✓ Correctly interpret a multiple choice nursing test question by using a quick 3-step method.
- ✓ Identify what a test question is really asking about.
- ✓ Apply a selection procedure to eliminate "distractors" (incorrect options).
- ✓ Compare possible answers in a logical way.
- ✓ Use test-taking strategies to select the best answer when you are unsure.
- ✓ Apply special guidelines for answering communication questions, questions that select nursing priorities, and questions that focus on the nursing process.
- ✓ Pace yourself on a timed exam.

How This Book Is Organized

You can "study smarter"—starting today!—by taking just a few moments to see how this book is organized.

If you haven't read the **Introduction,** this would be a good time to stop and read it, because it will give you a better idea of *how this book can help you. Of special interest* is the Q&A on the NCLEX exam.

Chapter One provides an explanation of *how to study and use the material in this book.*

It is very important to read **Chapter Two, "How to Study for a Nursing Exam."** This chapter shows you *how to "study smarter"*—starting on the first day of class—as well as *how to review material and prepare for a final exam.* In addition, there are valuable *time management tips* in this chapter to show you how to stay "on top" of your assignments and how to get the most out of your study time. Be sure to note that the study methods in this book use the *nursing process*—and Chapter Two is about special study methods for *nursing students.* So even if you have always been a good student, you will benefit from the special tips for the new challenges you will face in nursing school. NOTE: Be sure to read Chapter Two BEFORE you read the chapters on the test-taking strategies!

Chapters Three through Seven present the powerful *test-taking strategies* developed in the MEDS' test-taking workshops and Live NCLEX Review courses. BE SURE TO READ THESE CHAPTERS IN ORDER!

Chapter Three, "How Do I Avoid 'Reading Into' a Test Question?" explains the unique *"test-question logic"* used in nursing exams. Students "read into" a test question by assuming information that is not actually given. This can happen when you misinterpret the question. This chapter will show you a quick three-step method for understanding what each test question is really asking. *This is the most basic and the most important test-taking chapter.*

Chapter Four, "How Do I Choose Between the Two Best Options?" shows you how to use three powerful test-taking strategies. There is only one *best* option in each question. These strategies will help you to identify it!

Chapter Five, "Learning to Answer Communication Questions," provides some useful insight into what makes these questions tick. To succeed in your nursing courses and on the NCLEX, it is *essential* to be able to demonstrate that you can *communicate effectively with the client.* In this chapter you will learn some simple guidelines to follow when selecting your answer to a complex communication question.

Chapter Six, "Learning to Answer Questions that Select Priorities," will show you *how to apply priority-setting guidelines.* "What should the nurse do first?" "What is the priority nursing action at this time?" This chapter is *essential* for your success as a nursing student. Learn these guidelines now, and use them on your course exams. Priority-setting questions don't have to be so confusing!

Chapter Seven, "Learning to Answer Questions that Focus on the Nursing Process," shows you *how to use the nursing process as a problem solving and test-taking guideline.* You will also learn to identify key words in a question that are signals to apply the nursing process to select the correct answer. Nursing students tell us that this chapter explains a lot about how nursing exams work!

Chapter Eight, "How to Take a Timed Exam," shows you how to use a simple *pacing* method. When taking a timed exam, it is important to pace yourself so that you will have enough time to complete the exam and avoid getting stalled or "hung up" on any one question. Pacing strategy has been proven to decrease students' test-taking stress and anxiety—and increase their scores.

When you have completed the chapters on test-taking strategies, be sure to take the **"Final Exam"** in **Chapter Nine.** Use this 50-question practice exam to see for yourself how helpful your new test-taking skills can be. Be sure to time yourself and use your pacing strategy, too.

NOTE: Be sure to try using the *Test Smart* CD-ROM enclosed with this book

Using this CD-ROM, you can select either Open Book mode, to view the rationales instantly—or Assessment mode, with automatic scoring and a computerized Personal Performance Analysis.

Chapter Ten, "Final Exam Answers and Analysis," provides complete nursing rationales for each correct and incorrect answer to every question in the Final Exam. These complete rationales are hallmarks of MEDS Publishing nursing education materials and are included for maximum learning. Test-taking tips are also provided, so you can see exactly how to use the strategies you have learned.

Practice makes perfect! **Chapter Eleven, "Drill Questions on Fundamental Nursing Concepts,"** provides a good sampling of practice test questions arranged according to basic nursing topic. Use these questions to polish your new test-taking skills and to review for your nursing exams. Complete rationales are included in **Chapter Twelve**.

We hope this brief guided tour of *Test Question Logic for Beginning Nursing Students* has given you a good idea of what you will learn from this book and how you can use it. Whether you are studying this book in a nursing class or on your own, you are already well on your way to becoming a better nursing student and improving your scores on nursing exams.

Chapter 2

HOW TO STUDY FOR A NURSING EXAM

Isn't it true that you begin your preparation for a nursing exam *on the first day of class?* After all, don't you usually review your class notes when you review for the exam?

You are preparing for the exam when you take notes and ask questions in class. You are preparing for the exam when you read assigned chapters in your textbook. With a few tips on how to prepare well for class, taking good notes, and using the right review techniques, *you can save time and be more successful.*

The good news is that good students aren't born—they have a method!

Time Management: Preparing for Class

Students today are very busy. Many students complain that they never have time to read the text ahead of time. It is very important, however, to prepare for class. Even if you have *only a few minutes* to spend, a little preparation will go a long way.

If you will take just a few minutes to look at the chapter before you go to class, you will understand more—and you will save time later. In fact, studies have shown that it can cut your study time *in half.* So be sure to prepare!

A Quick Method for Preparing for Class

1. Previewing the Chapter

Think of this as watching "Coming Attractions" at your neighborhood movie theater!

First, look at the chapter and just read the section headings. DON'T STOP TO READ ANYTHING NOW! Your goal is simply to identify what content is being covered.

Then, look at any charts or illustrations, and read the captions.

Certainly you can make the time to do at least this much before class!

2. A Quick Read-Through of the Chapter

Next, read the chapter through once—quickly!

Identify basic concepts and the most important information. Look for words in bold print. At this point, your goal is to gain a GENERAL UNDERSTANDING of the content, not to memorize it! So relax, and just see what it is about. Trust yourself to read quickly. It actually increases your understanding and your memory. This fact is the basis of those expensive "speed-reading" courses. Try it—it works!

Don't get bogged down in difficult sections! After all, you haven't even heard the lecture yet.

Try to write down any questions you have at this time—but be very brief. This is an important learning technique. Your questions will probably be answered during the lecture. If not, you will be prepared to ask the instructor for an answer—and you will be sure to remember it.

3. A Quick Review of the Chapter

After you finish your first reading, take one more minute to look again at the headings and illustrations.

This quick review will significantly increase your longer-term memory. This is another tip from the speed-reading experts. Professionals in all fields as well as in the business world use this technique to be successful. Make this a habit!

How to Take Notes in Class

Your nursing instructor's goal when giving a lecture or other presentation is to make the content *easier to understand*. The instructor will include explanations and will clarify ideas and information included in your textbook.
When taking notes, your object should also be to *clarify*. Here are some basic guidelines for good note-taking:

Guidelines for Taking Good Class Notes

1. **Always be sure you know *what is being discussed*.**

   This may seem obvious. However, but it isn't always easy to state the subject of a discussion!

   Here are some possible topics related to the study of a health problem:

   - Incidence and Etiology
   - Pathophysiology
   - Signs and symptoms
   - Side effects and adverse effects of treatments
   - Complications
   - Nursing interventions, including prioritizing
   - Client teaching

   Previewing the chapter before class will definitely help you to follow the lecture!

2. **Be sure you understand the *rationale* for a treatment or intervention.**

   You can look at the textbook later for the details—but *always be sure to ask a question if there is something that you don't understand.*

   Asking a question can cut your study time in half!

3. **Make sure you understand the *priorities:* What is *most important*?**

   One clue would be any visual aids that the instructor uses, such as charts, illustrations, or notes written on the board.

4. **Listen for the answers to any questions you wrote down when you were preparing for the class.**

   If one of your questions is not answered during the lecture, be sure to take this opportunity to ask it.

5. **Stay focused on the topic, and try to be analytical.**

   Remember, your goal in taking notes is to clarify information.

   Note taking is not the same as taking dictation! Don't try to record everything that the instructor says.

   If you are having a lot of difficulty following the discussion in one of your classes, talk with the instructor about it. You can also try bringing a tape recorder—listening to the discussion again later may clarify critical points.

6. **If you do not understand something that is presented in class, be sure to ask a question.**

If something is not clear to you, it is probably unclear to others as well—especially if you have prepared for the class.

Never leave a classroom if you are unclear about the information! When you don't understand something, *always* ask a question.

7. **Quick Post-Class Review**

   Here's a special tip from study experts: After class or later that day (or the next day, if it is easier for you), be sure to *look over your notes, quickly. Make a note of anything that is unclear, so that you will be able to clarify the information later.*

   Repetition does wonders for your memory!

After Class: How To Study Nursing Content

You have previewed the chapter and taken notes in class. NOW IS THE TIME TO RE-READ THE MORE DIFFICULT SECTIONS OF THE TEXT MORE CAREFULLY.

As you go through the chapter, *still try to read quickly* and avoid becoming bogged down. It helps to write down any questions you have—and be sure to ask the instructor.

If you follow this method, you will be surprised how much more you remember when exam time comes around!

Having Trouble Memorizing Definitions and Formulas?

When you have to memorize something and it just doesn't stick, here are a few tips you can try:

1. **Look it up in another textbook or a nursing manual, and make sure that you UNDERSTAND it.** Pay special attention to any illustrations or charts. Maybe it will make more sense—or will be presented in a way that will stick in your mind. Use any special memory clues (mnemonic devices—like the "Five Rights" of administering medications) that will help spark your memory.
2. **Formulas:** The best way to learn formulas "inside out" is to PRACTICE USING THEM in practice questions that can be found in other textbooks, as well as in special collections of practice test questions. (See product index).

3. **Try making up your own "flash cards"** with the term, drug name or formula name on one side and the definition, drug information or calculation on the other. This way, instead of worrying about the information, you can carry the cards with you and look at them a few times throughout the day. Try to explain the meaning or give the drug information or formula without looking; then, check to see if you are right. When you have learned the information, save the cards for review at exam time! This technique isn't new, but it works.

Reviewing for the Exam

Now it's exam time! You have taken your class notes and have read your textbook carefully. How are you going to study for the exam?

Don't wait until the last minute! Take a calendar and plan what you will do to review, how long it will take and exactly when you will do it.

All the leaders of the Fortune 500 use personalized written plans for important projects. Putting your plan in writing is like writing your own personal guarantee of success! So write out your plan.

Then, set aside the time to review. Plan your other activities so that you will be able to make good use of your study time. If possible, plan to do your reviewing in the library, where you will not be interrupted.

See the next page for a helpful table titled "A Time-Saving Way to Review for a Nursing Course Exam".

A Time-Saving Way to Review for a Nursing Course Exam

1\. **Review your class notes.**

Pay special attention to rationales for nursing interventions. If the reason for an intervention is unclear, look it up in your textbook.

2\. **As you review your notes, keep in mind the phases of the nursing process:**

(1) What should the nurse **assess** (collecting data)?

(2) How should the nurse **analyze** and interpret this information to arrive at a nursing diagnosis?

(3) How should the nurse **plan** care for the client?

(4) What should the nurse keep in mind when **implementing** care?

(5) How should the nurse monitor and **evaluate** the client's response to therapy?

Your focus is on *understanding*, so try to use your own words.

4\. **Re-read any sections of the textbook that you found unclear.**

If you still have questions about the content, *write them down and ask your instructor!*

5\. **Then, use some of the reviewing aids that are available in your bookstore or learning lab.**

For example, MEDS publishes a complete set of audiotapes and videotapes for the review of all clinical areas, plus special topics such as pharmacology and safety. (More information about these materials is available from MEDS by calling 1-800-200-9191.) Reviewing aids are especially useful for final exams, when a great deal of content is to be covered at one time.

6\. **Answer a set of practice test questions about the content to be covered.**

This is extremely important! Practice questions assess and reinforce what you have learned and give you a chance to practice applying it. Practice questions reflect what goes on in the real world in clinical situations, and they help you to become more analytical. Chapter Eleven, "Drill Questions on Fundamental Nursing Concepts," includes a good selection of test questions separated according to topic. See the product index for MEDS "Q&A" books and software.

7\. **Special study tip: Form a study group with some fellow students.**

Teamwork increases brainpower—so study in teams with other good students if you can. When you explain things to others, you understand them better yourself! Group study is good for morale, too.

Using Practice Questions

Be sure to plan time during your review to *answer practice questions* about the covered nursing content! This is your best "plan of attack" for any exam.

Answering practice questions is as important as going over your notes or reviewing your text. This is because it gives you a chance to practice *applying* your newly acquired nursing knowledge.

As a rule of thumb, MEDS Publishing recommends that you plan to answer about 200 practice questions in preparation for a typical 50–question exam.

You will find "Q&A" (question and answer) books in your bookstore, as well as in your learning lab or library. Computerized practice tests are also available. MEDS offers Q&A books, software, and a series of Q&A review tapes.

When answering questions, be sure to time yourself and practice using pacing strategy (explained in Chapter Eight, "How to Take a Timed Nursing Exam"). Then, to assess your knowledge and your test-taking skills, be sure to check your answers and read the rationales! Be sure to assess the reason why you missed any questions that you answered incorrectly: Did you misunderstand or "read into" the question? Or, did you lack the required nursing knowledge to answer the question? Is there a test-taking strategy that would have helped you to select the correct answer?

When you have completed a set of practice questions, you may wish to review any content areas that gave you difficulty. You may also wish to return to *Test Question Logic for Beginning Nursing Students* to review how to answer particular types of questions, or how to use certain test-taking strategies.

The Payoff

Following these guidelines for organized, streamlined preparation and review will pay off in increased confidence, understanding, better use of your time, and improved test scores. Try it and see!

MEDS Best Study Tips

DO:

PREVIEW—READ-THROUGH—and REVIEW each day's assignment.

Take notes to CLARIFY.

Focus on RATIONALES and NURSING PRIORITIES.

USE THE NURSING PROCESS whenever possible. Ask yourself, "How would the nurse assess—analyze—plan—implement—evaluate" when caring for a client with a given disease, or when performing a procedure.

ASK QUESTIONS when you don't understand. Write down questions briefly when reading your text book.

Use MNEMONICS (memory devices) and make flashcards.

REVIEW QUICKLY after class.

SET ASIDE TIME EVERY DAY to preview, read and review.

Before the exam, prepare a WRITTEN STUDY SCHEDULE.

ANSWER PRACTICE TEST QUESTIONS.

DON'T:

Go to class without previewing

Get bogged down preparing for class

Try to memorize the textbook

Leave all your studying until the night before the exam

Chapter 3

HOW DO I AVOID "READING INTO" THE QUESTION?

It seems justified to lose points on an exam because you did not know the necessary information. However, it is extremely frustrating to score poorly on an exam just because you "read into" or misread the questions!

You can maximize your score on your nursing course exams and the NCLEX Exam by learning select **test-taking techniques and strategies.** This chapter will show you some techniques to help you to read and interpret test questions correctly and how to determine which options are possible answers.

Three test-taking techniques are described in this chapter. First, you will learn a technique for analyzing a test question by separating what the **introductory statement** in the question **tells** you, from what the **stem** of the question **asks.** Second, you will learn a technique for interpreting a test question by identifying the **four critical elements.** Third, you will learn a technique for **eliminating incorrect options**. Each time you answer a test question, you should use **all three** of these techniques!

Finally, this chapter will also demonstrate how to avoid the common errors made when students misread a question, and give you some helpful test-taking tips.

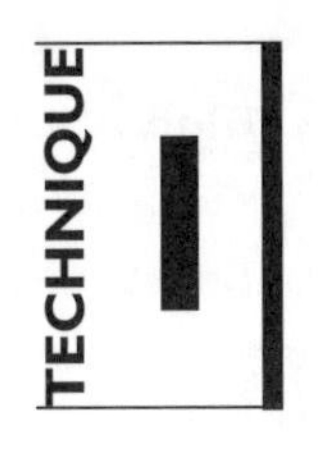

IDENTIFYING THE "INTRODUCTORY STATEMENT" AND THE "STEM"

The first step in analyzing a test question is to separate what the question **tells** you from what it is **asking**.

Each test question basically consists of three parts:

1. Introductory statement.
2. Stem, which asks you to select an answer.
3. Four options, from which you must select the answer.

The **introductory statement** in a test question may give you information about a clinical problem, present data, or it may state a nursing topic, such as a nursing intervention or a disease. The introductory statement always includes a *specific question* that you must answer using your nursing knowledge. The specific question in the introductory statement is referred to as the **stem** of the question. The stem asks you to solve a specific problem and select one of the four options as the answer.

Here is an example of an introductory statement which includes a clinical situation. The **stem** is in bold print:

> A client is receiving care at the clinic. Her doctor has prescribed an iron supplement and an increased intake of Vitamin C in her diet. **The nurse understands that the best rationale for increasing Vitamin C in the client's diet is to:**

As you can see, the introductory statement **tells** you about the client's health problem and **gives you the clinical information** you should consider in answering the question.

The **stem** is the portion of the test question that **asks** the nurse to solve a specific problem and select one of the four options. The stem in the question *asks you to choose the option which presents the best rationale for increasing Vitamin C* in the client's diet.

Here is another introductory statement, with the **stem** in bold print:

> During dinner, a client puts on his call light. When the nurse enters his room, she notices that he cannot talk and is grasping his throat with his hands. **What is the first nursing action in this situation?**

The stem is not always in a separate sentence. Sometimes the information in the introductory statement seems to "run into" or "overlap" the stem, as it does in the following question. When this happens, you can still separate what the question is **telling** you from what it is specifically **asking**. It may be helpful in a question like this to restate the question in your own words. The **stem** in the following introductory statement is in bold print:

> A client had a stroke two weeks ago. He is paralyzed on the left side. While getting him out of bed to sit in a wheelchair, **which nursing action is essential?**

Now compare this question to another question about the same client, and see what happens. The *new information* is in *italics,* and the **stem** is in **bold print:**

> A client had a stroke two weeks ago. He is paralyzed on the left side. *In transferring him to a wheelchair, the nurse notices a reddened area on his left hip.* **Which nursing action is essential?**

Notice that although the stem appears to remain the same, **the information about the clinical situation has been changed.** As you can see, it is very important to **read all the information in the introductory statement!** The second question about the client will have a *different answer* from the first question.

It is important to identify what the question *tells* you and what it *asks,* because:

- Incorrect options may "answer" something that is not actually being asked; and
- Incorrect options may include information which was not given in the case scenario.

Test questions which do not describe a clinical situation might ask you to select the option which best:

- Identifies a sign or symptom of a specific disease.
- Describes the difference between two diseases.
- Identifies a sign of a problem.
- Explains the rationale for a nursing intervention.
- Specifies the priority nursing action for a certain kind of situation.

You can think of a question *without* a description of a clinical situation as giving you a **subject**; then the stem of such a question asks you something about that subject.

Reading each question carefully will help you make the most of your nursing knowledge when taking an exam.

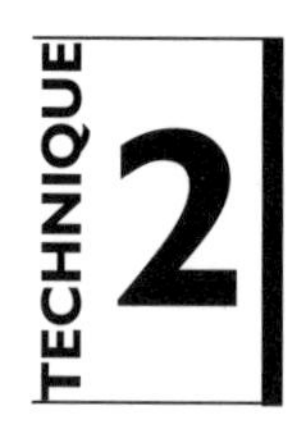

IDENTIFYING THE FOUR CRITICAL ELEMENTS

Learning to identify the **critical elements** in a test question is crucial to interpreting the question correctly.

The four critical elements in each test question are:

1. The key words.
2. The client.
3. The issue.
4. The type of stem.

To clarify a question's meaning, it is necessary to identify each of these elements.

1. What are the key words?

The key words are the important words or phrases in a question. Key words focus your attention on crucial ideas in the stem and in the options. Here are some phrases from questions with the key words in **bold** print:

- **Early** or **late** signs
- **Immediately** after surgery or in the **postoperative** period
- The **most likely** or **least likely** characteristics to occur
- The **initial** nursing action
- **After several days**
- **On the day of** admission

2. Who is the client in the question?

The client is the person who is the focus of the question. This is usually the person with the health problem described in the introductory statement—but this is not always true! The client in the question might be:

- The person with the health problem.
- A family member, friend or neighbor of the person with the health problem.
- Another client in the health care setting.
- Another member of the health care team.

It is crucial to identify the client in the question because the answer must relate to the client.

For example, the stem might ask you to select the nurse's most therapeutic response to a question asked by a client's wife. Since the nurse must respond to the wife, the wife is the client in the question.

Another question might ask how the nurse should respond to a concern about contagion expressed by another client sharing a room with your client. Then the client sharing the room becomes the client in the question.

3. What is the issue in the question?

The issue is the specific problem or subject that the question is asking about. For example, the issue might be:

- A drug (e.g., digoxin, Lasix)
- A problem (e.g., drug addiction, depression)
- A toxic effect of a drug (e.g., nausea, vomiting)
- A behavior (e.g., restlessness, agitation)
- A disorder (e.g., diabetes mellitus, ulcerative colitis)
- A procedure (e.g., glucose tolerance test, cardiac catheterization)

NOTE: The issue *always has something to do with the client in the question.*

4. What is the type of stem?

As you have already learned, the stem is the part of the question that asks you to solve a problem and select a response. To select the correct option, you need to determine the **type of stem.**

There are two types of stems:

A. TRUE RESPONSE STEMS

B. FALSE RESPONSE STEMS

A. TRUE RESPONSE STEMS

True response stems are questions **for which the answer must be an appropriate nursing action or an accurate explanation.** For example, a true response stem might ask you to identify:

- An appropriate nursing action.
- The most essential or highest priority nursing action.
- A safe nursing judgment.
- A therapeutic nursing response.

- An accurate rationale for a nursing action.
- An action or statement by the client indicating the success of the nurse's client teaching.
- A correct explanation of the difference between two disorders.

In the examples shown below, note the words in **bold** print. These words focus your attention on the "best" or "most appropriate" option. Here are some examples of **true response stems:**

- Which nursing action is **most** important?
- Which approach by the nurse would be **best**?
- The nurse would demonstrate the **best** judgment by taking which action?
- Which response by the nurse would be **most therapeutic**?
- **Initially,** the nurse **should:**
- The nurse understands that the **chief** purpose of the drug is to:
- The nurse should give **immediate** consideration to which symptom?
- In collecting data on admission, which objective sign observed by the nurse would be **indicative** of a fracture?
- Which comment by the nurse would indicate the **best** understanding of the client's needs?
- The nurse knows that the client **understands** how to care for his health problem when the client states:

B. FALSE RESPONSE STEMS

It may seem strange, but many test questions do ask you to select an answer which is wrong!

False response stems indicate that the best option will be the one which is an **inappropriate** nursing action or an **inaccurate** explanation—or the option which has something **unimportant** or otherwise **negative** about it.

The following are examples of **false response stems.** Note the negative word or phrase in **bold** print:

- At this time, which nursing action would be **inappropriate**?
- The nurse knows that which medication would be **contraindicated** for this client?
- The **least important** concern for the nurse to raise with the client at this time is:
- Which nursing action receives the **lowest priority** at this time?
- The nurse would identify that the client **required further instruction** in CPR if the client placed his hands:
- Which nursing action would demonstrate an **unsafe** nursing judgment?
- Which characteristic would the nurse identify as **least likely** to contribute to the client's hypertension?

ELIMINATING INCORRECT OPTIONS BASED ON THE TYPE OF STEM

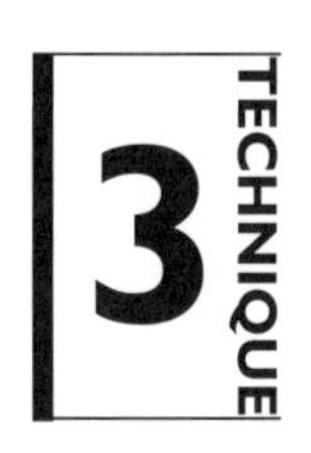

After you have identified the four critical elements in a test question, then you can begin to narrow your choices for selecting the correct option.

Most multiple choice questions you will find on your nursing course exams have four options. Of these, three are "distractors" and one is the correct answer.

> **"Distractors" are options that are designed to resemble the correct answer but, in fact, are not. They are intended to "distract" you from answering correctly.**

Here is a selection procedure which will help you to eliminate the distractors. First, follow these instructions—and then see Chapter 4 for some strategies you can use to narrow the choices even further.

1. First, decide whether the question has a **true response stem** or a **false response stem.**

2. Then read each of the four options to determine whether it is appropriate or accurate. For each option, write one of the following symbols:

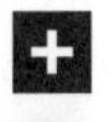

- + This option is **appropriate** (or accurate, etc.)
- − This option is **inappropriate** (or inaccurate, etc.)
- ? I am **not sure**.

3. If the question has a **true response stem,** make a decision about each option, as follows:

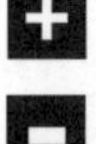

- + This option is **appropriate—<u>This might be the correct answer</u>.**
- − This option is **inappropriate—<u>This is a distractor</u>.**
- ? I am **not sure—<u>This is a possibility.</u>**

4. If the question has a **false response stem,** make a decision about each option as follows – and note that **you are looking for an inappropriate or incorrect option as the answer:**

- + This option is **appropriate—<u>so this is a distractor</u>.**
- − This option is **inappropriate—<u>so this might be the answer</u>.**
- ? I am **not sure—This is a possibility.**

HOW TO AVOID MISREADING TEST QUESTIONS

Misreading test questions is a major problem that hinders success on nursing exams. There are many ways in which a question can be misread!

Misreading a test question may happen because you:

- Incorrectly analyze what the question is really asking.
- Overlook important words such as "early" or "late," or "unsafe" or "inappropriate."
- "Read into" a question information that is not actually given in the case scenario.
- Incorrectly interpret a disorder (for example, mistakenly interpreting a complication of diabetes mellitus, such as ketoacidosis, as diabetes mellitus itself).

Here are some test-taking tips to avoid misreading test questions:

1. To avoid incorrectly analyzing what is being asked: Separate the case scenario and the stem, and identify the client, the issue, and the type of stem.

2. To avoid overlooking important words: Identify the key words.

3. To avoid "reading into" a question:
   Try to restate the question in your own words. Then eliminate any option which includes "new" information that was not given in the case scenario. You should also eliminate any option which requires you to make assumptions about the client involving information not presented in the case scenario.

4. To avoid misinterpreting disorders:
   Review carefully for the exam! Use the method outlined in Chapter Two to review for nursing course exams. Focus on any areas in which you have difficulty. Then, use your nursing knowledge and your test-taking techniques when you read each question.

A Guideline to Use When Narrowing the Options

- Make a decision about each option as you read it—you will save time!
- After you have eliminated an option, do not go back to it. Continue to work with the options that are remaining.
- Try to eliminate at least two options by using this selection procedure.
- If you are left with one + option and one ? option (with a true response stem), select the + as the correct answer. Remember to always go with what you know!
- Use this elimination procedure before making an "educated guess." Then, if you are left with two + options, you have a 50% chance of guessing correctly—but if you made a wild guess from all four choices, you would have only one chance in four of guessing correctly.

Practice Session: Identifying the Critical Elements and Eliminating Distractors

Here are some practice questions to try out your new test-taking skills.

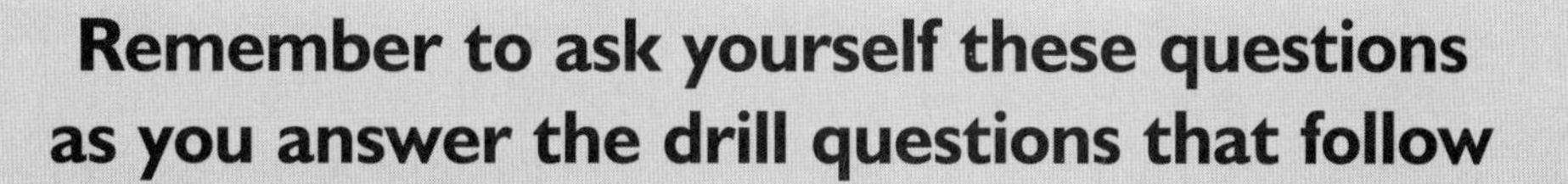

1. What are the key words?
2. Who is the client?
3. What is the issue?
4. Is this a true response stem or a false response stem?

Always be sure to determine whether the question has a true response stem or a false response stem. When you know the type of stem, then make a decision about each of the options by using the selection procedure.

After you have answered the question, read the Analysis. Note that the **key words** and the **correct answer** are in bold print.

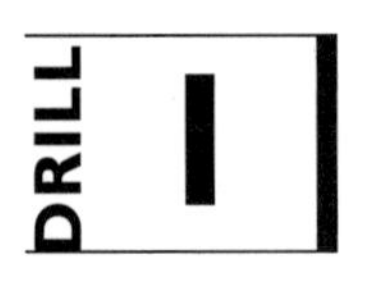

In preparing to give a client a bed bath, the nurse would:

A. Place the bed in the lowest position.
B. Expose the top side of the body, washing and drying quickly, then doing the same on the posterior side.
C. Gather all articles necessary for the bed bath and place them where they will be within easy reach of the nurse during the bath.
D. Use firm, scrubbing strokes to remove dirt and bacteria.

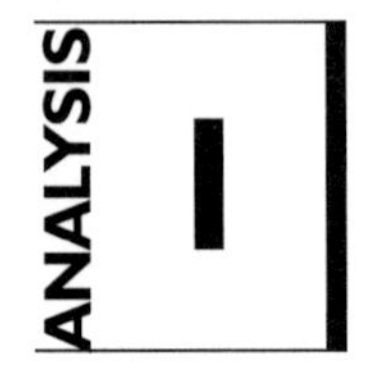

Critical Elements	
Key words:	See bold print.
Client:	Any client.
Issue:	Bed bath.
Type of stem:	True response stem.

Eliminate Options

In preparing to give a client a **bed bath**, the nurse would:

− A. Place the bed in the lowest position.
This unsafe (-) action is a distractor. The bed should be placed in a high position to protect the nurse from frequent bending of her back.

− B. Expose the top side of the body, washing and drying quickly, then doing the same on the posterior side.
This is inappropriate (-) and a distractor. Each area of the body should be exposed, washed, and dried separately, to avoid chilling the client and to provide privacy.

+ C. Gather all articles necessary for the bed bath and place them where they will be within easy reach of the nurse during the bath.
This is the only option which describes an appropriate (+) nursing action to facilitate bathing the client.

− D. Use firm, scrubbing strokes to remove dirt and bacteria.
This is an inappropriate (-) technique. The strokes should be firm but gentle—not "scrubbing"—to avoid injuring the skin.

2 DRILL

The nurse is preparing to give a morning medication. The first nursing action in this activity is to:

A. Read the label.
B. Check for the right dose.
C. Wash the nurse's hands.
D. Check for the right time.

2 ANALYSIS

Critical Elements	
Key words:	See bold print.
Client:	Any client.
Issue:	Administering medications.
Type of stem:	True response stem.

Eliminate Options

The nurse is **preparing** to give a morning **medication.** The **first** nursing action in this activity is to:

 A. Read the label.
Reading the label to identify the medication is an important part of avoiding medication errors. However, it is not the first thing that the nurse should do.

 B. Check for the right dose.
It is important to have the right dose to prevent over or under dosing the client. However, this is not the first step in preparing medications.

+ C. Wash the nurse's hands.
Yes! Handwashing is the first action prior to performing any nursing procedure.

? D. Check for the right time.
The time for administration of the medication is very important, but this is not the first thing that the nurse should do.

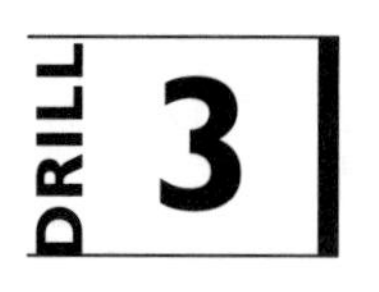

A client who has right sided weakness needs to be transferred from his bed to a wheelchair. In transferring the client, the nurse must remember to:

A. Keep the client at arm's length while transferring him.
B. Bend at the waist to get down to his level.
C. Maintain a straight back and bend at the knees.
D. Try to transfer the client alone, before determining that help is needed.

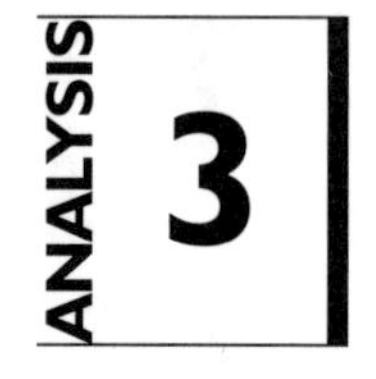

Critical Elements	
Key words:	See bold print.
Client:	Client with right-sided weakness.
Issue:	Transferring client from bed to wheelchair.
Type of stem:	True response stem.

Eliminate Options

A client who has **right sided weakness** needs to be **transferred from the bed** to a wheelchair. In transferring the client, the nurse must remember to:

− A. Keep the client at arm's length while transferring him.
This is incorrect. When lifting an object or a client, it is important for the nurse to hold the object or person close to the body, where the base of support is.

− B. Bend at the waist to get down to his level.
You should not bend at the waist, since all of the client's weight will be placed on the back muscle and possibly cause injury to the nurse.

+ C. Maintain a straight back and bend at the knees.
Correct! A straight back usually limits the amount of weight that is placed on the back muscles. Good body mechanics are essential in preventing injury to the nurse.

− D. Try transfer the client alone, before determining that help is needed.
No! This would be very unsafe! If a client or object appears to be too heavy for one person, always get help first rather than attempting the lift alone and risk injuring your back-and, in this case, the client.

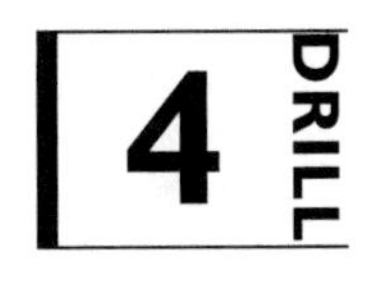

Client A and Client B are sitting in the day lounge. The nurse has medicat-tion to administer to Client A. When the nurse enters the lounge, Client B says to the nurse, "I see you found me to give me my pills." The best nursing response would be:

A. "I don't have any pills for you, Client B."
B. "Let me check your identification arm band, and I will check to see if you are supposed to receive any pills."
C. "Client A, I have pills for you to take, but none for Client B."
D. "Client A, would you please take these pills."

4 ANALYSIS

Critical Elements	
Key Words:	See bold print.
Client:	Client B.
Issue:	Administering medications/communication.
Type of stem:	True response stem.

Eliminate Options

Client A and Client B are sitting in the day lounge. The nurse has **medication** to administer to Client A. When the nurse enters the lounge, Client B says to the nurse, "I see you **found me** to give me my **pills**." The **best nursing response** would be:

? A. "I don't have any pills for you, Client B."
This response correctly identifies Client B as the client in the question, so it might (?) be the answer. However, this response does not adequately address the client's concerns, since he believes he is to receive medication.

\+ B. "Let me check your identification arm band, and I will check to see if you are supposed to receive any pills." ***This response correctly identifies Client B as the client (+) and properly addresses his concern (+) about medication.***

− C. "Client A, I have pills for you to take, but none for Client B."
Client A is the client in this question, because he has spoken to the nurse about a concern. This response is inappropriate (-) because the nurse's response must be addressed to the client in the question.

− D. "Client A, would you please take these pills."
Client B is the client in this question, because he has spoken to the nurse about a concern. The nurse's response must be addressed to the client in the question. With this response to Client A, the nurse ignores the client (-) in the question.

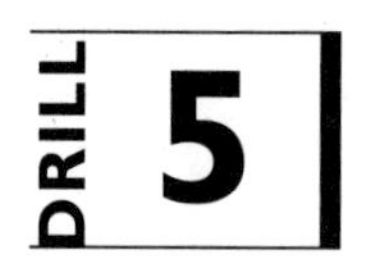

The nurse must lift a heavy object which is found in the hallway. Which is the best approach when the nurse must lift a heavy object?

A. Lift the object at arm's length so all of the arm muscles are being used.
B. Bend from the waist, using a wide stance, so that the leg muscles are used.
C. Maintain good body alignment and use the large muscles of the body.
D. Bend at the knees and use the large leg muscles when lifting the object.

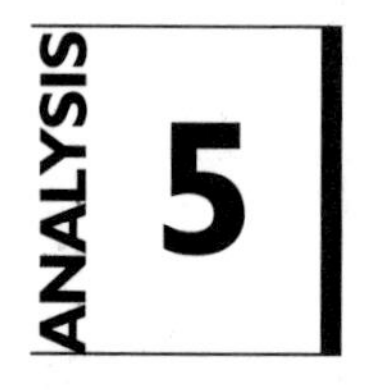

Critical Elements	
Key Words:	See bold print.
Client:	Any client.
Issue:	Error in name on identification bracelet.
Type of stem:	True response stem.

Eliminate Options

The nurse must lift a heavy object which is found in the hallway. Which is the **best** approach when the nurse must lift a **heavy** object?

− A. Lift the object at arm's length so all of the arm muscles are being used.
Incorrect. When lifting an object at arm's length, the muscles in the arm are stretched, which fatigues the muscles quickly. This position also results in poor balance, because the heavy object is outside the body's base of support.

− B. Bend from the waist, using a wide stance, so that the leg muscles are used.
Incorrect. Bending from the waist results in the use of small back muscles, which become stretched and easily injured.

+ C. Maintain good body alignment and use the large muscles of the body while lifting the object.
Correct! Using good body alignment provides a good base of support, which reduces back strain and helps maintain balance while lifting. Using the large muscles of the body, including the arms and legs, prevents muscle strain and fatigue. This is the safest approach for the nurse.

− D. Bend at the knees and use the large leg muscles when lifting the object.
Bending at the knees and using the large leg muscles to lift provides decreased risk for musculoskeletal strain. This is a correct action. However, this is not the best option because it is a less complete description of the best approach than one of the other options.

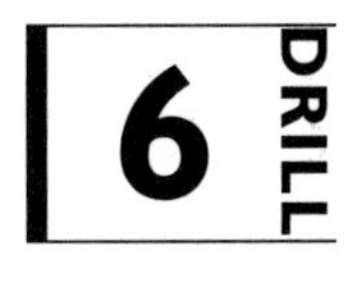

An elderly client was admitted to the hospital with pneumonia. He is receiving oxygen at 6 liters per mask. In obtaining vital signs, which nursing action is inappropriate?

A. Taking an axillary temperature.
B. Listening to his lungs when counting respirations.
C. Listening to an apical heart rate.
D. Taking an oral temperature.

6 ANALYSIS

Critical Elements	
Key words:	See bold print.
Client:	An elderly client with pneumonia, receiving oxygen per mask.
Issue:	Obtaining vital signs.
Type of stem:	False response stem.

Eliminate Options

An elderly client was admitted to the hospital with pneumonia. He is **receiving oxygen** at 6 liters **per mask.** In obtaining his **vital signs**, which nursing action is **inappropriate?**

+ A. Taking an axillary temperature.
This action is <u>appropriate (+)</u>, since the oral temperature of a client receiving oxygen therapy per nasal cannula or mask is not a reliable measurement. This question has a false response stem.

+ B. Listening to his lungs when counting respirations.
The lungs <u>should be auscultated (+)</u> because the client has pneumonia. You are looking for an <u>inappropriate</u> action.

+ C. Listening to an apical heart rate.
Because of the client's age, auscultating an apical heart rate is <u>important (+)</u> because it allows the nurse to assess for any abnormal heart sounds.

− D. Take an oral temperature.
The oral temperature of a client receiving oxygen therapy via nasal cannula or mask is <u>not a reliable measurement (-)</u>. Since the question has a false response stem, this option is the correct answer.

In this chapter, two important test-taking strategies were introduced. In addition to these strategies, here are some important points to remember.

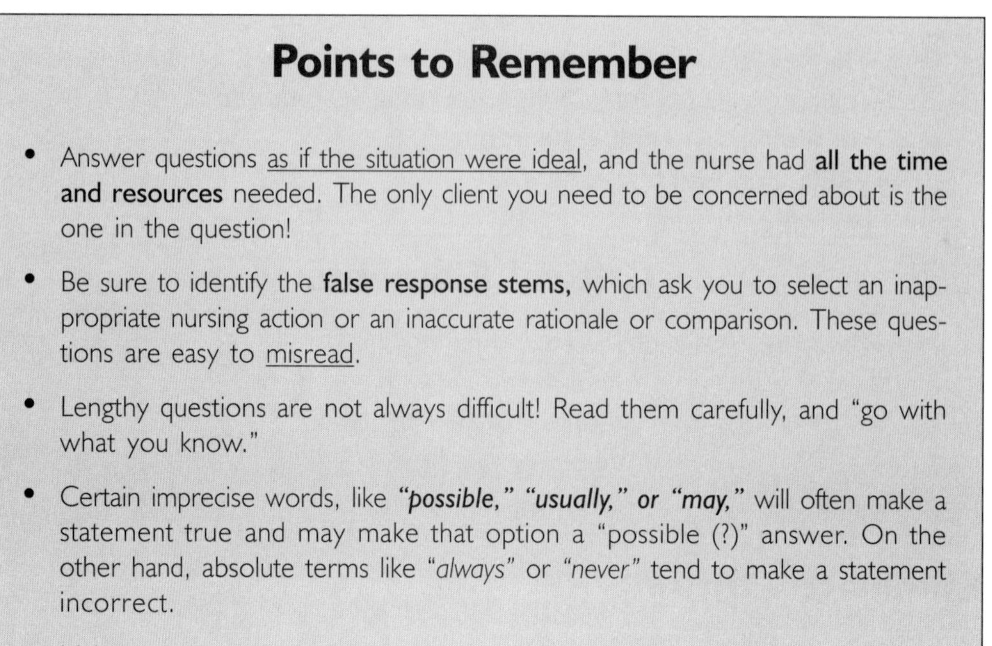

Points to Remember

- Answer questions as if the situation were ideal, and the nurse had **all the time and resources** needed. The only client you need to be concerned about is the one in the question!
- Be sure to identify the **false response stems,** which ask you to select an inappropriate nursing action or an inaccurate rationale or comparison. These questions are easy to misread.
- Lengthy questions are not always difficult! Read them carefully, and "go with what you know."
- Certain imprecise words, like ***"possible," "usually," or "may,"*** will often make a statement true and may make that option a "possible (?)" answer. On the other hand, absolute terms like *"always"* or *"never"* tend to make a statement incorrect.
- Make sure to read all of the options—and then select the best!

Chapter 4

HOW DO I CHOOSE BETWEEN THE TWO BEST OPTIONS?

Understand the Question!

The test-taking techniques presented in Chapter Three should be used on every question. You should ***always*** identify the critical elements, identify the type of stem, and eliminate distractors based on the type of stem. This three-step technique is the best way to determine what the question is asking, and which of the options are possible answers.

Eliminate Incorrect Options

As you learned in Chapter Three, you can often eliminate two or more options based on the type of stem. Identifying the type of stem is essential to selecting the correct answer. There is no substitute for this step.

STEP 3

Use Test-Taking Strategies

Even after eliminating the incorrect options, it is often hard to choose between the remaining two options. This can be very frustrating!

What can you do when two options appear to be equally correct? How can you decide which option is the best choice?

The problem, of course, is that you only receive credit for selecting the correct answer. You never receive any credit for identifying the best distractor! Although two options may *seem* to be equally good answers, there is always one option which is better and more correct.

NOTE

The three new test-taking strategies presented in this chapter are designed to help you choose between the two best options when you cannot decide using your nursing knowledge alone. If you are unable to choose the answer to a question on the basis of your nursing knowledge, you should apply one of these strategies—instead of just guessing at the answer.

Identify the Global Response

When more than one option appears to be correct, your best strategy is to look for a global response.

A global response is a more general statement which may also include correct ideas from other options.

This strategy works because the option that is a more comprehensive or general statement is a better answer than an option which may be correct but is more specific or limited. In "test question logic," the global response option is the best answer because it is more complete.

Practice Session: Identifying the Global Response

In each of the following questions, first use the three-step technique of (1) identifying the critical elements, (2) determining the type of stem, and (3) eliminating options which do not match the type of stem.

Then, compare the remaining options, and look for the global response option. Ask yourself if one of the possible options is more comprehensive or global than the other choices.

After you have selected your answer, read the Analysis. Note that the **key words** and the **answer** are shown in bold print.

DRILL I

A client returns with a Foley catheter after surgery. In providing catheter care, which is the best nursing approach?

A. Preventing infection and maintaining a patent catheter and drainage system.
B. Keeping the collection bag above the level of the bladder.
C. Using soap and water to clean the perineal area.
D. Maintaining a closed system without any kinks in the tubing.

ANALYSIS I

Critical Elements

Key words:	See bold print.
Client:	A post-surgical client.
Issue:	Catheter care.
Type of stem:	True response stem.

Eliminate Options

A client returns with a **Foley catheter after surgery.** In providing **catheter care,** which is the **best** nursing **approach**?

+ A. Preventing infection and maintaining a patent catheter and drainage system.
This is the best nursing approach in caring for a post-operative client with a catheter. Taking measures to prevent infection will protect the client from the most common complication in catheter care. Maintaining a patent catheter and drainage system will assure drainage of urine and prevent back flow of urine into the bladder. This is one of three which are appropriate nursing approaches (+) and possible answers. This option is the best because it is the most comprehensive.

− B. Keeping the collection bag above the level of the bladder.
This action is unsafe (-)! The collection bag must be kept ***below*** *the level of the bladder to prevent back flow of urine into the bladder.*

+ C. Using soap and water to clean the perineal area.
This action is appropriate (+) because it helps reduce the possibility of infection. However, this is not the "best nursing approach." Look for an option which is more global.

+ D. Maintaining a closed system without any kinks in the tubing.
This is an essential (+) nursing approach in catheter care. However, there is a more global option which is a more comprehensive statement of the "best nursing approach."

While getting an elderly client who is very weak out of bed and into a wheelchair, the best nursing approach initially is to:

A. Lock the wheels of the bed.
B. Place the equipment to provide the safest transfer that is possible for the client.
C. Align the wheelchair as close to the bed as possible, to prevent the client from falling to the floor.
D. Remove the leg support on the wheelchair on the side closest to the bed.

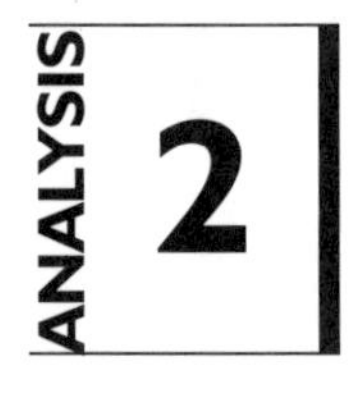

Critical Elements	
Key words:	See bold print.
Client:	A weak, elderly client.
Issue:	Transferring the client to a wheelchair.
Type of stem:	True response stem.

Eliminate Options

While getting an **elderly** client who is **very weak** out of bed and into a wheelchair, the best nursing approach initially is to:

+ A. Lock the wheels of the bed.
The wheels of the bed should be in the locked position to prevent it from moving. This is a safe (+) nursing action. However, there is another option which is a more comprehensive or inclusive statement of the best nursing approach. Read all of the options before selecting the best one!

+ B. Place the equipment to provide the safest transfer that is possible for the client.
This option is the best because it emphasizes ensuring the client's safety (+) and is a comprehensive statement about the initial nursing approach in transferring a client. It includes all aspects of placing equipment in preparing for the client's safe transfer.

+ C. Align the wheelchair as close to the bed as possible, to prevent the client from falling to the floor.
This is an appropriate (+) action which provides for the client's safety. However, there is another option which is more comprehensive statement of the best initial nursing approach.

+ D. Removing the leg support on the wheelchair on the side closest to the bed.
This is an appropriate (+) action, since it provides unobstructed access to the wheelchair. However, this is not the best approach initially. Look for an option which is a more comprehensive or general statement.

3 DRILL

In a long-term care facility, the nurse finds an elderly client on the floor. After having the client examined by the physician, the most important nursing action is to:

A. Call the family and ask them to stay with the client.
B. Provide for the safety and protection of the client.
C. Apply wrist and leg restraints to prevent the client from falling from the bed.
D. Obtain an order for medication to sedate the client.

3 ANALYSIS

Critical Elements	
Key words:	See bold print.
Client:	An elderly client.
Issue:	Client found on floor.
Type of stem:	True response stem.

Eliminate Options

In a long-term care facility, the nurse finds an **elderly client** on the **floor. After** having the client examined by the **physician,** the **most important** nursing action is to:

? A. Call the family and ask them to stay with the client.
Incorrect. Having a member of the family stay with the client may be a possibility if it can be arranged. This provides for the client's safety and allows some mobility for the client while in bed. However, this is not the best option.

+ B. Provide for the safety and protection of the client.
Yes! This option means that the nurse will provide all appropriate interventions that address the safety needs of the client. This global response option is the best because it is a more comprehensive statement about providing for the client's safety.

C. Apply wrist and leg restraints to prevent the client from falling from the bed.
No! Application of a vest restraint may be appropriate to ensure the safety of the client, but leg and wrist restraints would be inappropriate because they do not allow for the client's mobility and are likely to cause agitation. This is not the least restrictive option for providing for this client's safety and therefore cannot be the first nursing action in this clinical situation.

D. Obtain an order for medication to sedate the client.
Incorrect. Sedating a client often makes the client more confused and more likely to behave inappropriately. Try to identify another measure which would be more appropriate for this client.

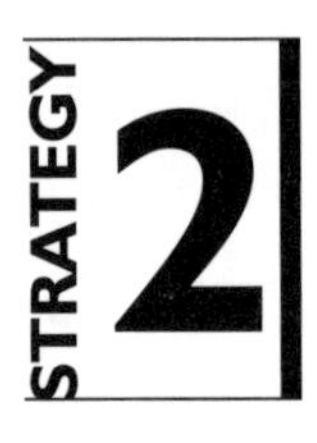

Eliminate Similar Distractors

When you don't know the answer and can't identify a global response option, your second strategy is to eliminate similar distractors.

In "test question logic," there can be only one best option. Therefore, if two options essentially say the same thing or include the same idea, then neither of them can be the answer. The answer has to be the option that is different.

This strategy may be difficult to understand. However, the following questions will help to clarify how it works. This is an excellent strategy to learn and use!

Practice Session: Eliminating Similar Distractors

Read and answer the following questions, eliminating the options that are similar.

First, review the questions by identifying the four critical elements, and narrow your choices. Then practice using the similar distractor strategy and look for the option that is different.

After you have answered the question, read the Analysis. The **key words** and the **answer** are in bold print.

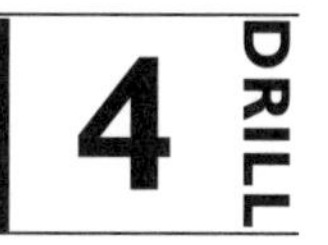

One of the most important nursing actions in the care of the elderly is to:

A. Avoid drying agents when providing skin care.
B Encourage the client to perform as many activities of daily living as possible.
C. Gently apply moisturizing lotions to pressure areas.
D. Apply powder to moist folds in the skin.

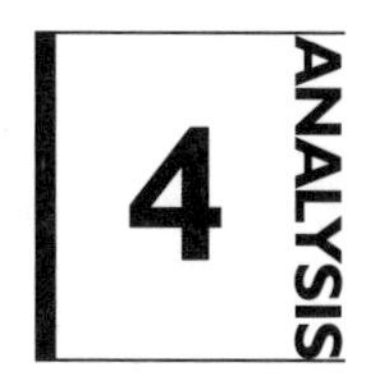

Critical Elements	
Key words:	See bold print.
Client:	Any elderly client.
Issue:	Care of the elderly.
Type of stem:	True response stem.

Eliminate Options

One of the **most important** nursing actions in the care of the **elderly** is to:

+ A. Avoid drying agents when providing skin care.
The skin of the elderly is dry. Soap and other drying agents can cause further drying and cracking of the skin, which permits entry of bacteria. Avoiding drying agents is an appropriate (+) nursing action. Before selecting this option, read the other choices and look for a nursing action that is more important in the care of the elderly.

+ B. Encourage the client to perform as many activities of daily living as possible.
Performing the activities of daily living is important (+) because it directly promotes the nursing goal of maintaining the health and functioning of the aging client. Encouraging the geriatric client to be as independent as possible also promotes a sense of self worth. Because the other three options are all related to care of the skin, they are similar distractors and should be eliminated. Each of these actions is appropriate, but none of them is the most important nursing action in the care of the elderly. This is the option which is different.

+ C. Gently apply moisturizing lotions to pressure areas.
The skin of the elderly is dry, and drying and cracking of the skin permits entry of bacteria. Applying moisturizing lotions is an appropriate (+) nursing action which helps prevent skin breakdown. However, this option is similar to option A—so eliminate these two,

and look for another option which describes a nursing action that is more important in the care of the elderly.

D. Apply powder to moist folds in the skin.
Powder can help alleviate moisture in particular areas of the skin and help prevent skin breakdown. This is an appropriate (+) nursing action in care of the elderly; however, it is not the most important. Like options A and C, this option is about skin care.

DRILL 5

A newly diagnosed adult diabetic is doing a return demonstration of the proper technique for insulin injection. He draws up the correct dose of insulin using the proper technique, but when he is ready to inject the needle, he hesitates and says, "I'm not sure I can do this." Which response by the nurse would be best initially?

A. "I'll show you again how to inject the needle."
B. "I'll inject the needle for you this time."
C. "You're doing fine so far. Give it a try."
D. "Why are you so nervous? Do you need help?"

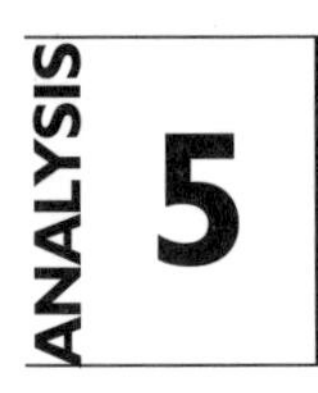

Critical Elements	
Key words:	See bold print.
Client:	A newly diagnosed adult diabetic.
Issue:	The nurse's initial response to an unsure client doing a return demonstration.
Type of stem:	True response stem.

Eliminate Options

A **newly diagnosed adult diabetic** is doing a **return demonstration** of the proper technique for insulin injection. He draws up the correct dose of insulin using the proper technique, but when he is ready to inject the needle, he hesitates and says, "I'm **not sure** I can do this." Which response by the nurse would be best **initially?**

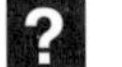

A. "I'll show you again how to inject the needle."
This response is a possibility (?), since this nursing action may sometimes be appropriate in client teaching. However, the case scenario states that the client is using the proper technique in this return demonstration. This response focuses on the nurse doing the procedure rather than on the client doing the procedure. Remember, the purpose of nursing is to help the client maintain an optimal level of functioning.

? B. "I'll inject the needle for you this time."
This is also a possibility (?), but this is similar to option A in that the nurse does the procedure.

\+ C. "You're doing fine so far. Give it a try."
This is the correct answer because it focuses on the nurse encouraging the client to do the procedure for himself. This answer is client-centered.

− D. "Why are you so nervous? Do you need help?"
"Why" responses are always non-therapeutic (-). This response blocks communication by making the client feel defensive. This response is not therapeutic because it focuses on the client's nervousness and need for help. Being nervous and unsure is an appropriate feeling for this newly diagnosed adult diabetic. The nurse's response should enhance the client's feelings of competency.

Look for Similar Words

STRATEGY 3

If you don't know the answer and have tried the first two strategies, the next strategy to try is Strategy Three. This strategy isn't as reliable as the other two strategies, but if you don't know the answer it is better than guessing.

What you will do in this strategy is to *look for a similar word or phrase used in the stem or case scenario, and in one of the options.* If you find a word, feeling, or behavior that is repeated in one of the options, that option may be the correct answer.

Again, although looking for similar words is not as reliable as the first two strategies in this chapter, it is helpful when you can't decide on the best answer and the other two strategies cannot be used.

PRACTICE SESSION: Looking for Similar Words

To answer the following drill questions, first identify the four critical elements and eliminate incorrect options based on the type of stem. Then, read the remaining options and look for a word or phrase that is similar to a word or phrase in the stem or case scenario.

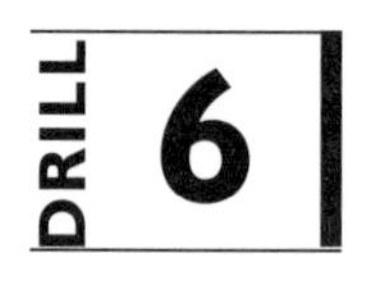

An obese client has been placed on a high-protein, low-calorie diet by his physician. Which nursing action is most appropriate?

A. Explain to the client that he will have to change his eating habits.
B. Explain the importance of exercise when dieting.
C. Explain to the client what types of foods are permitted on a low calorie, high protein diet.
D. Tell the client that if he doesn't stay on this diet he will continue to gain weight.

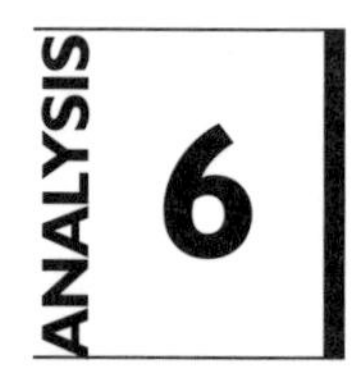

Critical Elements	
Key words:	See bold print.
Client:	An obese client.
Issue:	High-protein, low-calorie diet.
Type of stem:	True response stem.

Eliminate Options

An **obese** client has been placed on a **high protein, low calorie diet** by his physician. Which nursing action is **most** appropriate?

+ A. Explain to the client that he will have to change his eating habits.
Although it is true (+) that the client will have to change his eating habits, this option does not provide much useful information for the client. Consider the other options before selecting the best one.

? B. Explain the importance of exercise when dieting.
It is true that exercise enhances the diet process by burning up calories. This action might be a possibility (?). However, there is no indication that exercise is included in this client's care plan. Do not "read into" the question! Note that this option does not address the issue of the question, which is a high-protein, low-calorie diet. This cannot be the answer.

+ C. Explain to the client what types of foods are permitted on a low-calorie, high-protein diet.
This nursing action is appropriate (+). Providing the client with knowledge concerning the types of foods that he can eat will help him to be more compliant. If you did not know the answer to this question, the words "high protein, low calorie diet" in this option and in the case scenario are a clue that this might be the correct answer.

[-] D. Tell the client that if he doesn't stay on this diet he will continue to gain weight.
This statement is non-therapeutic (-) and provides no useful information. Also, the nurse does not know that the client is gaining weight at this time. Do not "read into" the question!

7 DRILL

A client tells the nurse that his last name is not spelled right on his identification bracelet. The appropriate nursing action is to:

A. Tell the client that as long as his medical record numbers are correct, the mistake is not a problem.
B. Ask the client for the correct spelling, and change his name in his chart.
C. Notify the admitting office of the error and obtain a correct identification bracelet for the client.
D. Notify the physician of the error.

7 ANALYSIS

Critical Elements	
Key words:	See bold print.
Client:	Any client.
Issue:	Name incorrect on ID bracelet.
Type of stem:	True response stem.

Eliminate Options

A client tells the nurse that his last **name** is not spelled right on his **identification bracelet**. The **appropriate** nursing action is to:

[-] A. Tell the client that as long as his medical record numbers are correct, the mistake is not a problem.
This nursing action would be unsafe (-). The client's identification bracelet should be corrected. However, it is possible that his name also appears incorrectly in his medical chart and other hospital records, so these records will also have to be checked. Also, the case scenario does not state that the medical record numbers are correct. Do not read into the question.

[?] B. Ask the client for the correct spelling, and change his name in his chart.
The nurse should ask the client about the correct spelling, so this option might appear to be a possibility (?). However, it is not correct procedure for the nurse to change the client's name in his chart. Other hospital records as well as the client's identification bracelet

must also be corrected. When part of an option is inappropriate, the entire option is inappropriate. This cannot be the answer.

C. Notify the admitting office of the error and obtain a correct identification bracelet for the client.
The admitting office must be informed of the error, and the client's identification bracelet should show his name correctly. This is an <u>appropriate (+)</u> nursing action that will provide for the client's safety. If you were unsure of the answer, the repetition of the words "identification bracelet" from the case scenario would be a clue that this is a possible answer. Note, however, that the word "spelling" occurs in the case scenario and in option B, so this strategy should be used only when you have no other clues and the other strategies do not apply.

D. Notify the physician.
This action is <u>inappropriate (-)</u>. The spelling of the client's name is not a medical problem. If the admitting office determines that an error has been made in identifying the client, and it is determined that the client has received inappropriate care, the physician would be notified at that time. Do not "read into" the question.

DRILL 8

A client is admitted to the hospital for evaluation of inadequate circulation to her lower extremities. The doctor orders a tub bath at the client's request. In assisting the client with her bath, which nursing action would be unsafe?

A. Place a rubber mat on the bottom of the tub.
B. Fill the tub approximately half full.
C. When the client steps into the bath, ask her if the water is the right temperature for her.
D. Obtain all of the necessary supplies and place them within easy reach of the client.

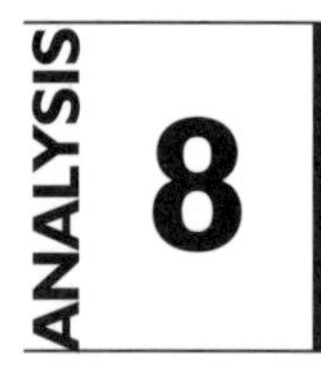

Critical Elements

Key words:	See bold print.
Client:	Client with insufficient circulation in the extremities.
Issue:	Tub bath.
Type of stem:	False response stem.

Eliminate Options

A client is admitted to the hospital for evaluation of **inadequate** circulation to her **lower** extremities. The doctor orders a tub bath at the client's request. In assisting the client with her bath, which nursing action would be **unsafe**?

+ A. Place a rubber mat on the bottom of the tub.
A rubber mat provides for the client's safety (+) by helping to prevent slipping on a slippery tub bottom. However, this question has a false response stem. You are looking for something the nurse should not do.

+ B. Fill the tub approximately half full.
Since water is displaced when the client sits in the tub, filling the tub about half full will prevent the water from running over, which could result in a fall from water on the floor. This is an appropriate (+) nursing action. However, this question has a false response stem.

− C. When the client steps into the bath, ask her if the water is the right temperature for her.
This question has a false response stem, and this nursing action would be unsafe (-). For the safety and comfort of the client, the nurse should regulate the water temperature at 105° to 110° F (40° to 43° C). A client with poor circulation in the lower extremities will not be able to accurately detect feelings of hot and cold when they step into a tub. This happens to be the only option which uses the word "bath," so the strategy of looking for similar words would work in this question. However, the word "tub" is repeated in all of the other options. Note that the other three options are actions the nurse would take (alone) in preparing the tub and equipment, before the client enters the tub. The strategy of eliminating similar distractors would identify this option as the best choice because it is different.

+ D. Obtain all of the necessary supplies and place them within easy reach of the client.
The equipment should be available to the client, within easy reach. This action provides for the client's safety (+) because the client may slip and fall trying to reach the equipment. However, this question has a false response stem.

Points to Remember:

- If you are unable to answer using your nursing knowledge alone, then apply strategies!
- When more than one option appears correct, look for:

(1) A global response, or

(2) Similar distractors that you can eliminate, or

(3) A similar word or phrase used in both the case scenario (or stem) and one of the options.

Chapter 5

LEARNING TO ANSWER COMMUNICATION QUESTIONS

Why Are There So Many Communication Questions On Nursing Exams?

Students are often surprised to find so many questions involving communication on their nursing exams. It is important to understand that the nurse's constant interaction with clients and others in the health care setting makes therapeutic communication skills an integral part of professional nursing.

One reason that good communication skills are so necessary is that they are essential for the nurse to practice *safely.* If you cannot communicate therapeutically with the client and others in the health care setting, it is difficult to practice safely.

Another reason is that communication skills are essential in *achieving your nursing goal* of helping the client attain and maintain an optimal level of functioning. To achieve your nursing goal, you must always be in a *therapeutic role.* In other words, the nurse must have an excellent command of the communication principles necessary to build and maintain a therapeutic relationship with the client.

Communication skills have long been recognized as vital at all levels of nursing practice. Today there are communication questions on every type of certification exam in nursing practice, including the NCLEX exam and the specialty levels.

Nursing exams are used to measure your ability to practice safely and effectively. You must be able to communicate therapeutically in order to practice safely and to achieve your nursing goal.

Why Do Some Communication Questions Look Like Psych Questions?

The client in a test question may be described as confused, angry, anxious, grieving, or upset in some other way. Other questions may describe client behaviors that indicate that there is an emotional issue. You are correct in identifying an emotional or psychological issue in these kinds of questions. However, these questions are usually *communication* questions, *not* questions that deal with psychiatric disorders.

As you know, clients in the health care setting may be experiencing a variety of emotional stresses, including dysphoria related to a disease process, privacy concerns, fear of medical procedures, anxiety concerning possible outcomes, and fear of death. Clients also experience stress from hospitalization itself, from separation from their families and friends, and from temporary or permanent loss of their independence, their daily routines and even their occupation. The client may also be experiencing stress relating to developmental tasks.

The emotional needs of clients must be of concern to the nurse *in all the clinical areas and in any clinical setting,* not just in psychiatric nursing. The nurse must know how to deal with clients' emotional needs *in order to establish and maintain a therapeutic relationship with the client.*

The nurse also needs good therapeutic communication skills *to safely provide routine care and carry out nursing procedures.* Performing assessment activities is an obvious example. Other nursing actions requiring awareness of client needs and therapeutic communication are:

- Explaining procedures to the client.
- Obtaining the client's cooperation implementing nursing interventions.
- Achieving success in client teaching.

The nurse will also use therapeutic communication skills in cooperating with other members of the health care team and in evaluating client care.

To communicate therapeutically, the nurse must always be alert for emotional clues and must know how to interpret the client's verbal and nonverbal behavior. Many test questions include these clues. To answer this kind of test question, you must know how to use therapeutic communication tools.

Learning how to interpret communication questions—and how to answer them correctly—will increase your score on nursing exams.

Using "Test Question Logic" in Communication Questions

As you learned in Chapter Three, test questions have their own special logic, and it is always important to identify the **critical elements** in a question. This can be a little more difficult in communication questions, however!

The first thing you have to do is **identify the *client*** in the question. Here is the catch: The client in a communication question is *not necessarily* the person with the health problem!

The client in a communication question may be a relative, another client, or even another nurse with whom the nurse must communicate in the health care setting. The client in the question is the person that the nurse must respond to. So look for the person in the introductory statement who has said something, or done something, that requires a response by the nurse. The **stem** of the question may also indicate who the client in the question is.

Second, identify the **issue** in the question. *The issue always concerns the client.* The client's issue may be a **problem** of concern to the client, or **feelings** that the client expresses to the nurse or that the nurse observes. To identify the issue, ask yourself, "What is the client's issue or concern?" Look at what the client is doing in the introductory statement, and what the client is saying to the nurse. For example, the introductory statement may identify that the client is *angry,* or that the nurse finds the client *crying.* Be especially alert for key words. They are good clues to selecting the correct answer. Remember—*the correct answer in a test question must relate to the issue.*

Third, always identify the **type of stem.** Although it is less common for a communication question to have a false response stem, some communication questions are written this way. For example, a question might ask you which response by the nurse would be *least appropriate* or have *lowest priority* at this time.

Eliminating Distractors in Communication Questions

There is a special way to eliminate incorrect options in a communication question.

In a communication question, the correct answer is a nursing response that is *therapeutic*—because the nurse must *always* be in a therapeutic role. To communicate therapeutically, the nurse uses communication tools—and avoids communication blocks. If the question has a true response stem, you are looking for a therapeutic response. Your strategy then is to *eliminate all options which include communication blocks.*

Here is an important test-taking tip: If a response includes both a tool and a block, it CANNOT be the correct answer.

Any option which is partly correct
but partly incorrect or inappropriate
should be ruled out.

Communication Tools and Blocks

Communication tools are mechanisms that enhance communication, while **blocks** are responses that interfere with communication. When you answer communication questions, remember that the *tools* are the correct answers in questions with true response stems. Here are some nursing statements which are examples of the therapeutic communication tools:

Therapeutic Communication Tools

Communication Tools	Examples of Statements
Being silent	Sitting quietly with the client.
Offering self	"Let me sit with you."
Showing empathy	"You are upset."
Focusing	"You say that . . ."
Restatement	"You feel anxious?"
Validation/clarification	"What you are saying is . . .?"
Giving information	"Your room is 423."
Dealing with the here and now	"At this time, the problem is . . ."

When answering test questions, keep in mind that **blocks are the distrac** and **tools are the answers** (in questions with true response stems). Example of **communication blocks,** which prevent therapeutic communication, are shown below.

Communication Blocks

Communication Blocks	Examples of Statements
Giving advice	"If I were you, I would . . ."
Showing approval/disapproval	"You did the right thing."
Using cliché and false reassurance	"Don't worry. It will be all right."
Requesting an explanation	"Why did you do that?"
Devaluing client feelings	"Don't be concerned. It's not a problem."
Being defensive	"Every nurse on this unit is exceptional."
Focusing on inappropriate issues or persons	"Have I said something wrong?"
Placing the client's issues "on hold"	"Talk to your doctor about that."

To sum up: If the question has a true response stem, you can eliminate any option that includes a communication block. *Remember that it is a communication block to address an inappropriate issue or person.* Instead, look for responses that address the client's issue. These communication concepts are very important on nursing exams!

Prioritizing Communication Responses

There may be more than one option that uses a therapeutic communication tool and addresses the client's issue. To select the nurse's **first, best** or **most therapeutic** response, you need to know how to set priorities.

One useful guide to use in selecting nursing priorities in a communication question is *communication theory.* Communication theory identifies that it is a priority to *address the client's feelings.* Addressing the client's feelings is a *client-centered* nursing response. If the client is upset, the nurse should address the client's feelings *before* attempting to present or clarify information.

Look at the introductory statement carefully. Is there a need for the nurse to address the client's feelings at this time? If so, this takes priority over other therapeutic responses like giving information.

tors

introductory statement, the nurse may address the client's
ıe communication tools of *showing empathy* ("It must be
estatement* ("You are angry that . . ."), or just sitting with the
lent,* which shows the client that the client's feelings are
the client is worth the nurse's time.

ommunication priority can be identified using the *nursing*
ıurse in the question have enough *information* to respond
ern? If not, the nurse must *assess* further. *Validation/clarifi-*
riate communication tool at this time.

Finally, the nurse must be aware that the client's statement or behavior may indicate that there is a *physical problem.* In that case, the nurse would address that possibility first, before investigating a possibly psychological cause.

Note: You will find more information on these priority setting guidelines in Chapter 6.

Using Test-Taking Strategies in Communication Questions

If you are not sure of the answer, you can also use these three test-taking strategies from Chapter 3:

1. **Strategy One: Look for a global response option.**
   A nursing response which is more global is probably the best answer.
2. **Strategy Two: Eliminate similar distractors.**
   Two nursing responses which use the same idea can be eliminated.
3. **Strategy Three: Look for similar words in the stem.**
   If you have no other clue to the answer, look for a nursing response that uses a similar word from the stem or case scenario of the question.

SUMMARY:

Your Winning Strategy for Communication Questions

To select the correct option in a communication question:

1. Identify the critical elements:
   Identify the client in the question, the key words, the client's issue, and the type of stem.

2. **Eliminate incorrect options using communication tools and blocks:** If the question has a true response stem, rule out any nursing response that fails to addresses the client's feelings and/or concerns, and any response that uses a communication block.
3. **Consider whether the nurse needs to address the client's feelings at this time.**
4. **If you do not know the answer, use a test-taking strategy.**

Doesn't this make sense? Try answering the drill questions, and see for yourself.

Your increased confidence in answering communication questions will give you a competitive edge on your nursing exams!

PRACTICE SESSION: Communication Questions

Read and answer the following questions, and look for an option that enhances communication.

Remember to identify the critical elements, especially the **client** in the question. When you know the type of stem, narrow your choices by eliminating incorrect options.

After you have answered the question, read the Analysis. The key words and the correct answer are in bold print.

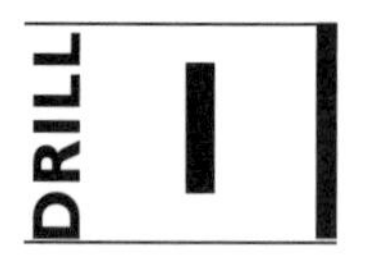

An elderly male client is admitted to the hospital. His son asks the nurse what he should do concerning his father's hearing problem. The nurse's best response to the son is:

A. "As people get older, they tend to have hearing problems."
B. "Your father will need to be seen by a specialist."
C. "I would ask your father how he feels about his hearing loss."
D. "What kind of hearing problem does your father have?"

ANALYSIS I

Critical Elements

Key words:	See bold print.
Client:	The son.
Issue:	The son's concerns about his father's hearing.
Type of stem:	True response stem (therapeutic response).

An elderly male client is admitted to the hospital. His **son** asks the nurse what he should do concerning his **father's hearing problem.** The nurse's best response to the son is:

Eliminate Options and Identify Tools and Blocks:

A. "As people get older, they tend to have hearing problems."
This response tells the client that hearing problems are common in older people. This kind of a response tends to devalue the client's concerns (-). Also, the nurse does not know that the client's father's hearing problem is related to aging.

B. "Your father will need to be seen by a specialist."
The nurse needs more information about the father's hearing problem. With this response, the nurse is putting the client's concerns on hold (-). To be therapeutic, the nurse's response should address the client's concerns.

C. "I would ask your father how he feels about his hearing loss."
The nurse is giving advice, which blocks communication. This response also focuses on the father's feelings, not his hearing problem. While addressing the client's feelings is a priority, we have no information to indicate that the father's feelings are a problem. This is an inappropriate issue (-). To respond to the son's concerns, the nurse needs more information about his father's hearing problem.

D. "What kind of hearing problem does your father have?"
The nurse is communicating therapeutically by addressing the client's concerns. The nurse is assessing by asking the client for more information about his father's hearing problem. The nurse is using the communication tool of <u>clarification (+)</u>.

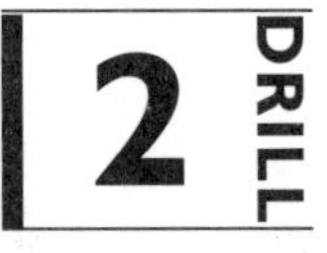

A client is in the hospital because of severe weight loss and refusal to eat. The physician orders the insertion of a nasogastric tube for feeding. The nurse finds the client with the tube removed. The client tells that nurse that he "doesn't need that thing." The most appropriate nursing response is:

A. "You shouldn't have done that! Now I have to put it down again."
B. "Why did you pull that tube out? Do you want to die?"
C. "Tell me what you don't like about the tube."
D. "Your doctor is going to be really upset with you for doing this."

2 ANALYSIS

Critical Elements	
Key words:	See bold print.
Client:	A client with severe weight loss who refuses to eat.
Issue:	Client's removal of nasogastric tube.
Type of stem:	True response stem (therapeutic response).

Eliminate Options and Identify Tools and Blocks:

A client is in the hospital because of severe weight loss and refusal to eat. The physician orders the insertion of a **nasogastric tube for feeding.** The nurse finds the client with the tube removed. The client tells that nurse that he "**doesn't need** that thing." The most appropriate nursing response is:

A. "You shouldn't have done that! Now I have to put it down again."
This response <u>focuses on the nurse's being inconvenienced (-)</u> by the client's actions. "You shouldn't have done that!" is a <u>judgmental (-)</u> statement which is non-therapeutic and therefore not appropriate.

B. "Why did you pull that tube out? Do you want to die?"
This response is <u>judgmental (-)</u> because it implies that the client did something wrong and that he did it because he wants to die. The

response is also a "why" question (-), which blocks communication by putting the client on the defensive.

C. **"Tell me what you don't like about the tube."**
This response allows the client to tell the nurse how he feels about the tube and what it means to the client. It promotes therapeutic communication and does not pass judgment on the client's actions.

D. "Your doctor is going to be really upset with you for doing this."
This response is not client centered (-). It focus on the an inappropriate person—the doctor. It also expresses the opinion of the nurse, which is not important. This response is judgmental because it implies that the client did something that is wrong. This option is not therapeutic because it does not promote the expression of the client's feelings.

DRILL 3

A female client is scheduled for cardiac bypass surgery in the morning. She says to the nurse, "I don't think I'm going to have the surgery. Everybody has to die sooner or later." The most therapeutic nursing response is:

A. "If you don't have the surgery, you will most likely die sooner."
B. "There are always risks involved with surgery. Why have you changed your mind about the operation?"
C. "Cardiac bypass surgery must be very frightening for you. Tell me how you feel about the surgery."
D. "I will call your doctor and have him come in and talk to you."

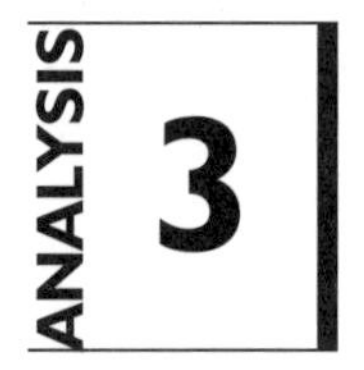

Critical Elements

Key words:	See bold print.
Client:	Female client scheduled for cardiac bypass surgery.
Issue:	Concern about surgery.
Type of stem:	True response stem (therapeutic response).

A female client is **scheduled for cardiac bypass surgery** in the morning. She says to the nurse, "I don't think I'm going to have the surgery. **Everybody has to die** sooner or later." The most therapeutic nursing response is:

Eliminate Options and Identify Tools and Blocks:

− A. "If you don't have the surgery, you will most likely die sooner."
This response devalues the client's feelings (-) and is a block to any further communication!

− B. "There are always risks involved with surgery. Why have you changed your mind about the operation?"
The first part of this response addresses the procedure but not the client's fear. The second part may appear to address the client's feelings, but the nurse is requesting an explanation using a "why" question (-). This can be intimidating and is a communication block. An option which is even partly non-therapeutic should be eliminated. Finally, to be therapeutic, the response should address the client's feelings.

+ C. "Cardiac bypass surgery must be very frightening for you. Tell me how you feel about the surgery."
The nurse's response shows empathy and focuses on the client's feelings in a non-threatening way by using the communication tool of clarification.

− D. "I will call your doctor and have him come in and talk to you."
This response fails to address the client's feelings and puts the issue on hold (-). This response is non-therapeutic.

4 DRILL

A male nurse has received a doctor's order to catheterize one of his female clients. The client says, "I'm not going to allow a male nurse to catheterize me." The nurse's best response is:

A. "Your doctor is a male. Would you let him catheterize you?"
B. "I've done this many times with no problems."
C. "You can explain to your doctor why the catheter wasn't inserted."
D. "You appear to be upset. Let me find a female nurse to help with the procedure."

4 ANALYSIS

Critical Elements

Key words:	See bold print.
Client:	A female client.
Issue:	Refusal to be catheterized by a male nurse.
Type of stem:	True response stem (therapeutic response).

Eliminate Options and Identify Tools and Blocks:

A male nurse has received a doctor's order to catheterize one of his female clients. The client says, "I'm not going to allow a **male nurse** to **catheterize** me." The nurse's best response is:

− A. "Your doctor is a male. Would you let him catheterize you?"
This response is defensive (-), focuses on an inappropriate person (the doctor) (-), focuses on an inappropriate issue (whether the client would allow the doctor to catheterize her) (-), and devalues the client's feelings (-). This response places the client on the defensive and is not therapeutic.

− B. "I've done this many times with no problems."
This response is defensive (-), focuses on an inappropriate person (the nurse)(-), focuses on an inappropriate issue (the nurse's competency(-), and does not address the client's feelings or concern (-). This response is not therapeutic for the client.

− C. "You can explain to your doctor why the catheter wasn't inserted."
This response is defensive (-), focuses on an inappropriate person (the doctor) (-), and aggravates the problem (-). With this response, the nurse will fail to see that the required procedure is performed, which might endanger the client. This response is not professional.

+ D. "You appear to be upset. Let me find a female nurse to help with the procedure." ***This statement shows empathy (+), responds to the client's concern (+), and offers a possible solution to the problem in this situation. The nurse is recognizing the client's right to request to have a female nurse present for this type of procedure. This is the best of the four options in this question. The other options are not client centered, are defensive, and focus on an inappropriate person.***

DRILL 5

A male client is admitted to the hospital for surgery after finding a lump in his right testicle. He asks the nurse, "Do you think that the doctor will find cancer?" The most appropriate nursing response is:

A. "Most lumps found in the testicles are benign."
B. "It must be difficult for you not to know what the doctor will find."
C. "I think that you should discuss this with your doctor."
D. "It might be, but the doctor won't know until the surgery is performed."

5 ANALYSIS

Critical Elements

Key words:	See bold print.
Client:	Client with undiagnosed lump in testicle.
Issue:	Fear of cancer.
Type of stem:	True response stem (therapeutic response).

Eliminate Options and Identify Tools and Blocks:

A male client is admitted to the hospital for surgery after finding a **lump in his right testicle.** He asks the nurse, "Do you think that the doctor will find **cancer**?" The most appropriate nursing response is:

A. "Most lumps found in the testicles are benign."
This may be an accurate statement, but it does not allow the client to express his fears (-) concerning cancer. This response blocks communication between the client and the nurse. To be therapeutic, the nurse should encourage the client to express his feelings.

B. "It must be difficult for you not to know what the doctor will find."
This response uses empathy (+) and promotes communication by allowing the client to express his feelings.

C. "I think that you should discuss this with your doctor."
Referring the client's concern to the doctor puts the client's concern on hold (-) and is not a therapeutic nursing response. The client's feelings and concern needs to be addressed by the nurse.

D. "It might be, but the doctor won't know until the surgery is performed."
This response puts the client's concerns on hold (-). It does not help the client to explore his feelings and is not a therapeutic nursing response.

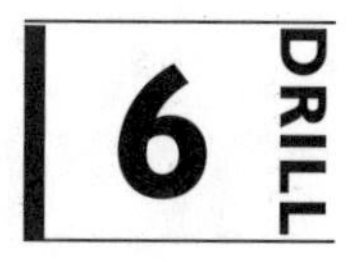

A client is admitted to the hospital with abdominal pain. She overhears her doctor and her nurse discussing cancer of the liver. Later, she says to her nurse, "Having cancer of the liver must be a terrible thing." Which is the best nursing response?

A. "Yes, it is a terrible disease."
B. "What made you think about cancer of the liver?"
C. "Any kind of cancer is terrible, but you can't live without a liver."
D. "Yes. A client on this floor has it and it is very sad for everyone."

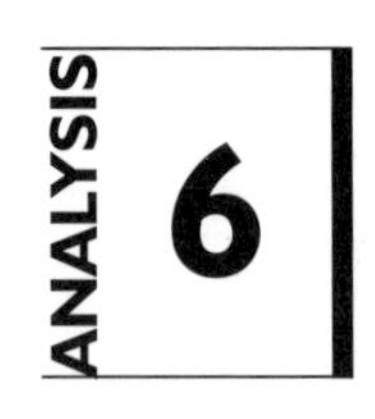

Critical Elements

Key words:	See bold print.
Client:	A client with abdominal pain.
Issues:	Fear of cancer.
Type of stem:	True response stem (therapeutic response).

Eliminate Options and Identify Tools and Blocks:

A client is admitted to the hospital with abdominal pain. She overhears her doctor and her nurse discussing cancer of the liver. Later, she says to her nurse, "Having **cancer** of the liver must be a **terrible** thing." Which is the best nursing response?

− A. "Yes, it is a terrible disease."
This response is an accurate factual statement, but it does not encourage further communication (-). The client has an obvious concern, or she wouldn't have mentioned the subject. The nurse needs more information about the client's concern.

+ B. "What made you think about cancer of the liver?"
By asking this question, the nurse enhances therapeutic communication by using the tool of clarification (+), to identify the reason for the client's concern about cancer of the liver. The case situation tells you that the client overheard her doctor and her nurse talking about a client. The client may think that the conversation concerned her. (Note that the words "cancer of the liver" occur in the case situation and in this option, which is a clue that this might be the correct answer.)

− C. "Any kind of cancer is terrible, but you can't live without a liver."
This response by the nurse does not really address the client's feelings or concern (+), and it does not help the nurse to identify or clarify why the client is talking about this particular illness. The nurse needs more information, and this response may deter the client from pursuing this topic any further.

− D. "Yes. A client on this floor has it and it is very sad for everyone."
This response does not address the client in the case scenario (-)—it addresses the other client on the floor and "everyone" who is sad. Therefore, this response is not therapeutic. This response can also be interpreted as a breach in confidentiality for the client who has the cancer. This is an inappropriate response by the nurse.

7 DRILL

The nurse is teaching a female client about self breast exam. The client tells the nurse that she doesn't understand why she is being taught this, since she doesn't plan on doing it anyway. The best response by the nurse is:

A. "Self breast exam is taught to women in order to detect any lumps or changes in the breast which can be an early sign of cancer, because early treatment has a higher rate of cure."
B. "You're right. If you don't plan on doing the exams, then I don't need to show you how to do it."
C. "If you don't plan on doing the exam yourself, then you should have your doctor do it at your annual check up."
D. "You have the right to do whatever you choose. It is your body."

7 ANALYSIS

Critical Elements	
Key words:	See bold print.
Client:	Female.
Issue:	Self breast exam.
Type of stem:	Asks for a therapeutic response.

Eliminate Options and Identify Tools and Blocks:

The nurse is teaching a female client about self breast exam. The client tells the nurse that she **doesn't understand** why she is being taught this, since she **doesn't plan** on doing it anyway. The best response by the nurse is:

+ A. "Self breast exam is taught to women in order to detect any lumps or changes in the breast which can be an early sign of cancer, because early treatment has a higher rate of cure."
This response by the nurse provides the client with information (+) concerning the rationale for self breast exam. This response provides the client with information that allows her to make an informed choice. Giving information is an important therapeutic communication tool!

− B. "You're right. If you don't plan on doing the exams, then I don't need to show you how to do it."
In this response the nurse has become defensive, which is a block to communication because it also places the client on the defensive. This approach focuses on an inappropriate person (the nurse) (-), and fails to promote the nurse's goal in this important area of client teaching.

C. "If you don't plan on doing the exam yourself, then you should have your doctor do it at your annual check up."
Having a physician perform an exam annually is a good validation action but does not take the place of monthly self-exams. This is not an appropriate response since it does not address the need for regular breast examination (-) to detect early changes and implies that this is an acceptable recommendation. It also fails to encourage further explanation of the client's statement (-). (Note also that Options C and D are similar in supporting the client's decision not to do the self-exams. Similar distractors should be eliminated.)

D. "You have the right to do whatever you choose. It is your body."
This statement is factually correct; clients should have choices concerning their health care. However, the nurse has a responsibility for client teaching so that the choices will be ***informed*** *choices. This client has made a decision without the benefit of an explanation of the rationale for the intervention. This response does not encourage any further communication (-) and is not therapeutic for the client.*

A confused elderly female client has wet herself and is standing in the hospital corridor in a puddle of urine. She has trouble getting to the bathroom in time. She looks ashamed. She says to the nurse, "I want to go outside for a walk now." What is the most appropriate response by the nurse at this time?

A. "Before we go for a walk, perhaps we can make a list that will help you make your bathroom trips easier."
B. "Right now, let me wipe up the urine on the floor, and let's get a change of clothing. I am sure that this problem is upsetting for you."
C. "This has been a problem for you. Let's see if we can find a solution together."
D. "Wetting yourself is very upsetting. Yes, let's take a walk."

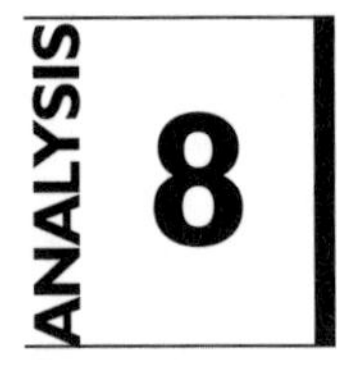

Critical Elements

Key words:	See bold print.
Client:	A confused elderly female client.
Issue:	Puddle of urine on the floor and client's wet clothes.
Type of stem:	True response stem (therapeutic response).

Eliminate Options and Identify Tools and Blocks:

A **confused elderly female client,** has **wet** herself and is standing in the hospital corridor in a **puddle of urine.** She has trouble getting to the bathroom in time. She looks **ashamed.** She says to the nurse, "I want to go outside for a walk now." What is the **most appropriate** response by the nurse at this time?

− A. "Before we go for a walk, perhaps we can make a list that will help you make your bathroom trips easier."
The issue in this question is a wet client standing in a puddle of urine. This response does not address the current problem (-). Also, since the client is confused, making a list is not appropriate (-) because she couldn't remember.

+ B. "Right now, let me wipe up the urine on the floor, and let's get a change of clothing. I am sure that this problem is upsetting for you."
With this response, the nurse is dealing with the here and now (+) by helping the client focus on her current need, which is dry clothes, and is informing the client that she is going to wipe up the urine off the floor. The nurse is also showing empathy (+). This response is therapeutic for the client and provides for the safety of the client and others on the unit. (Note that the words "urine on the floor" in this option are similar to the words "puddle of urine" in the question. This is a clue that this may be the correct answer.)

− C. "This has been a problem for you. Let's see if we can find a solution together."
The client is feeling uncomfortable, and this response fails to address her immediate need (-) for dry clothes and a safe environment. The client is also confused, and she is feeling ashamed. Discussing possible solutions to the problem of not getting to the bathroom in time will not be helpful (-).

− D. "Wetting yourself is very upsetting. Yes, let's take a walk."
In this response, the nurse is showing empathy. However, this response fails to address the client's basic need at this time for dry clothes and a safe environment (-). An option which is partly wrong cannot be the correct answer.

NOTES

Chapter 6

LEARNING TO ANSWER QUESTIONS THAT SELECT PRIORITIES

Demonstrating Your Nursing Judgment

Nursing exams test your ability to demonstrate good nursing judgment in applying and analyzing nursing knowledge. For this reason, many test questions require decision making.

Decision-making questions very often involve **setting priorities:** "What should the nurse do first?" "What is the best nursing response?" Questions that require selecting priorities are often difficult to answer! However, they are usually easy to recognize.

Here are some typical stems found in priority-setting test questions:

- What is the nurse's **initial** response?
- What is the **essential** nursing action?
- What is a **vital** consideration in planning the client's nursing care?
- The nurse would give **immediate** attention to which questions?
- The **priority** nursing action is to:
- Which response demonstrates the **best** nursing judgment?
- The nurse would identify which information as **most** important?

A <u>false response stem</u> might ask you to:

- Identify the nursing action which **receives lowest priority** at this time.
- Select the **least important rationale** for a nursing intervention.
- Select the option which identifies the **least appropriate** nursing action or nursing response.

Priority-setting Guidelines

There are **four priority setting guidelines** that you can use to help answer multiple choice questions which select priorities:

1. **The Nursing Process,** as you know, identifies that the nurse must always *assess* before planning or implementing any nursing action. Assessment comes first, because the nurse must obtain the necessary information before taking action.

2. **Maslow's Hierarchy of Needs** identifies that the client's "lower level" or basic *physiological needs and safety needs* must be satisfied *before* "higher level" psychosocial needs can be addressed. Physiological needs come first. When no physiological needs are apparent, safety needs receive priority.

3. **Communication Theory** tells us that for communication to be effective and therapeutic, the nurse must first address the client's *feelings.* This is important in establishing and maintaining a therapeutic relationship with the client. Also, if the client is upset, it is difficult to obtain information from the client, or to give the client necessary information. When prioritizing possible nursing responses in a communication question, *look to see whether the nurse needs to address the client's feelings at this time.*

4. **Teaching/Learning Theory** identifies that *motivation* is the key to successful client teaching. The nurse must first determine that the client is motivated to learn and to care for his or her health needs.

How Will I Know Which Guideline to Use in a Question?

Selecting the appropriate priority-setting guideline to use in a question is the hardest part! After that, all you have to do is select the option that addresses the important priority.

To determine which guideline to use, it is important to *identify the critical elements and then read all four options.* This will give you a better idea of which guideline is most applicable to the situation, and to the choices you are asked to compare. The key words are also a good clue.

If you are unsure which guideline to use in a question, first ask yourself if the introductory statement *includes enough information* for the nurse to decide what to do. If more information is needed, the *nursing process* identifies that *assessment receives priority.* The nurse must always assess first! Then, look for an option that includes an assessment action. (There is more information about using the nursing process in Chapter Seven.)

If the nurse has enough information, use Maslow's theory and try to identify an option which responds to an *urgent physiological need.* Remember the ABC'S! Maslow's theory is often the best guideline in questions which involve a sudden emergency or describe a situation which is life-threatening for the client. If there is no urgent physiological need, look for an option which responds to a *safety* concern. Safety is a priority nursing consideration at all times! In Maslow's theory, the "lower level" physiological and safety needs receive priority over the "higher level" psychosocial needs.

In *communication* questions, remember that the correct answer always addresses the client in the question and uses a therapeutic communication tool (see Chapter Five to review strategy for communication questions). When selecting the nurse's first or best response, see if there is a need for the nurse to *address the client's feelings* at this time—and look for a therapeutic nursing response that addresses the client's feelings.

If the question concerns *client teaching,* look to see if one of the options focuses on the client's *motivation.* If the client is not motivated to care for his or her health problem, client teaching will probably not be successful.

How to select a priority setting guideline will become clear once you have seen a few sample questions.

idelines Used to Select Priorities

cess	*Assessment* comes first.
eory of Needs	*Physiological needs* come first; when no physiological needs exist, *safety needs* receive priority.
ion Theory	Focus on the client's *feelings* first.
Teaching/Learning Theory	Focus on *motivation* first.

PRACTICE SESSION: Selecting Priorities

In each of the following questions, you will need to decide which of the guidelines in the table above provides the rationale for the correct answer.

First, identify the four critical elements in the question—the key words, the client, the issue, and the type of stem. Then eliminate incorrect options according to the type of stem. (A false response stem would ask you to select the option that receives lowest priority.)

To select priorities, read the four options. Try to decide if there is enough information in the introductory statement. If there is no need for more assessment, try to identify an option that addresses an urgent physiological or safety need.

If the question concerns communication or client teaching, look for an option that addresses the client's feelings or motivation. Always be sure to read all the options before selecting the one that receives highest priority!

If you are unsure of the answer, try using one of the test-taking strategies you learned in Chapter Four: looking for a global response option, eliminating similar distractors, and looking for similar words in the question.

After you have answered the question, read the Analysis. Note that the key words and the answer letter are marked in bold print.

DRILL

A client, 21 years old, is admitted to the hospital because of extreme weight loss. It is noted on the admission assessment that the client believes that she is overweight at 88 pounds. What aspect of care should the nurse consider her first priority?

A. Assessing the client's nutritional status.
B. Obtaining a psychiatric consult.
C. Planning a therapeutic diet for the client.
D. Talking to the family members to find out more about the client's self concept.

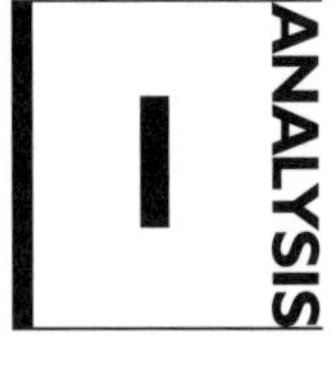

Critical Elements	
Key words:	See bold print.
Client:	Client with extreme weight loss.
Issue:	Extreme weight loss.
Type of stem:	True response stem (high priority).

Eliminate Options and Select Priorities:

A client, 21 years old, is admitted to the hospital because of **extreme** weight loss. It is noted on the admission assessment that the client believes that she is overweight at 88 pounds. What aspect of care should the nurse consider her first **priority**?

+ A. Assessing the client's nutritional status.
The client's nutritional status should receive first priority because nutrition is a basic physiological need (+). If the client's nutritional needs are not met, the situation may be life threatening.

? B. Obtaining a psychiatric consult.
Obtaining a psychiatric consult may be an appropriate intervention (?), but with only the information given in this case situation it would not take priority at this time. Can you identify a basic ***physiological*** *need for this client?*

+ C. Planning a therapeutic diet for the client.
The client will need adequate nutrition. Nutrition is a basic physiological need (+) and a high priority. However, ***planning*** *nursing interventions should come* ***after*** *one of the other options in this question. What should the nurse do first?*

? D. Talking to the family members to find out more about the client's self-concept.
Obtaining further information from the family may be appropriate (?), but it is not the priority action in this situation. Can you identify a basic ***physiological*** *need which should be addressed first?*

DRILL 2

An elderly male client with chronic obstructive pulmonary disease (COPD) is receiving oxygen per nasal cannula at 2 liters per minute. At 3:00 PM, the nurse assesses that the client appears to have made a good adjustment to hospitalization. At 5:00 PM the nurse finds the oxygen cannula on the floor. The client is angry and says, "It's about time you got here. Where am I? Where is my breakfast?" Which consideration would receive the nurse's immediate consideration?

A. Has the oxygen cannula been off long enough to cause hypoxia?
B. Is the client's anger related to being hospitalized?
C. Does the client need a clock in the room to keep track of time?
D. Is the client accustomed to eating dinner very early in the day?

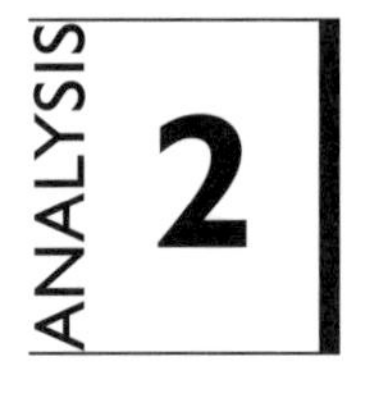

Critical Elements	
Key words:	See bold print.
Client:	An elderly male client with COPD.
Issue:	Oxygen cannula on floor, client confused.
Type of stem:	True response stem (high priority).

Eliminate Options and Select Priorities:

An elderly male client with chronic obstructive pulmonary disease (COPD) is receiving oxygen per nasal cannula at 2 liters per minute. At 3:00 PM, the nurse assesses that the client appears to have made a good adjustment to hospitalization. At 5:00 PM the nurse finds the **oxygen cannula on the floor.** The client is angry and says, "It's about time you got here. **Where am I? Where is my breakfast?"** Which consideration would receive the nurse's immediate consideration?

+ A. Has the oxygen cannula been off long enough to cause hypoxia?
This is a priority consideration because the focus is on an immediate physiological need (+). A low flow of oxygen is necessary to maintain the hypoxic drive for a client with COPD. Due to his confused behavior and lack of oxygen for a period of time, the

client may be exhibiting manifestations of acute respiratory insufficiency. This is a life threatening situation. Maslow's Theory identifies that physiological needs receive first priority.

– B. Is the client's anger related to being hospitalized?
This is a lower priority concern for the nurse because it focuses on a ***psychological*** *explanation (-) for the client's anger and ignores the client's confusion ("Where am I?"). It must first be determined if his confused behavior is due to a* ***physiological*** *need.*

– C. Does the client need a clock in the room to keep track of time?
This is another low priority consideration. This ***psychological*** *rationale (-) for the client's confused behavior related to the time of day would be explored only after clarifying that his more general confusion is not due to a respiratory insufficiency.*

– D. Is the client accustomed to eating dinner very early in the day?
This is another low priority consideration. Physiological rationales for the client's confusion should be explored before any possible psychological rationales for his anger (-). This option is similar to Option C because both focus on the time of day. Also, B, C and D are all similar because they are concerned with possible psychological rationales. Similar distractors can be eliminated.

3 DRILL

A hospitalized elderly female client is to receive an x-ray. The nurse enters the client's room, and asks if the client is ready to go to x-ray. She nods her head "yes." The next **priority** nursing action is to:

A. Explain the x-ray procedure to the client.
B. Help the client into a wheelchair, so that when the transporter arrives the client will be ready.
C. Ask if the client has any questions.
D. Look at the client's identification bracelet.

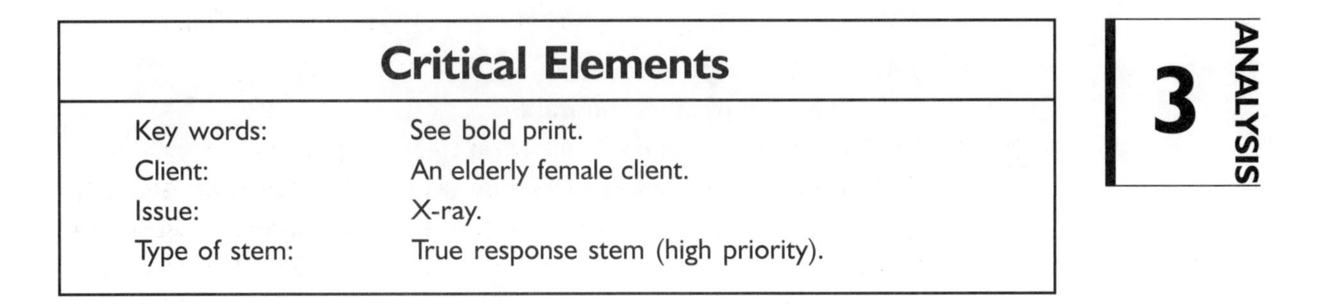

Critical Elements

Key words:	See bold print.
Client:	An elderly female client.
Issue:	X-ray.
Type of stem:	True response stem (high priority).

3 ANALYSIS

Eliminate Options and Select Priorities:

A hospitalized elderly female client is to receive an x-ray. The nurse enters the client's room, and asks if the client is ready to go to x-ray. She nods "yes." The next **priority** nursing action is to:

? A. Explain the x-ray procedure to the client.
Incorrect. Although the x-ray procedure should be explained to the client, this is not the priority nursing action at this time. When answering a priority-setting question, try to identify an action that addresses physiological needs or the safety of the client.

− B. Help the client into a wheelchair, so that when the transporter arrives the client will be ready.
No, this is not correct. Having the client ready for the transporter is very considerate; however, another option takes priority over this. Try to identify an action that addresses physiological needs or the safety of the client.

? C. Ask if the client has any questions.
Answering any questions is an appropriate nursing action; however, this is not the priority action at this time.

\+ D. Look at the client's identification bracelet.
Excellent! The nurse must always check the client's identification before performing any nursing action. Once the client's identity is determined, the nurse can then proceed with the other options. This is the priority action because it provides for the safety of the client.

DRILL 4

A 15-year-old female client is being seen in the family planning clinic. She says to the nurse that she is nervous and has never had a pelvic examination before. The best response by the nurse initially is:

A. "All you have to do is relax."
B. "It is only slightly uncomfortable."
C. "What part of the exam makes you nervous?"
D. "If you want birth control pills, then a pelvic exam is required."

Critical Elements	
Key words:	See bold print.
Client:	A 15-year-old female client.
Issue:	Concern about pelvic examination.
Type of stem:	True response stem (high priority).

Eliminate Options and Select Priorities:

A 15-year-old female client is being seen in the family planning clinic. She says to the nurse that she is **nervous** and has never had a pelvic examination before. The **best response** by the nurse **initially** is:

− A. "All you have to do is relax."
This statement is not therapeutic because it does not address the client's concerns (-). It also blocks communication by using cliché and false reassurance (-). This cannot be the correct answer.

− B. "It is only slightly uncomfortable."
This response devalues the client's concern (-) and fails to encourage the client to clarify her concern about the exam. This option cannot be the answer.

+ C. "What part of the exam makes you nervous?"
This response recognizes the client's feelings (+) and uses the tool of clarification (+) to encourage the client to tell the nurse more about her concerns. This response is therapeutic for the client. Note that this is a communication question. Communication theory identifies that focusing on the client's feelings is the priority.

− D. "If you want birth control pills, then a pelvic exam is required."
Be careful! There is no information in the introductory statement that the client wants birth control pills. Do not "read into" the question! This response by the nurse addresses an inappropriate issue (-) and might be interpreted as expressing disapproval by the nurse (-). This response also fails to address the feelings or concerns that the client has shared with the nurse. This cannot be the answer!

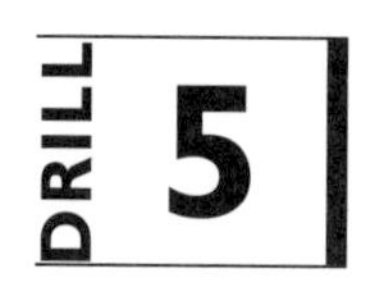

The nurse is caring for a postoperative client. The nurse is informed during report that the client has not voided for eight hours. The initial nursing action would be to:

A. Assist the client to the bathroom.
B. Place the client on a bed pan and pour warm water over her perineum.
\C. Palpate and percuss the client's bladder.
D. Catheterize the client.

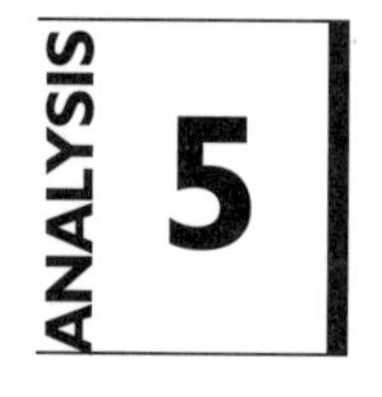

Critical Elements

Key words:	See bold print.
Client:	A postoperative client.
Issue:	Client who has not voided in 8 hours.
Type of stem:	True response stem (high priority).

The nurse is caring for a **postoperative** client. The nurse is informed during report that the client **has not voided for eight hours.** The **initial** nursing action would be to:

Eliminate Options and Select Priorities:

? A. Assist the client to the bathroom.
This nursing action is a possibility (?). Assisting the client to the bathroom may be helpful if the client needs to urinate. However, this information needs to be obtained before action is taken.

− B. Place the client on a bed pan and pour warm water over her perineum.
This action is probably not appropriate (-) in this introductory statement, because there is no information that the client is not ambulatory. Placing the client on a bed pan is not always conducive to urinating. If the client is allowed out of bed, sitting on the toilet while pouring warm water over the perineum can facilitate the client to void. More importantly, the nurse must assess that the client has the need and an urge to void before this intervention is implemented.

+ C. Palpate and percuss the client's bladder.
This assessment action is the priority (+) in this introductory statement. The nurse needs more information. Assessing the client's bladder provides information concerning the need to void. This is the only option that provides for assessment of the client.

D. Catheterize the client.
The nurse does not have enough information, so this action would be inappropriate (-) at this time. This cannot be the initial nursing action. Catheterizing the client should only be done after it has been determined that the client has a full bladder and is unable to void. The nurse must assess first.

6 DRILL

The nurse has completed pre-discharge teaching for an elderly female client who is being discharged from the hospital after treatment for poor circulation to her lower extremities. Which action by the client would the nurse identify as the most important indication of the success or failure of the pre-discharge teaching?

A. The client puts on stockings with elastic tops and tells the nurse that she does not like other kinds of hosiery.
B. The client tells the nurse that she will get a thermometer to measure the temperature of the bath water.
C. The client asks her husband to take her sandals home, and bring a pair of shoes to the hospital for her to wear home.
D. The client tells the nurse that she is going to have to have a hard time remembering to keep her legs uncrossed.

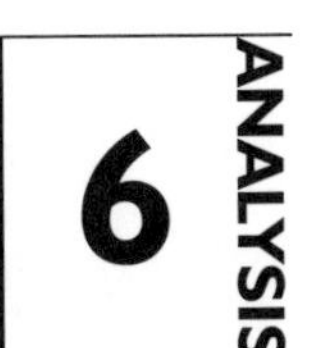

Critical Elements	
Key words:	See bold print.
Client:	An elderly female with poor circulation of the lower extremities.
Issue:	Success of pre-discharge teaching.
Type of stem:	False response stem.

Eliminate Options and Select Priorities:

The nurse has completed pre-discharge teaching for an elderly female client who is being discharged from the hospital after treatment for **poor circulation** to her lower extremities. Which action by the client would the nurse identify as the **most important** indication of the **success or failure** of the pre-discharge **teaching?**

A. The client puts on stockings with elastic tops and tells the nurse that she does not like other kinds of hosiery.
Elastic tops on stockings decrease circulation and should be avoided by clients with circulation problems. This action and

statement by the client are "most important" because they indicate that the client is not motivated (-) to care for her health care needs. Teaching/learning theory identifies that motivation is the priority. Note that this question has a false response stem, so the answer must be an action that is not appropriate for a client with circulation problems. This is the only option which describes an incorrect action.

+ B. The client tells the nurse that she will get a thermometer to measure the temperature of the bath water.
A client who has poor circulation has a decreased sense of temperature. This statement indicates that the client has successfully learned (+) what the nurse taught her. This is a true statement. Because this question has a false response stem, this option cannot be the correct answer.

+ C. The client asks her husband take her sandals home, and bring a pair of shoes to the hospital for her to wear home.
This statement by the client indicates proper understanding (+) of pre-discharge teaching. Clients with poor circulation need to wear shoes that protect their feet from injury. This action by the client indicates to the nurse that learning has taken place.

? D. The client tells the nurse that she is going to have a hard time remembering to keep her legs uncrossed.
Crossing the legs at the knees impairs circulation and should be avoided by the client. This statement by the client indicates to the nurse that the client does understand (+) the discharge instructions. If you thought this statement by the client indicated a lack of understanding or unwillingness to avoid crossing her legs, you were "reading into" the question. The client has understood and is thinking about the effort required to follow this instruction.

Chapter 7

LEARNING TO ANSWER QUESTIONS THAT USE THE NURSING PROCESS

How Do Test Questions Use the Nursing Process?

Test questions on nursing exams present clinical problems and ask you to solve them using the nursing process.

The nursing process is the method by which the nurse solves clinical problems and applies nursing knowledge. To become a professional nurse, it is necessary not only to acquire a lot of nursing knowledge, but to know how to identify and solve clinical problems. Questions on nursing exams use the nursing process because it is fundamental to the practice of nursing.

THE FIVE PHASES OF THE NURSING PROCESS

1. Assessment
2. Analysis
3. Planning
4. Implementation
5. Evaluation

In Chapter Two, you learned special study tips that use the nursing process. To test your ability to apply nursing knowledge and make safe nursing decisions, nursing exams include questions that use all five categories or phases of the nursing process. A test question that uses the nursing process will involve *nursing behaviors associated with one or more of the five phases.*

How Will I Know Which Phase of the Nursing Process to Use in a Question?

When reading a test question, look carefully at the introductory statement to see what information you are given about the client—and *what the nurse is doing, is preparing to do, or has already done.* This is your main clue. For example, if the question tells you that the nurse is assessing the client—or is taking vital signs, interviewing a client, or doing other assessment activities—then the question uses the assessment phase.

Also, be sure to identify the *issue* in the question. Try to state your understanding of the situation and information presented so far. Look for nursing behaviors in the options that address the issue in the question. This will become clear with a few examples and a little practice.

When preparing for any nursing exam, it is very helpful to *practice answering test questions that use the nursing process*—questions with introductory statements that present clinical scenarios and ask you to make nursing decisions. Answering practice questions gives you a chance to practice applying your nursing knowledge and your decision making skills. In fact, learning how to answer test questions using the nursing process can actually sharpen your decision making and critical thinking skills—and make you a better nurse as well as a better test-taker!

Where Can I Find Practice Questions that Use the Nursing Process?

We're glad you asked! In this chapter, you will review the five phases of the nursing process and have a chance to try some drill questions that reflect each category. Be sure to note the specific nursing activities associated with each category of the nursing process. All the questions in the Final Exam in Chapter Nine (and the computerized Final Exam on the CD-ROM included with this book) use the nursing process. Chapter Eleven includes additional nursing process test questions classified according to fundamental nursing subjects.

MEDS Publishing offers "Q&A" (question and answer) books and software with practice problem-solving questions and detailed answers, known as rationales. These materials explain the "why" or the logic behind both the correct and incorrect answers.

Using Q&A books and software on different clinical areas is an excellent way to reinforce your nursing knowledge, practice applying it in different settings, polish your problem-solving skills and your command of the nursing process, and assess your progress. When taking a practice test, be sure to record and check your answers, calculate your score, and see if you can explain the answers and any mistakes you made.

Check with your school or local library or bookstore for these MEDS software and book titles: *Test-Taking Beginning Students: A Critical Thinking Tutorial; The Complete Q&A for the NCLEX-RN, The Complete Q&A for the NCLEX-PN* (both with CD-ROM); *Learning System Online; NCLEX-RN Gold, and NCLEX-PN Gold.* Or call 800-200-9191.

ASSESSMENT QUESTIONS

In the assessment phase, the nurse is collecting data. This is the first phase of the nursing process, because the nurse must always *assess first.*

Nursing Behaviors Associated with the Assessment Phase of the Nursing Process

- Gathering objective and subjective data (e.g., taking vital signs, reading lab values, asking the client how he or she is feeling).
- Identifying signs and symptoms.
- Evaluating environments.
- Identifying the nurse's reaction.
- Verifying data.
- Communicating information.

When answering prioritizing questions that ask what the nurse should do *first,* check to see if the nurse in the question has enough information. If not, look for an option that includes an assessment behavior.

Tips for Questions that Focus on Assessment

- If you see terms in the question like "observe," "monitor," "check," "obtain information" or "find out," these refer to the assessment process.
- Remember to <u>assess first</u>, before planning or implementing nursing care.
- Know your vital signs and normal lab values!
- When assessing, be sure to focus on the *issue* of the question. For example, is it a drug, a disorder, or an early sign of a complication?

Practice Session: Assessment Questions

Read and answer the following assessment questions. *Always* identify the critical elements and use your test-taking strategies! When you know the type of stem and the issue, make a decision about each option as you read it by using the selection procedure, keeping in mind the nursing behaviors included in assessment. After you have answered the question, read the analysis. The **key words** and the **correct answer** are in bold print.

NOTE: The practice sessions on the other four categories of the nursing process in this chapter all require similar problem solving and test-taking methods.

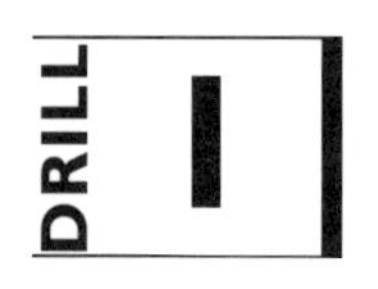

A male client returns from the recovery room to the surgical unit following surgery. Upon his arrival in the client care unit, what is the initial focus of the nurse's assessment?

A. Urine output.
B. Vital signs.
C. Pain in the incision.
D. Status of the dressing.

Critical Elements

Key words:	See bold print.
Client:	A male client returning after surgery.
Issue:	Initial focus of postoperative nursing assessment.
Stem:	True response stem.

Eliminate Options

A male client is returning from the recovery room to the surgical unit **following surgery**. Upon his arrival in the client care unit, which parameter would be the **initial** focus of the nurse's **assessment?**

? A. Urine output.
This is a possibility (+), since postoperative assessment of urine output is necessary to measure renal, circulatory, and genitourinary function. However, this would not be the initial focus for postoperative assessment. When answering questions that require prioritizing, remember to read all options before selecting the answer.

+ **B. Vital signs.**
This is the initial focus (+) of the nurse's assessment. At this time the nurse needs to gather objective data about the client's condition. This is a critical situation in which it is necessary to implement the ABC guideline. First, the airway and breathing are monitored by observing the rate of respirations. Next, the circulation is assessed by monitoring the pulse rate and the blood pressure.

? C. Pain in the incision.
This is an appropriate assessment and possible (?) option, but not the focus of the initial assessment. It is necessary to manage and monitor postoperative pain since the greatest postoperative pain occurs during the first 12 to 36 hours. Potent drugs may depress the respiratory rate and increase tracheal secretions. Management of pain is necessary for client comfort and prevention of postoperative atelectasis and pneumonia. However, this is not the highest priority.

? D. Status of the dressing.
This is another possibility (?), since it is necessary to observe the dressing for amount, type, odor and consistency of the drainage. Any drainage is marked and noted on the dressing. This is another important assessment, but it is not the initial focus.

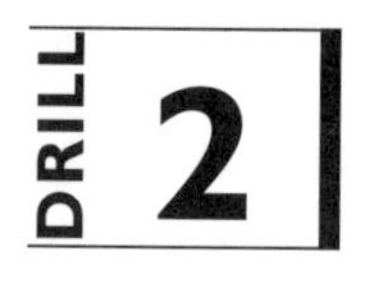

The nurse is monitoring a client who is receiving an intravenous infusion for signs of infiltration. In assessing an IV site which has become infiltrated, the nurse knows that which finding is unexpected?

A. The infusion rate slows or stops while the tubing is not kinked.
B. The area around the injection site feels warm to the touch.
C. Swelling, hardness, or pain is found around the needle site.
D. Blood fails to return in the tubing when the bottle is lowered.

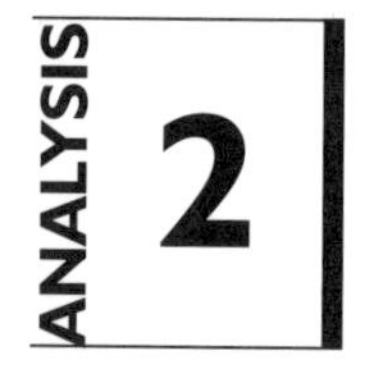

Critical Elements	
Key words:	See bold print.
Client:	Any client receiving IV infusion.
Issue:	Signs of infiltration.
Type of stem:	False response stem.

Eliminate Options

The nurse is monitoring a client who is receiving an intravenous infusion for **signs of infiltration.** In assessing an IV site which has become infiltrated, the nurse knows that which finding is **unexpected?**

+ A. The infusion rate slows or stops while the tubing is not kinked.
This finding is indicative (+) of an infiltration—and you are looking for a finding that is unexpected in an infiltration. When infiltration occurs, the IV fluid enters the subcutaneous space and the flow of the IV fluid decreases or may even stop. The area around the venipuncture site swells from the tissue fluid. Note that this assessment question has a false response stem!

− B. The area around the injection site feels warm to the touch.
Since this false response stem asks for a finding which is not expected (-) in an infiltration, this is the correct response. IV fluid is cool, which causes the area around the venipuncture site to be cool. A warm skin temperature indicates phlebitis, not an infiltration.

+ C. Swelling, hardness, or pain located around the needle site.
This is an expected finding (+) when an infiltration occurs. Swelling occurs as the fluid seeps into the tissue spaces. This is objective data that the nurse would observe when assessing an infiltration of an IV. As the edema continues, the discomfort and pain increase.

D. Blood fails to return in the tubing when the bottle is lowered.
This is another expected finding (+) in an infiltration. If the IV is patent when the bottle is lowered, the blood in the vein will flow into the IV tubing. When the needle is dislodged from the tissue, blood will fail to return in the tubing when the bottle is lowered. This is not the answer, because the question has a false response stem.

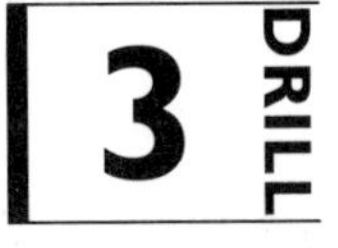

A client puts her call light on and tells the nurse that she has to urinate. The client has had a Foley catheter in place since her surgery two days ago. The appropriate nursing action is to:

A. Remind the client that she has a Foley catheter in place and does not need to go to the bathroom.
B. Replace the Foley catheter with a new catheter.
C. Explain to the client that the urge to void is a common occurrence for clients who have urinary catheters.
D. Check the catheter and tubing for kinks and note the urine output in the drainage bag.

3 ANALYSIS

Critical Elements	
Key words:	See bold print.
Client:	A client with a Foley catheter.
Issue:	Urge to void.
Type of stem:	True response stem.

Eliminate Options:

A client puts her call light on and tells the nurse that she **has to urinate**. The client has had a **Foley catheter** in place since her surgery two days ago. The **appropriate** nursing action is to:

A. Remind the client that she has a Foley catheter in place and does not need to go to the bathroom.
Incorrect! Although a Foley catheter is in place, it may not be patent, which can result in distention of the bladder and cause the client to feel the urge to void. This action does not meet the client's needs. The nurse must determine the cause of the client's urge to void.

B. Replace the Foley catheter with a new catheter.
Incorrect. A new catheter might be necessary to meet the client's needs, but the nurse must first determine the cause of the client's urge to void.

- C. Explain to the client that the urge to void is a common occurrence for clients who have urinary catheters.
  Incorrect. The urge to void usually occurs upon initial insertion of the Foley catheter, not two days afterwards. There are several possible reasons for the client having urgency, and the nurse must attempt to discover the cause in order to meet the client's needs. Notice that this option is very similar to option A—and neither is correct.

+ D. Check the catheter and tubing for kinks and note the urine output in the drainage bag.
  Correct! Assess first! Before replacing the catheter or offering an explanation to the client, the nurse needs more information. The Foley catheter may not be patent, which can result in distention of the bladder and cause the client to feel the urge to void. Checking the equipment is the best nursing action, since data will be obtained which will assist the nurse with problem solving. The nursing process is the best strategy in answering this kind of question.

ANALYSIS QUESTIONS

Questions that focus on the analysis phase of the nursing process are the most difficult questions. They require an understanding of the principles of pathophysiology, pharmacokinetics, and psychopathology, as well as growth and development.

Nursing behaviors associated with the analysis phase of the nursing process include:

- Interpreting data.
- Validating data.
- Organizing related data.
- Recording data.
- Identifying a nursing diagnosis.

When answering an analysis question, be sure you have correctly identified the *issue* of the question, and focus on the *nursing rationale.* For example, the rationale for bed rest for a client with pneumonia is different than for a client with a myocardial infarction.

Tips for Questions that Focus on Analysis

- Identify the issue in the question.
- Take care not to "read into" the question! Do not assume information that is not given in the question.
- Focus on nursing rationales.

Practice Session: Analysis Questions

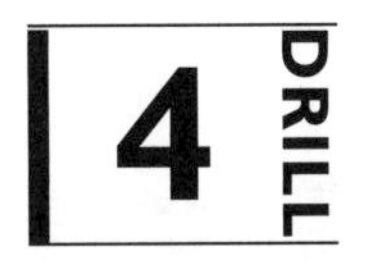

The nurse is performing a developmental evaluation of a two-year-old client. Which observation would the nurse consider a good indicator of normal development for this child?

A. Having command of a vocabulary of six words.
B. The ability to walk up and down stairs without help.
C. The ability to dress and undress.
D. The ability to point at what he/she wants.

4 ANALYSIS

Critical Elements	
Key words:	See bold print.
Client:	Any two-year-old.
Issue:	A normal developmental characteristic.
Type of stem:	True response stem.

Eliminate Options

The nurse is performing a developmental evaluation of a **two-year-old** client. Which observation would the nurse consider a good indicator of **normal** development for this child?

A. Having command of a vocabulary of six words.
This is not normal (-). A two-year-old has a vocabulary of about 200 to 300 words. An 18-month-old child has a vocabulary of about 10 words. This is a very difficult question!

+ B. The ability to walk up and down stairs without help.
This is a good indicator of normal (+) psychomotor development. An 18-month-old walks upstairs, but a two-year-old manages to walk up and down the stairs.)

– C. The ability to dress and undress.
This is an inappropriate (-) expectation for a two-year-old. This describes an older child of about three to four years old. A two- to three-year-old is only able to undress, not dress himself.

– D. The ability to point at what he/she wants.
This is not normal (-) communication ability for a two-year old. This describes a one-year-old infant. Because of increased language ability, a normal two-year-old does not need to point.

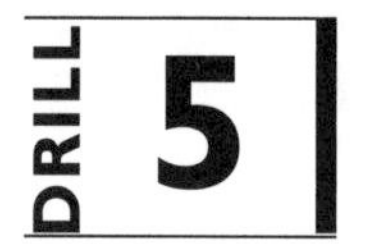

In preparing a preoperative teaching plan, the nurse would give top priority to:

A. Active range of motion exercises.
B. A rationale for various tubes, IV's, etc.
C. The need to record vital signs frequently.
D. Coughing and deep breathing exercises.

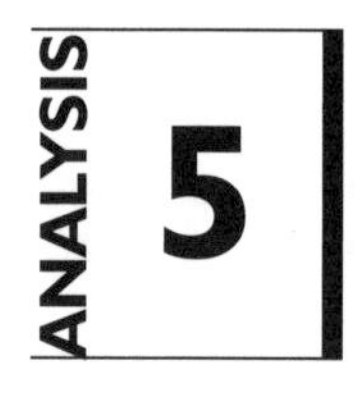

Critical Elements	
Key words:	See bold print.
Client:	A preoperative client.
Issue:	Preoperative teaching.
Type of stem:	True response stem (high priority).

Eliminate Options

In preparing a **preoperative** teaching plan, the nurse would give **top priority** to:

A. Active range of motion exercises.
This is inappropriate (-) for inclusion in the preoperative teaching plan, since passive—not active—range of motion exercises, are usually performed after surgery.

+ B. A rational for various tubes, IV's, etc.
This is appropriate (+) information to include in preoperative teaching, since knowing the reason for procedures and equipment helps to relieve anxiety. However, when selecting the highest priority, be sure to review all options before making your selection.

− C. The need to record vital signs frequently.
This is inappropriate (-), since this is a nursing priority, not a teaching priority for the client.

+ D. Coughing and deep breathing exercises.
Teaching skills that involve the client's cooperation in the postoperative period are a priority (+) preoperatively. To set priorities for preoperative teaching, the nurse must identify—using analysis skills—that the client will be at risk for pulmonary complications. Pulmonary complications are common postoperatively. Teaching the client to cough and deep breathe properly helps eliminate mucous plugs, which cause atelectasis in the postoperative period. Because this option addresses a physiological need, it is a higher priority than option B.

PLANNING QUESTIONS

Questions that address the planning phase of the nursing function are usually fairly easy to recognize because they concern the nursing care plan—including how it is developed and modified.

Nursing behaviors associated with the planning phase of the nursing process include:

- Stating goals and setting priorities for a nursing care plan.
- Selecting nursing interventions for a nursing care plan.
- Stating expected outcomes of nursing care.
- Modifying nursing care plans.
- Cooperating with other health personnel for delivery of client care.
- Recording relevant information.

Remember, the goal of nursing is to help the client attain and maintain an optimal level of functioning. So even though they are easy to recognize, planning questions may be quite difficult to answer because nursing care plans deal with all aspects of nursing care for a client—from routine comfort measures and privacy

to critical client monitoring measures in postop care.
Planning questions might ask you to:

- Select the most appropriate goal for a client's care plan—or an *inappropriate* goal. ***WARNING! Many planning questions have false response stems!***
- Identify the most important or *lowest priority* nursing intervention.
- Select an appropriate *or inappropriate* nursing intervention.
- Identify an expected *or unexpected* outcome of an intervention.
- Plan how and when to work with other health care professionals, e.g., a nutritionist or physical therapist, in providing care for a client.

Tips for Questions that Focus on Planning

- The answer involves something that is included in the *nursing* care plan, rather than in the *medical* plan. The exam is about NURSING, so focus on the nursing action rather than on the medical action.
- When planning specific care, highlight the *issue* of the question.
- Be careful not to "read into" the question. Assuming information that is not given may cause you to select an inappropriate nursing intervention—or overlook a necessary one!
- When the question asks you to select priorities, remember Maslow's Hierarchy of Needs.

Practice Session: Planning Questions

DRILL 6

An elderly, confused client is on bed rest. In planning nursing care for this client, which nursing intervention will not effectively provide for this client's safety?

A. Provide regular toileting.
B. Explain to the client that she should use the call light if she needs to get up.
C. Place the side rails in the up position and check on the client often.
D. Initiate the proper use of restraints.

Critical Elements

Key words:	See bold print.
Client:	A confused, elderly client on bed rest.
Issue:	Safety (preventing falls).
Type of stem:	False response stem.

Eliminate Options:

An elderly, **confused** client is on **bed rest.** In planning nursing care for this client, which nursing intervention will **not** effectively provide for this client's **safety**?

+ A. Provide regular toileting.
No, wrong choice—this is an important and necessary nursing action. When a confused, elderly client has the physiological need to void or have a bowel movement, an attempt is usually made to find a bathroom. This attempt may result in a fall for the confused client, who may not be able to perceive danger. Since this question has a false response stem, the correct answer is something that will NOT help prevent a fall.

− B. Explain to the client that she should use the call light if she needs to get up.
Excellent! Since the client is confused, as identified in the introductory statement, she is not likely to remember instructions concerning the use of the call light. This action is not likely to prevent a fall, and does not provide for the client's safety. This question has a false response stem, so the answer is something that will NOT prevent a fall.

+ C. Place the side rails in the up position and check on the client often.
Wrong choice. The side rails should be in the up position to prevent the client from falling out of bed, and to serve as a reminder to the client to remain in bed. You are looking for a nursing action that will NOT help prevent a fall.

+ D. Initiate the proper use of restraints.
Wrong choice. Note that this option specifies the PROPER use of restraints. If the client is assessed and it is determined that she needs to be restrained in order to avoid injury, then restraints may be applied and the physician notified of the situation.

In planning nursing care for a 12-month-old hospitalized client, which activity would the nurse include in order to meet the client's developmental needs?

A. A cradle gym across crib.
B. Push-pull toys.
C. Finger paints.
D. A stick horse.

Critical Elements

Key words:	See bold print.
Client:	A 12-month-old hospitalized client.
Issue:	Developmental needs.
Type of stem:	True response stem.

Eliminate Options:

In planning nursing care for a **12-month-old** hospitalized client, which activity would the nurse include in order to meet the client's **developmental** needs?

A. A cradle gym across crib.
Incorrect. Although this encourages fine motor skills, you have not matched the age of the client with the activity that is needed to improve skills. This could also be a safety issue, since the child may be able to stand and could strangle on the cradle gym.

B. Push-pull toys.
Great, correct choice! Walking is the skill that is being perfected at this age, and push-pull toys will encourage the client to walk unaided.

C. Finger paints.
Incorrect. Reread the question and think about the skill level of this age child.

D. A stick horse.
Incorrect. This is beyond the ability of the client and could be a safety concern.

8 DRILL

An elderly client is in a nursing home and confined to bed. In planning care for this client, the nurse knows that the most essential nursing intervention to prevent skin breakdown and decubitus ulcers is to:

A. Massage all bony prominences with lotion.
B. Keep the skin clean and dry.
C. Turn the client at least every two hours.
D. Place an egg crate mattress on the bed.

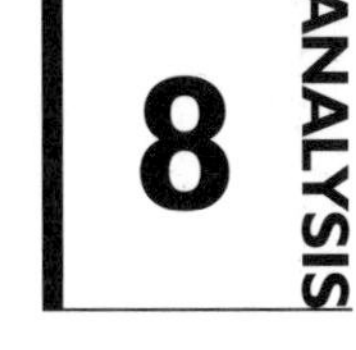

Critical Elements

Key words:	See bold print.
Client:	Elderly client confined to bed.
Issue:	Prevention of skin breakdown.
Type of stem:	True response stem (high priority).

An elderly client is in a nursing home and confined to **bed**. In planning care for this client, the nurse knows that the **most essential** nursing intervention to **prevent skin breakdown** and decubitus ulcers is to:

A. Massage all bony prominences with lotion.
This is not the best choice. Massage of the bony prominences helps in preventing skin breakdown, but massage alone will not eliminate breakdown if the client is left in one position for long periods of time.

B. Keep the skin clean and dry.
This is not the best choice. Clean, dry skin is helpful in the prevention of skin breakdown. Nevertheless, if the client has clean, dry skin but the client is not moved frequently, skin breakdown still will occur.

C. Turn the client at least every two hours.
This is the best choice. Turning the client frequently is the most important nursing intervention. This measure alternates the areas where the pressure of the mattress decreases circulation and tends to cause skin breakdown.

D. Place an egg crate mattress on the bed.
This is not the best choice. An egg crate mattress will help alleviate some of pressure on the skin, but the client must be turned in order to eliminate pressure at a particular site.

IMPLEMENTATION QUESTIONS

Implementation questions focus on the nurse's role in initiating and carrying out planned nursing interventions in a safe manner; responding to client questions, comments and needs; identifying contraindications and unexpected outcomes; taking emergency measures in life-threatening situations; and requesting assistance from other health care team members when appropriate.

Nursing behaviors associated with the implementation phase of the nursing process include:

- Providing care to achieve therapeutic goals.
- Providing care to optimize achievement of health goals by the client.
- Performing or assisting in performing activities of daily living.
- Transferring and ambulating clients.
- Identifying developmental factors and client risk factors when implementing care.
- Identifying and responding to life-threatening situations.
- Using proper body mechanics, taking safety precautions, and observing infection control measures.
- Counseling and teaching clients or families.
- Using therapeutic communication skills to establish and maintain a therapeutic relationship.
- Supervising and checking the work of the staff.
- Recording and exchanging information.

You will notice that many implementation questions on your exams are *communication* questions. This is because implementation includes explaining, teaching, instructing, or responding to the client while giving care. (Refer to Chapter Five for strategies)

Tips for Answering Implementation Questions

- **Safety first!** Check the introductory statement for any life-threatening signs or symptoms, then for any safety hazards or special client risk factors (e.g., contraindications, impaired mobility, sensory deficits, impaired or undeveloped cognitive ability, reduced level of consciousness). Remember that the nurse has the authority to implement life-saving measures in an emergency.
- Remember to *identify the client—and wash your hands*—before implementing any nursing measure.
- Make sure that the intervention is *within the domain of nursing,* and that the question specifies a physician's order if needed for a procedure.
- Remember that the nurse *must always be in a therapeutic role* when communicating with the client, the client's family, and others in the health care setting. Nursing responses must be *client centered* and respectful of the client's feelings.

Practice Session: Implementation Questions

9 DRILL

A postoperative client returned to the unit eight hours ago. Temperature is now 102.4° F. The dressing is dry and intact. The client has not yet been out of bed, and she has complained of incisional pain and was medicated with Demerol about 30 minutes ago. What should the nurse do first?

A. Give the client Tylenol 650 mg P.O. immediately.
B. Report the elevated temperature to the physician.
C. Do a physical assessment of the client's chest.
D. Send a urine specimen to the lab for culture.

9 ANALYSIS

Critical Elements

Key words:	See bold print.
Client:	A client 8 hours postop.
Issue:	Signs of postoperative complications.
Type of stem:	True response stem (high priority).

Eliminate Options

A **postoperative** client returned to the unit **eight hours ago**. Temperature is now **102.4° F.** The dressing is dry and intact. The client has **not yet been out of bed,** has complained of **incisional pain** and was medicated with **Demerol** (meperidine) about **30 minutes ago**. What should the nurse **do first?**

? A. Give the client Tylenol 650 mg P.O. immediately.
This is a possibility (-), since the client does have an elevated temperature which needs to be medicated—but is this the priority at this time? What is the issue in this question? What should the nurse do first? Review the other options to see if another action would receive higher priority.

? B. Report the elevated temperature to the physician.
This is a possibility (-); certainly, this temperature needs to be reported. However, again, look to see if another action would take priority.

+ C. Do a physical assessment of the client's chest.
This action is the nursing priority (+) in this clinical scenario because the elevated temperature is a sign of a possible postoperative complication in a client who was immobilized by surgery and a medication. Eight hours after surgery, the nurse assessed the client to have an elevated temperature. A temperature in the first 24 hour period is usually due to a pulmonary problem. At this time, more data needs to be collected about the client's lungs. First, a physical assessment of the chest is needed. Then information about the elevated temperature and the physical chest assessment needs to be reported to the physician. This question requires an analysis of the assessment data, and priority setting.

? D. Send a urine specimen to the lab for culture.
This is another possibility (?); however, a urine infection would occur about 48 hours after surgery and is unlikely at this time. In addition, note that this option represents a medical action and not a nursing action. Avoid actions that are not within the domain of nursing!

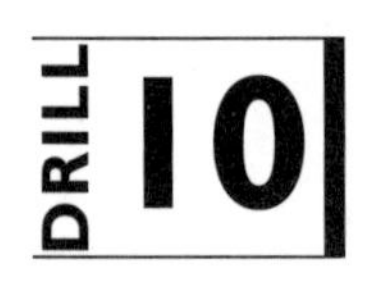

An elderly client with Alzheimer's disease is admitted to the hospital. His daughter says to the nurse, "I really feel guilty about leaving my father, but I need to go home." Which is the best response?

A. "Your father is well cared for here."
B. "Your worried feelings are normal."
C. "When you are getting ready to leave, tell me. I will sit with your father."
D. "Can I call another family member to stay with him?"

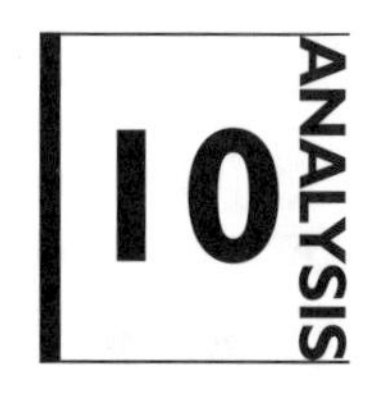

Critical Elements

Key words:	See bold print.
Client:	The daughter.
Issue:	Daughter's feelings about leaving father alone in hospital.
Type of stem:	True response stem (therapeutic communication).

Eliminate Options:

An elderly client with Alzheimer's disease is admitted to the hospital. His daughter says to the nurse, "I really **feel guilty** about **leaving** my father, but I need to go home." Which is the best response?

− A. "Your father is well cared for here."
This response may sound good, but it is not therapeutic (-). The client in this test question is the daughter! This response blocks therapeutic communication by falsely reassuring her; it may also sound defensive.

− B. "Your worried feelings are normal."
This response devalues the client's feelings (-). Also, this response does not answer the client's concern about leaving her father.

+ C. "When you are getting ready to leave, tell me. I will sit with your father."
In this response the nurse offers to help the daughter by sitting with the father. In this response, the nurse is using the therapeutic communication tool of offering self (+).

− D. "Can I call another family member to stay with him?"
This response is not therapeutic for the daughter (-). By suggesting getting someone else to sit with the father, the nurse makes the daughter feel all the more guilty about leaving.

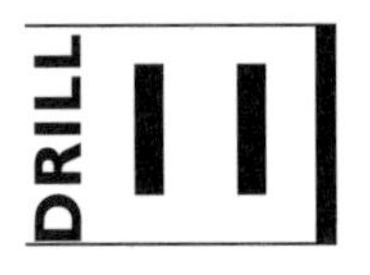

A client is scheduled for surgery and asks the nurse if she can put on some makeup before going to surgery. Which would be the best response by the nurse?

A. "Only a light application of makeup is allowed."
B. "Hospital policy states that all makeup must be removed before surgery."
C. "I will check to find out the regulations."
D. "Makeup will interfere with the ability to see your skin color during surgery."

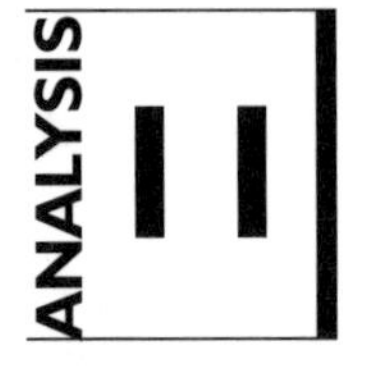

Critical Elements

Key words:	See bold print.
Client:	A client scheduled for surgery.
Issue:	Wearing makeup in surgery.
Type of stem:	True response stem (therapeutic communication).

Eliminate Options:

A client is scheduled for **surgery** and asks the nurse if she can put on some **makeup** before going to surgery. Which would be the **best response** by the nurse?

[-] A. "Only a light application of makeup is allowed.
This is not correct information (-). Makeup of any kind masks the color of the skin or nails. Assessment of the circulatory system is monitored by observing the color of the skin, nails and mucosa.

[?] B. "Hospital policy states that all makeup must be removed before surgery."
This information is correct, so this response might be a possibility (?). However, using hospital policy as an explanation is never very helpful. Clients deserve a better explanation. Using hospital policy for an answer is like "passing the buck." It never really answers the question being asked.

[-] C. "I will check to find out the regulations."
This response is not appropriate (-) because the nurse should know this information. With this response, the nurse is "passing the buck."

[+] D. "Makeup will interfere with the ability to see your skin color during surgery."
Makeup colors the skin and masks the ability to assess the circulatory status. Before surgery, all makeup must be removed, including any colored nail polish. This nursing response is therapeutic (+) because it addresses the client's concern and provides correct information.

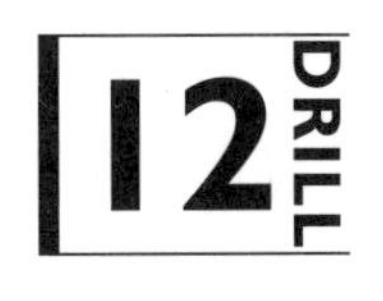

A client is hospitalized for a surgical procedure. The most important nursing intervention when administering the preoperative medication is:

A. Have the client void before going to the operating room.
B. Put the side rails up, and instruct the client to remain in bed.
C. Ask the client if she has signed all of the admission forms for the surgery.
D. Have the family leave, since the medication will decrease the client's inhibitions and she may say or do something that is out of character for her.

12 ANALYSIS

Critical Elements	
Key words:	See bold print.
Client:	A preoperative client.
Issue:	Preoperative medication.
Type of stem:	True response stem.

Eliminate Options:

A client is hospitalized for a surgical procedure. The **most** important nursing intervention when administering the **preoperative** medication is:

A. Have the client void before going to the operating room.
Incorrect. Although it is standard preoperative care to have clients void prior to surgery, the nurse should have the client void before administering the preoperative medication. The stem of the question asks about administering the preoperative medication— not about preoperative preparation of the client. This option does not address the issue in the question.

B. Put the side rails up, and instruct the client to remain in bed.
Correct! Preoperative medications may cause the client to become disoriented, drowsy, and unsteady when walking. Preoperative medications are identified as a priority risk factor, because they impair the client's ability to perceive and respond to danger. It is very important that the side rails are up and the client remain in bed in order to protect the client from an injury caused by a fall.

C. Ask the client if she has signed all of the admission forms for the surgery.
Incorrect. Asking the client is not an appropriate nursing action! The necessary forms should be signed prior to surgery, but the client does not know what forms are required by the hospital. It is the nursing staff's responsibility to check the forms for completion.

D. Have the family leave, since the medication will decrease the client's inhibitions and she may say or do something that is out of character for her. *No, this is not an appropriate nursing action. Although preoperative medications can alter a person's behavior, educating the family about the possible side effects is more appropriate than separating the family at this time, when support for the client is important.*

EVALUATION QUESTIONS

Evaluation questions focus on the process of determining whether therapy has been effective and whether nursing interventions have been successful in meeting the client's needs.

Nursing behaviors associated with the evaluation phase of the nursing process include:

- Comparing actual outcomes with expected outcomes of therapy.
- Determining the impact of nursing actions.
- Verifying that tests or measurements were performed correctly, and collecting additional data when needed.
- Evaluating the client's understanding of information presented and the client's motivation to care for his or her health problem.
- Re-assessing client needs and modifying the nursing care plan accordingly.

Evaluation questions may ask how the nurse should monitor or make a judgment concerning a client's response to therapy or a nursing action. Note that some evaluation questions may have a false response stem. For example, a question may ask for a client's statement that indicates inaccurate information or lack of motivation.

Tips for Answering Evaluation Questions

1. Focus on the **issue** in the question. Be aware that the issue in the question may *not* be the same as the client's medical diagnosis. The question may concern just one of several goals in the nursing care plan.
2. When evaluating the client's response to care, keep in mind the rationale or purpose of the care being evaluated.
3. Since re-assessment is critical in the evaluation phase, be sure to know your vital signs and normal lab values.
4. Don't "read into" the question! Ask yourself if the nurse has enough information for the evaluation, or if additional information is needed.

Practice Session: Evaluation Questions

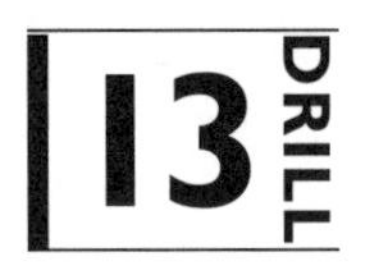

A client has been diagnosed with iron deficiency anemia. The nurse knows that the client has understood information about recommended diet for her anemia when she identifies which of the following food categories as good dietary sources of iron?

A. Fresh fruits.
B. Milk and cheese.
C. Organ meats.
D. Whole grain breads.

13 ANALYSIS

Critical Elements

Key words:	See bold print.
Client:	A client with iron deficiency anemia.
Issue:	Good dietary sources of iron.
Type of stem:	True response stem.

Eliminate Options:

A client has been diagnosed with **iron deficiency anemia**. The nurse knows that the client has understood information about recommended diet for her anemia when she identifies which of the following food categories as good **dietary sources of iron**?

A. Fresh fruits.
Incorrect. Fruits provide the body with a rich source of Vitamins A and C.

B. Milk and cheese.
Incorrect. Dairy products are good sources of calcium and high quality complete protein, not iron.

C. Organ meats.
Right choice! A diet rich in organ meats provides iron, which is what the client needs to improve her anemia. This question focuses on evaluation of client teaching.

D. Whole grain breads.
Incorrect. Whole grain breads are rich in carbohydrates and dietary fiber, not iron.

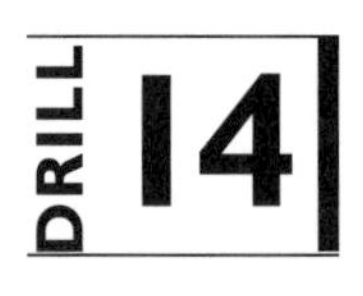

An elderly client is experiencing a decrease in his white blood cell count and is placed on protective precautions for infection. Which of the following comments by the client indicate to the nurse that he understands his condition and the precautions?

A. "I have never been so aware that germs are everywhere around us."
B. "I didn't realize that I am so contagious that I need a private room."
C. "Everyone who touches me washes their hands like I am really contaminated."
D. "I might make my sister's baby sick, so I told her not to visit."

Critical Elements	
Key words:	See bold print.
Client:	Elderly client with decreased white blood cell count.
Issue:	Protective precautions.
Type of stem:	True response stem.

Eliminate Options:

An elderly client is experiencing a **decrease in his white blood cell count** and is placed on **protective precautions** for infection. Which of the following comments by the client indicate to the nurse that he **understands** his condition and the precautions?

+ A. "I have never been so aware that germs are everywhere around us."
Correct evaluation! This comment indicates an understanding of the need for precautions, which are implemented to protect the client from infection.

− B. "I didn't realize that I am so contagious that I need a private room."
This is not the answer. The client's condition is not contagious. Protective precautions are implemented to protect the client from infection, not to prevent the spread of a contagious disease. This comment indicates that the client does not understand his condition or the need for precautions.

− C. "Everyone who touches me washes their hands like I am really contaminated."
Incorrect. The client is not contaminated with a contagious disease. Strict hand washing is done to protect the client from infection. This comment indicates that the client does not understand his condition or the need for precautions.

D. "I might make my sister's baby sick, so I told her not to visit."
The client's condition is not contagious. The sister and her baby are not at risk for developing an illness as a result of visiting the client.

15 DRILL

The nurse would interpret which finding as an indication of improvement in an infant who is receiving treatment for dehydration?

A. Weight gain of three ounces in 24 hours.
B. Specific gravity increased to 1.028.
C. Cool skin with tenting.
D. Frequent stooling.

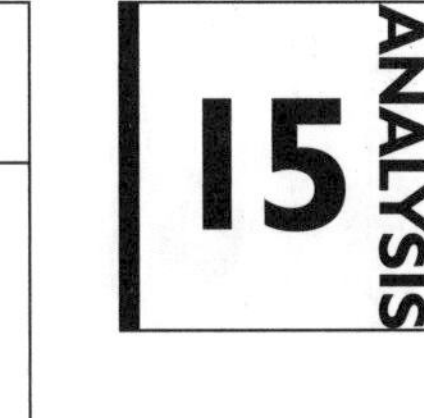

Critical Elements

Key words:	See bold print.
Client:	Infant being treated for dehydration.
Issue:	Rehydration.
Type of stem:	True response stem.

Eliminate Options:

The nurse would interpret which finding as an indication of **improvement** in an infant who is receiving treatment for **dehydration?**

A. Weight gain of three ounces in 24 hours.
Correct. Weight gain is the best indicator of rehydration in infants and small children.

B. Specific gravity increased to 1.028.
Incorrect. This indicates dehydration.

C. Cool skin with tenting.
Incorrect. Cool skin and tenting are signs of dehydration. The skin is cool and less elastic due to the decrease in circulating volume.

D. Frequent stooling.
Incorrect. This answer doesn't tell you anything about hydration status, but you might suspect that if stooling continues, dehydration may worsen or at least will not improve.

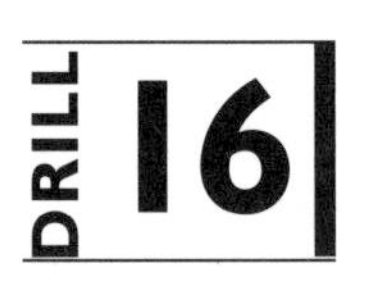

A client is scheduled for surgery in the morning. Before surgery, the preoperative teaching plan included deep breathing and coughing. To best evaluate the effectiveness of preoperative teaching, the nurse should ask the client:

A. "Do you understand what we have just discussed about deep breathing and coughing?"
B. "Do you think that you will need to have a sedative to help you sleep tonight?"
C. "Will you demonstrate for me the correct method of deep breathing and coughing?"
D. "Do you have any questions concerning your scheduled surgical procedure?"

Critical Elements

Key words:	See bold print.
Client:	Preoperative client.
Issue:	Preoperative teaching.
Type of stem:	True response stem.

Eliminate Options:

A client is scheduled for surgery in the morning. Before surgery, the preoperative teaching plan included deep breathing and coughing. To **best evaluate** the effectiveness of **preoperative teaching**, the nurse should ask the client:

? A. "Do you understand what we have just discussed about deep breathing and coughing?"
Incorrect. This question asks the client about the content of the preoperative teaching in the form of a closed question, which requires only a "yes" or "no" answer. The client could answer "yes" regardless of the true state of his understanding. This is not the best question to ask.

− B. "Do you think that you will need to have a sedative to help you sleep tonight?"
Incorrect. This test question asks you to select a question that the nurse should ask to evaluate preoperative teaching. In this option, the nurse is asking about the need for a sedative, not about the client's understanding of preoperative teaching. Although the ques-

tion is an appropriate question for the nurse to ask at this time, it is not the correct answer because it does not relate to the issue in the question.

+ C. "Will you demonstrate for me the correct method of deep breathing and coughing?"
Excellent! This question asks the client about the content of the preoperative teaching by requesting a return demonstration. If the preoperative teaching has been effective, the client will be able to do the return demonstration. If additional teaching is required, the client will be unable to do the return demonstration properly. This is the best question for evaluating the effectiveness of preoperative teaching.

− D. "Do you have any questions concerning your scheduled surgical procedure?"
Incorrect. This question is an appropriate question for the nurse to ask at this time. It is not the correct answer, however, because the test question asks you to select a question that the nurse should ask to evaluate preoperative teaching. In this option, the nurse is asking about the client's understanding of the surgical procedure. The client's questions concerning the surgical procedure should be referred to the doctor.

NOTES

Chapter 8

HOW TO TAKE A TIMED NURSING EXAM

The Importance Of Pacing Technique

Taking a timed exam is a stressful experience. Today most nursing programs give timed exams. If you are often among the last students to finish when taking a nursing exam, you may find this very stressful.

Have you ever been the last one left in the room when taking an exam? How many times have you been half way through an exam when the person next to you finished the exam and left? These experiences can be intimidating.

Pacing technique is your best strategy for reducing this stress. It will also increase your concentration and keep you from becoming stalled on any one question.

Nursing exams are not speed reading contests! You do not get extra points for finishing faster than anyone else. Use the pacing strategy, and work at your own best rate.

Practice Makes Perfect

Your preparation for a nursing exam should include *answering practice test questions* about the covered nursing content. When answering practice questions, be sure to use pacing technique.

Did you know that as your skill in answering test questions increases, so does your concentration, reading speed, and comprehension? Using your test-taking strategies, using pacing technique, and answering lots of practice questions will all increase your score on nursing exams.

Practice makes perfect—there is no other way!

How To Pace Yourself On An Exam

To pace yourself during an exam, first go through the entire exam and answer only those questions that you can answer quickly and easily. By answering the easy questions first, you are assured of getting credit for everything that you do know.

After you finish answering all the easy questions, return to the more difficult ones. Experience has also shown that when you return to the difficult questions, you will be able to answer at least half of those questions correctly. Part of the reason is that during an exam you will often have a "memory jog" when answering one question that helps you remember information needed to answer other questions.

Steps for Pacing Strategy

1. Immediately after you are allowed to begin, check the time. Make sure your watch is working! If not, use the clock in the room.
2. Figure what time it will be at the end of the time allowed for the exam.
3. Look for the number of the last test question. Then, CALCULATE THE NUMBER OF THE HALF-WAY TEST QUESTION.
4. On an exam with no more than 60 questions, identify the test question that is 5 past half way. On longer exams, identify the question that is 10 past half way. For example, if the exam contains 50 questions and you have an hour to answer them, you should be answering test question #30 (#25 + 5) at the 30-minute mark. If the exam has 100 questions and you have two hours, you should be answering question #60 at the end of the first hour.
5. Begin answering the questions, *spending less than one minute per test question.* Do not allow any question to immobilize you!
6. Use your test-taking strategies to select the best options whenever possible, if you cannot answer a question using your nursing knowledge alone. Select the best option, and move on to the next question.

7. On a paper-and-pencil exam, skip and do not answer the following:
   a. Questions that you do not understand.
   b. Questions for which you cannot choose between the two best options, when your test-taking strategies do not seem to apply.
8. On a paper-and-pencil exam, write down the question number of each question that you do not know the answer to (using the paper provided for your math calculations). Then these questions will be easy to locate when returning to them later.
9. When half the time has elapsed, you should be answering the question that you targeted for your half-way mark:
   a. If you are not yet at that question, you must work more quickly during the second half of the exam.
   b. If you are past that question, you may work a bit more slowly during the second half.
10. Continue to answer questions until you have attempted every question.
11. Return to those questions that you did not answer the first time through. Remember that you can probably answer at least half of those questions correctly!
12. Be sure to use your test-taking strategies to optimize your score.

Points to Remember

Pace yourself when answering practice questions.
Pace yourself during the exam!

When You Finish An Exam—Should You Take Another Look?

Take all the time that you are given! If you find that you finish with time left over, it is a good idea to reread the exam. You may find an error because you misread something in a question.

However, you should remember to *change an answer* *ONLY* *if you have misread the question, or if other questions help you clarify information.*

Point to Remember

After finishing the exam, be sure to make use of all the time you have left. Reread the exam!

Do You Constantly Change Your Answers?

One of the most common problems in taking multiple choice tests is changing from correct answers to *incorrect* ones. This can even cause some students to fail exams.

Test-taking anxiety or nervousness is one reason why students change answers. When you become nervous while answering a difficult question, this anxiety causes you to lose self confidence. When you lose self confidence, even if you have some idea about the question, you feel that you cannot trust your own judgment. You may end up choosing the opposite of your first hunch or "gut feeling." This can cost you important points on an exam.

One important test taking strategy is to always *go with your "gut feeling."* This means that you may select an answer for a reason that you are not sure of. Maybe you just like one choice better than another, and it may be difficult to say why. Trust yourself and choose the answer that you like. And don't change your answer later, unless you have a concrete reason for doing so.

You will also increase your self confidence by answering many practice questions. Prove to yourself how many times your "gut" feelings are correct during your practice sessions.

Point to Remember

Never change answers unless you misread a part of the question, or you are able to clarify information.

What If You Cannot Answer A Large Number Of Questions?

When you have finished answering the questions that you think you know, return to and answer all the remaining questions. *Make sure you answer all the questions on the exam the best you can—even if there are 10 or more that you may not know.* Use your test-taking strategies . . . Go with your gut feelings . . . And guess if you have to! This is the only way to maximize your score.

Think of it this way: On a multiple choice exam in which there are four choices, you can often eliminate two of the choices. If it is difficult to choose between the two remaining choices, take the answer that is more appealing for whatever reason. In any case, *when you can narrow it down to two choices, you have a 50-50 chance of being correct when guessing—not just one chance in four!* Most importantly, you do not *lose* any points by choosing a wrong answer. So never leave any question unanswered.

The test-taking strategies which help you select the best of two close choices are discussed in the preceding chapters. Take the time to read and practice these important strategies. If you are unable to apply your nursing knowledge on a question and cannot use one of the test-taking strategies, then you will have to guess. Guessing is your last option. But it is better to guess than to leave any question unanswered! Just go with your "gut feeling"—and go on to the next question.

Do You Have Trouble Concentrating When Taking an Exam?

Concentration during an exam is crucial. Your ability to concentrate helps you to notice the key words, focus on rationales for nursing actions, and select priorities.

As explained in the introduction, *answering practice test questions* will increase your familiarity with different types of questions and improve your ability to concentrate on the information in the question and the issue. With a little practice, students frequently report that after they start answering the first few questions they forget that anyone else is in the room!

Poor concentration can cause you to misread the question and answer incorrectly. As an informed test-taker, you should learn to identify signs of poor concentration so that you can identify in yourself those signals that prevent you from answering questions correctly.

Here are some common distractions that you may experience when you are losing your concentration

- You feel a sudden physical discomfort such as a neckache or backache.
- You get a real craving for food.
- You hear noise from another test-taker (e.g., someone chewing gum).
- You feel extremely tired.
- You read the same question many times over.
- You listen to someone in the room tap a foot or pencil.
- You start to think about your vacation.

If you notice these kinds of distractions occurring during an exam, take a few minutes to breathe deeply, and then get back on track.

When You Take Your Next Exam, Remember . . .

You have studied hard and reviewed carefully. You have also learned test-taking techniques and strategies, and you have practiced taking a timed exam. These efforts will pay off!

As a skilled test-taker, you can maintain your concentration, pace yourself, and make confident choices. With these skills and abilities, *you can make the most of your nursing knowledge* when taking a nursing exam.

Chapter 9

HOW TO PREPARE FOR THE NCLEX EXAM

Are you ready for the *TQLogic for Beginning Nursing Students* Final Exam?

You have your choice of using this chapter OR of answering the questions in computerized format, using the *Test Smart* CD-ROM enclosed with this book.

To use the "paper-and-pencil" exam in this chapter, you will need a sheet of paper on which to record your answers and some scratch paper, in case you wish to make any notes while taking the exam.

Allow yourself 50 minutes to complete the exam. You will need a wristwatch so that you can use the pacing strategy.

To use *Test Smart* on CD-ROM follow the installations instructions enclosed with the book. Allow 100 minutes to complete the exam.

To achieve your best score, take this exam when you are well rested. A relaxed, positive attitude helps. Make sure that you have eaten well. And make sure that you have a comfortable chair.

Tips for the Final Written Exam

1. Read each question carefully. If you are taking the exam on paper, circle or underline important words.
2. Be sure to identify all four of the critical elements. Be extra sure you have correctly identified the *client* in a communication question.
3. Remember that only one answer in each question is correct, and you receive credit only for correct answers. You are looking for the best option in each question.
4. When you know the type of stem and the issue in the question, make a decision about each option as you read it, by using the selection procedure (+, -, or ?).
5. If you cannot decide which option is the best, use a test-taking strategy. If none of the strategies helps, follow your gut feeling—and if you don't know, guess! Most exams have no penalty for wrong answers.
6. If you are taking the exam on paper, be sure to record all your answers! (The computerized exam includes automatic scoring.) You may also wish to mark any questions you answered using one of the strategies.
7. Pace yourself! This exam has 50 questions, and the time allowed is 50 minutes. Find the question that is halfway-plus-five (Question 30), and try to finish this question at the end of 25 minutes. Use your test-taking strategies when necessary, and use your time wisely!
8. If you are using the paper-and-pencil version, answer the easy questions first, and then go back to the difficult ones.
9. Concentrate during the exam, and be sure to use relaxation techniques as needed.
10. When you are finished, don't forget to check your answers, and read the rationales to make sure you understand *why* your answers are right or wrong.

The Computerized Final Exam

Welcome to *Test Smart—Test Question Logic for Beginning Nursing Students*. *Test Smart* may be used in Assessment or Practice mode.

In Assessment mode, the computer automatically "remembers" each answer you select and scores and assesses your success in using the test-taking techniques and strategies you have learned in this book. After displaying your score, the program will show you the questions you answered incorrectly and let you view the rationales.

Please note that the computerized exam does NOT allow you to skip questions or to return to previously answered questions; once you have "entered" your answer, you cannot change it. However, you can use the pacing strategy and your test-taking strategies to avoid becoming "hung up" on difficult questions.

In Practice mode, the program lets you instantly view rationales while reading questions.

Good luck! Start the final exam here or log on to your computer and see the instructions on the CD-ROM.

1. A six-month-old male infant with AIDS has a nursing diagnosis of "altered growth and development" on the care plan. Which of the following nursing interventions will most enhance the growth and development of the child?

1. Encourage the child to eat whatever he wants.
2. Provide therapy to help the child meet developmental milestones.
3. Provide nutritional supplements in addition to an adequate diet.
4. Weigh and measure the infant on a frequent basis.

2. A client has undergone surgery to correct a bowel obstruction. He has returned from the recovery room with an indwelling urinary catheter. For several hours the urinary output has been adequate. The nurse notes, however, that the catheter has drained no urine during the last hour. What action should the nurse take first?

1. Offer the client 100 cc of oral fluids each hour.
2. Irrigate the catheter according to the postoperative orders.
3. Call the physician and request an increase in IV fluid rate.
4. Monitor the vital signs every 15 minutes for one hour.

3. A client is admitted to the hospital in respiratory distress. The doctor orders oxygen per mask and the client to be placed in high Fowler's position. Which nursing action is most important for this client?

1. Support and align the hands with the forearms.
2. Use handrails.
3. Raise the head of the bed to allow for greater lung expansion.
4. Support the feet at right angles to the lower legs.

4. While the nurse is caring for a seven-month-old female infant, she aspirates a small toy. She begins to cough and becomes cyanotic, and then no sound is made. At this time, the best nursing action is to:

1. Perform a chest thrust.
2. Turn the client prone and administer back blows.
3. Stimulate further coughing.
4. Perform a modified Heimlich maneuver with one hand.

5. An elderly client is admitted with a broken right arm and contusions to the left wrist following an automobile accident. The nurse is preparing to feed the client. Which of the following nursing actions is least effective in preventing aspiration?

1. Offer small bites of food.
2. ✓ Order pureed foods.
3. Have the client use her dentures while eating.
4. ✓ Allow enough time for the client to chew the food well before offering more.

6. To monitor a client for the most common complication arising from the administration of total parenteral nutrition, the nurse should:

1. Weigh the client at the same time each day using the same scale.
2. Keep accurate records of total intake and total output.
3. Determine the increase or decrease in body weight each day.
4. Take the client's temperature at least every four hours.

7. A hospitalized client has just found out that her mother has died of a heart attack. She is crying and has her face buried in the pillow. The best nursing action is to:

1. Return in 15 minutes to see how the client is doing.
2. Sit with the client for a little while.
3. Tell the client that she will feel better in the morning.
4. Share with the client that you lost your mother within the last year and that you know how she feels.

8. An elderly client is admitted to the hospital for surgery after finding a lump in his right testicle. He asks the nurse, "Do you think the doctor will find cancer?" The best response by the nurse initially is:

1. "Most lumps found in the testicles are benign."
2. "It must be difficult for you not to know what the doctor will find."
3. "I think that you should discuss this with your doctor."
4. "It might be, but the doctor won't know until the surgery is performed."

9. A 76-year-old client was admitted to the hospital for surgery for a fractured hip. The client says to the nurse, "I guess I've lived long enough, and my number's up." How should the nurse respond initially?

1. "You are in really good shape for your age."
2. "This is just a minor setback. You will be on your feet in no time."
3. "You feel that your life is ending?"
4. "The doctors and nurses are going to take good care of you while you are here. There's nothing to worry about."

10. A daughter has come to take her mother home from the hospital after a colostomy. The daughter tells the nurse that she doesn't know how she is going to care for her mother's colostomy. The nurse's most helpful response to the daughter is:

1. "Your mother can take care of her colostomy without difficulty."
2. "What part of your mother's care are you concerned about?"
3. "A home health nurse will be stopping by tomorrow. If you have any questions, you can ask her."
4. "It is quite simple. I'll make sure that her colostomy bag is clean before she leaves."

11. A client is scheduled for a mastectomy in the morning. Her daughter is visiting her and says to the nurse, "I should call my brother and sister and have them here in the morning, just in case something goes wrong." The most helpful nursing response is to:

1. Ask the mother if she would like her children there in the morning.
2. Suggest to the daughter that she ask her mother how she feels about that.
3. Say to the daughter, "If your brother and sister want to be here, they are welcome."
4. Ask the daughter what she knows about her mother's surgery and diagnosis.

12. An 84-year-old married man is admitted from his home to a skilled nursing facility with a diagnosis of Alzheimer's disease. While speaking with the admitting nurse, his wife begins to cry and says, "I never thought it would come to this. I feel so guilty bringing him here." Which nursing response is best?

1. "You have done all you could. We will take good care of him here."
2. "This has been a difficult time for you. Let's find a quiet place where we can talk."
3. "Admitting your husband was the right decision. He requires more care then you can provide at home."
4. "What are you feeling guilty about?"

13. A client is admitted to the hospital. He has been on bed rest at home and has been incontinent of urine. His wife has been caring for him, and there is a strong odor of urine. The wife says that she is sorry and embarrassed about the unpleasant smell. Which response by the nurse is therapeutic?

1. "It must be difficult to care for someone who is confined to bed. How have you been able to manage?"
2. "Don't worry about it. He will get a bath, and that will take care of the odor."
3. "A lot of clients that are cared for at home have the same problem."
4. "When was the last time that he had a bath?"

14. A general anesthesia has been given for multiple tooth extractions on a three-year-old child. He returns crying, but awake, from the recovery room. What approach by the nurse is most likely to be successful?

1. Assess the child, examining the mouth first.
2. Assess the child, leaving the mouth until last.
3. It really makes no difference what is done first.
4. Medicate the child for pain first.

15. The nurse's clinical assessment of a two-year-old child who is poorly nourished is most likely to include:

1. Mother's statement that the child is a "picky eater."
2. Height and weight in the 25th percentile.
3. Observing that the child is slender and active.
4. Dry, colorless hair and pale skin.

16. A mother expresses concern about her infant's lack of eye muscle control at two days of age because her neighbor's daughter is mentally retarded and her eyes cross the same way. What is the nurse's best reply?

1. "You should probably talk to the doctor about your concerns."
2. "Newborns all lack the ability to control eye movement until they are three to four months of age."
3. "I will take the baby back to the nursery and assess other neuromuscular activity."
4. "It's nothing to worry about."

17. A mother watches the nurse in the pediatrics ward place her toddler in a highchair for a meal. After placing the client in the highchair, what nursing action would be most essential initially?

1. Pour a small amount of milk into the glass.
2. Ask the mother to feed the child.
3. Belt the child securely to the chair.
4. Cut the child's food into bite size pieces.

18. An 82-year-old client is admitted to the hospital for hip replacement surgery. She appears alert and cooperative, although in great pain. While doing an assessment, the nurse learns she is disoriented to time and believes she is in a hotel. The nurse identifies acute confusion as a nursing problem. Of the following, which does the nurse understand would least impact the client's confusion?

1. Her age.
2. Relocation to the hospital.
3. Her physical pain.
4. Bed confinement.

19. A client has right-sided paralysis following a stroke. He is not able to talk but can make gestures to make himself understood. To effectively communicate with the client, the nurse should:

1. Speak very loudly to the client.
2. Speak quickly to the client, since his attention span may be short.
3. Use gestures while speaking slowly.
4. Wait until the family comes in, so they can interpret his behavior.

20. A client in a long-term care facility has been given a cane to assist her with ambulation. In caring for this client, which of the following would place the client at risk?

1. Inspect the rubber tip often and replace it if appears to be worn.
2. Place the cane on the side of the weak leg.
3. Position the cane to support and balance the client with decreased strength in one of the lower extremities.
4. Keep the cane within easy reach when sleeping or sitting.

21. An elderly female client has been in the hospital for a week on bed rest. She complains of elbow pain. The best nursing action is to:

1. Place elbow pads on the client.
2. Examine the elbow.
3. Call the physician for an order for pain medication.
4. Reposition the client so that she is more comfortable.

22. The nurse is preparing to transfer a client from a bed to a chair. To avoid back injury to the nurse, the safest technique is to:

1. Bend at the waist while maintaining a wide stance, lift the client to a standing position, and then pivot the client toward the chair.
2. Have the client lock his or her hands around the nurse's neck, so that the client will feel more secure during the transfer.
3. Place the bed in an elevated position so that the client's hips are at the same level as the nurse's hip, resulting in the center of gravity being the same for both individuals.
4. Bend at the knees, while maintaining a wide stance and straight back, with the client's hands on the nurse's shoulders and the nurse's hands at the client's axillae.

23. The nurse would demonstrate a good understanding of safe body mechanics by avoiding which of the following actions?

1. Move muscles quickly, using short tugs in order to avoid muscle fatigue.
2. Use the longest and strongest muscles of the body whenever possible.
3. Lean toward objects being pushed, such as a stretcher.
4. Carry objects close to the body without touching your clothing.

24. A male client sustained a fracture of the tibia and fibula while playing football. A long leg cast has been applied, and the client is admitted to the orthopedic unit. In providing nursing care for the client, which of the following is a vital consideration?

1. Elevation of the leg in the cast on a pillow will minimize edema.
2. Healing of a fractured bone requires an extended period of time.
3. A long period of immobility may lead to atrophy of the muscle.
4. Analgesics may be needed for pain associated with the fracture.

25. A client has been incontinent of loose stool and is complaining of a painful perineum. The most appropriate initial nursing action is to:

1. Notify the physician to obtain an order for the loose stools.
2. Check the client's perineum.
3. Turn the client every two hours.
4. Increase the client's fluid intake to prevent dehydration.

26. A teenage client had an appendectomy. When the nurse offers meperidine (Demerol) for postoperative pain, the client says, "No, I don't want to get hooked." Which is the most appropriate nursing response?

1. "You are right. Why take a chance?"
2. "Tell me what you mean by getting hooked."
3. "You will not get addicted for the short amount of time that you will be in the hospital."
4. "The Demerol will make you more comfortable, not make you an addict."

27. An elderly client has a draining pressure sore. The culture of the drainage reveals staphylococci. The best nursing action is to:

1. Reinforce the pressure dressing with a sterile towel before ambulating the client.
2. Wear gown and gloves when changing the client's bed linen.
3. Use sterile technique when changing the dressing on the pressure sore.
4. Discourage the client's use of his personal effects until they have been sterilized.

28. Before administering an injection, the nurse performs aseptic handwashing. This technique includes:

1. Avoiding soap, since it causes drying of the skin.
2. Using paper towels to turn the faucet on and off.
3. The use of lotion to prevent drying.
4. Holding arms and hands upright so that all organisms will drain away from hands while washing.

29. An infant is in respiratory isolation. The nurse can most effectively prevent the spread of pathogens via droplet infection by:

1. Wearing a gown and mask when feeding the client.
2. Using sterile gloves when changing her diapers.
3. Having the baby wear a mask when in the playroom.
4. Using enteric precautions when caring for the baby.

30. An infant with AIDS is being prepared for discharge. The nurse is instructing the grandmother, who will care for the infant, in methods of home care. Which statement made by the grandmother represents the

greatest safety hazard?

1. "I know that handwashing is an important preventive measure."
2. "I'll use disposable diapers, discarding them in separate plastic bags."
3. "Blood spills should be washed up immediately with hot soapy water."
4. "Gloves should be worn by whoever changes the baby's diapers."

31. A client seen at the clinic is to receive an injection. When preparing to administer a medication for injection from an ampule, which nursing action would place the client at risk?

1. Score the neck of the ampule with a file. ✓
2. Protect the thumb and fingers with a gauze square ✓ or alcohol wipe.
3. Snap the neck of the ampule toward the body when breaking the top free from the ampule.
4. Insert the needle into the ampule without touching the needle to the edges of the ampule. ✓

32. A new order is written for ear drops for a three-year-old child. The nurse knows in preparing for the procedure, the lowest priority is to:

1. Anticipate the need for assistance to restrain. ✓
2. Check the child's name bracelet, before administration. #1
3. Explain the purpose of the medication to the child. ✓
4. Check which ear is to receive the drops prior to administration. ✓

33. The nurse is assessing a young child with asthma in order to determine the usefulness of a metered dose inhaler. The nurse assesses that the use of the inhaler is discouraged by the:

1. Child's inability to follow directions. ✓
2. Family's poor financial situation.
3. Size of the medication particles.
4. Severity of the child's disease.

34. A client has returned after major surgery and is complaining of pain. The physician ordered morphine sulfate to control her pain. Before administering the medication, the nurse would first:

1. Discuss the side effects with the client.
2. Take the client's vital signs.
3. Provide mouth care.
4. Have the client turn, cough and deep breathe.

35. A client is to receive eye drops. Which of the following nursing actions best prevents injury to the eye during administration?

1. Apply gentle pressure over the opening to the nasolacrimal duct.
2. Hold the tip of the container above the conjunctival sac.
3. Instruct the client to look upward. ✓
4. Deposit the drops into the conjunctival sac.

36. The nurse has been assigned to care for a recently diagnosed diabetic client who is resistant to learning self-injection of insulin. The client insists that the nurse administer all the injections. What is the appropriate nursing response in dealing with the client's resistance?

1. "You won't be able to go home unless you learn to give yourself the insulin injection."
2. "I will have to tell your doctor that you refuse to give yourself the insulin injections. I'm sure she will be angry with you."
3. "Don't worry about it. Your daughter can come over to your house every morning to give you the insulin injections."
4. "It is important that you learn to give yourself the insulin injections. What can I do to help you overcome your fear of giving the injections?"

37. While caring for a client 24 hours following surgery, the priority nursing action is to:

1. Monitor his comfort level.
2. Encourage the client to verbalize his fears.
3. Observe safety precautions.
4. Instruct the client in self-care skills.

38. An 88-year-old client is admitted to the hospital for surgery. The nurse places the bed in the low position and puts the call light within easy reach. He is scheduled to have surgery in the morning. The most important nursing action during the admission of this client is to:

1. Explain the surgical procedure to the client and family.
2. Explain to the client how to use his call light if he needs the nurse.
3. Tell the client and his family about visiting regulations.
4. Teach the client how to deep breathe and cough.

39. A client is scheduled for an abdominal hysterectomy. In order to prevent pneumonia from developing postoperatively, the most important nursing action is to:

1. Teach the client how to deep breathe and cough before surgery.
2. Inform the client that even though she will have pain after surgery, she will have to move from side to side in bed.
3. Tell the client that if she does not ambulate soon after surgery that there is a good chance that she may develop complications.
4. Tell the client that it is very important that she deep breathe and cough often after surgery to prevent complications.

40. In preparing a client for surgery, the preoperative checklist has been completed, and the nurse has just administered the preoperative injection. What would the nurse do next?

1. Take the client to the bathroom to void.
2. Dim the overhead and bedside lights.

3. Review deep breathing and coughing exercises.
4. Put the side rails up on both sides of the bed.

41. In assessing postoperative clients for manifestations of early hypovolemic shock, the nurse notes that an initial observation would most likely be:

1. Thirst.
2. Warm, flushed skin.
3. Irritability.
4. Bradycardia.

42. A 15-year-old client has had an appendectomy. As the nurse prepares to give discharge instructions, the best approach is to:

1. Instruct both parents.
2. Explain to the client and one parent.
3. Explain to only one parent.
4. Instruct any family member.

43. While taking vital signs, the nurse notices an irregularity in the heart rate. Which nursing action is best?

1. Request the assistance of another staff member and take an apical/radial pulse.
2. Count the apical pulse rate for one full minute and describe the irregularity in the chart.
3. Call the doctor and request an order for a Holter monitor recording for the next day.
4. Take the pulse at each peripheral site and count the rate for 30 seconds.

44. A confused elderly client is found wandering around the ward wearing a bathrobe and cotton socks. He also is bumping into walls as he walks. What is the priority nursing action?

1. Take the client's shoes to him and assist him in putting them on.
2. Accompany the client to his room and obtain a baseline assessment.
3. Ask the client to return to his room and rest until he feels better.
4. Tell the client to be careful of any wet spots on the floor.

45. The day after abdominal surgery, a 10-year-old girl is lying quietly in bed when the nurse makes rounds. The last rounds were made four hours ago, and she was last medicated six hours ago. At this time, the nurse should first:

1. Encourage her to turn, cough, and deep breathe.
2. Assess the need for pain medication.
3. Ambulate her to the door.
4. Ask her if she is hungry, and provide fluids.

46. A client is ordered to have a hypothermic or cooling blanket applied because of a very high body temperature. When caring for this client, which of the following is the least appropriate nursing action?

1. Check the client's body temperature frequently.
2. Place a layer of cloth, such as a bath blanket, between the client and the cooling blanket if the cooling blanket does not have a protective covering.
3. Keep the cooling blanket in place until the client's body temperature is a couple of degrees below the desired level recommended by the physician.
4. Remove the cooling blanket when the client's body temperature is a couple of degrees above the desired level recommended by the physician.

47. An elderly client is admitted to the hospital with chest pain. His daughter tells the nurse that he has certain routines for his personal hygiene and for taking his medicine. Your most appropriate nursing response is to:

1. Assure the daughter that everything possible will be done to accommodate her father's needs.
2. Ask the daughter what routines and medicines her father uses at home.
3. Inform the daughter that the hospital has policies that have to be followed, and that you will provide the best care for her father.
4. Tell the daughter that she should inform the doctor about her father's routines so that orders can be written to meet the client's needs.

48. The nurse is preparing the staffing assignment. An infant on the unit has AIDS and cytomegalovirus (CMV). Which staff person should the nurse assign as the primary care giver for this child?

1. An experienced practical nurse who is six months pregnant.
2. A male graduate nurse, recently oriented to pediatrics.
3. An experienced nurse's aide who is healthy.
4. A licensed practical nurse with eczema.

49. The nurse tells the client that she is going to be catheterized for a urine specimen. The client pulls the covers to her neck. She glances at the open door and says, "Someone might see me out there!" At this time, the best nursing action is to:

1. Explain the procedure to the client.
2. Obtain some assistance, since the client does not appear to be comfortable and may be resistant to the procedure.
3. Close the door and assure the client that you will cover her as much as possible during the procedure.
4. Gather all of the needed equipment before starting the procedure.

50. Following a colostomy, a client and his wife have been taught to perform a colostomy irrigation. Which behavior by the client would best indicate readiness for discharge?

1. The client's wife verbalizes all steps in the irrigation procedure.
2. The client performs the irrigation following written instructions.
3. The client and his wife attend all classes given about colostomy care.
4. The client asks appropriate questions about irrigations.

CONGRATULATIONS!
You have reached the end of the Final Exam.

Now, turn to Chapter Ten to score your exam, assess your progress, and read the rationales.

If you wish, you may take another Final Exam on the enclosed CD-ROM, *Test Smart*, using either Practice mode, to view all the rationales, or Assessment mode.

NOTES

Chapter 10

FINAL EXAM: ANSWERS & ANALYSIS

Before you turn the page and look for the answers to the Final Exam, read the following tips. And remember, the more test questions you answer during your review practice sessions, the better you will become at taking nursing exams. It's true—practice makes perfect! And there is no other way.

Making the Most of Your Final Exam Results

1. If you answered a question incorrectly, *determine whether you did not know the material or just misread the question.* If you misread a question, identify the **critical element** that was overlooked. You need to minimize the questions you are answering incorrectly because of misreading!
2. When you review the answers to the questions—using either this chapter or the Answers and Analysis post-test section on the accompanying *Test Smart* CD-ROM—be sure to read the rationales: It is possible to answer a question *correctly* using an *incorrect* rationale! (In your practice sessions, always review the rationales.)
3. Try to determine how many questions you answered correctly *by using one of the three test-taking strategies.* When you are unsure of an answer, eliminating incorrect options and using test-taking strategies can increase your score dramatically!
4. Use this Assessment Scale to assess your progress:

Score	Recommendation
Less than 65%	OOPS! Don't get discouraged! Spend some time reviewing the basic concepts and strategies in Chapters 3 and 4, and try again.
65-75%	Good work. Try reviewing the "Test-Taking Tips" and "Points to Remember," and keep practicing.
75-85%	Very good. You are becoming a good strategist! Keep answering practice questions until the exam.
85%+	Superior work!! Continue to apply these principles, and try to ace the exam!

5. After calculating your score and analyzing your answers, you should continue to practice answering questions and assessing your progress. You can use the questions in Chapter Twelve to help prepare for your nursing exams.

6. If you were not able to use the *Test Smart* CD-ROM enclosed with this book, you may wish to try using a computer in your learning lab. MEDS Publishing also offers other Q&A review software that incorporates the special features of the enclosed *Test Smart* CD-ROM. Remember, the more test questions you answer, the more successful you become!

We hope *Test Question Logic for Beginning Nursing Students* has revolutionized your approach to taking an exam, and to studying and reviewing nursing content.

CONGRATULATIONS—you have acquired an important new professional skill!
GOOD LUCK ON YOUR NURSING EXAMS!

STRATEGY: MASLOW

1. A six-month-old male infant with AIDS has a nursing diagnosis of "altered growth and development" on the care plan. Which of the following nursing interventions will most enhance the growth and development of the child?

1. Encourage the child to eat whatever he wants.
2. Provide therapy to help the child meet developmental milestones.
3. Provide nutritional supplements in addition to an adequate diet.
4. Weigh and measure the infant on a frequent basis.

1. *INCORRECT. This is not the best answer because it will not ensure that his nutritional needs are met. What is the specific question asked in the stem of this question?*
2. *INCORRECT. Think about Maslow's Hierarchy of Needs. Which need has priority here?*
3. ***CORRECT. The issue in this question is altered growth and development. Maslow's Hierarchy of Needs identifies that physiological needs take priority. If this child is behind in measurable ways on growth and development, his nutritional needs cannot be met by food alone. He needs extra supplements to help him fight infection and grow.***
4. *INCORRECT. This doesn't answer the question. These are assessments or means of evaluating responses, but they do not imply action toward improving or correcting the alteration in growth and development.*

STRATEGY: MASLOW

2. A client has undergone a surgery to correct a bowel obstruction. He has returned from the recovery room with an indwelling urinary catheter. For several hours the urinary output has been adequate. The nurse notes, however, that the catheter has drained no urine during the last hour. What action should the nurse take first?

1. Offer the client 100 cc of oral fluids each hour.
2. Irrigate the catheter according to the postoperative orders.
3. Call the physician and request an increase in IV fluid rate.
4. Monitor the vital signs every 15 minutes for one hour.

1. *INCORRECT. The issue in this question is a sudden stop in urine output from the catheter following the surgery. This is probably the result of an occluded catheter. Increasing oral fluids without removing the obstruction in the catheter will just cause the client to be uncomfortable.*
2. ***CORRECT. A sudden stop in urine output from the catheter following the surgery is probably the result of an occluded catheter. Irrigation will remove the obstruction from the catheter.***

> ***TEST-TAKING TIP:*** Note that the word "catheter" appears in the stem of the question and in the correct answer.

3. *INCORRECT. A sudden stop in urine output from the catheter following surgery is probably the result of an occluded catheter. Increasing IV fluids without removing the obstruction in the catheter will just cause the client to be uncomfortable.*
4. *INCORRECT. Monitoring the vital signs is not relevant because there is no indication in the introductory statement that the vital signs are not stable.*

STRATEGY: ISSUE

3. A client is admitted to the hospital in respiratory distress. The doctor orders oxygen per mask and the client to be placed in high Fowler's position. Which nursing action is most important for this client?

1. Support and align the hands with the forearms.
2. Use handrails.
3. Raise the head of the bed to allow for greater lung expansion.
4. Support the feet at right angles to the lower legs.

1. *INCORRECT. Supporting and aligning the hands prevents potential contractures of the wrist. This action is not inappropriate, but it does not address the issue in the question, which is respiratory distress.*
2. *INCORRECT. Handrails aid in preventing contractures by maintaining the fingers and thumbs in a functional position. This option does not address the issue in the question, which is respiratory distress.*

> ***TEST-TAKING TIP:*** The purpose of this action is the same as for options 1 and 4. Options which use similar ideas can be eliminated.

3. ***CORRECT! The elevation of the head of the bed allows for greater lung expansion and decreased respiratory effort. This option correctly addresses the issue in the question, which is respiratory distress. This action identifies an immediate physiological need.***

> ***TEST-TAKING TIP:*** Raising the head of the bed is included in high Fowler's position, which the doctor's order specifies. Go with what you know!

4. *INCORRECT. Supporting the feet prevents foot drop and contractures at the ankle. This option does not address the issue in the question, which is respiratory distress.*

> ***TEST-TAKING TIP:*** The purpose of this action is the same as for options 1 and 2. Options which use similar ideas can be eliminated.

STRATEGY: CLIENT

4. While the nurse is caring for a seven-month-old female infant, she aspirates a small toy. She begins to cough and becomes cyanotic, and then no sound is made. The best nursing action is to:

1. Perform a chest thrust.
2. Turn the client prone and administer back blows.
3. Stimulate further coughing.
4. Perform a modified Heimlich maneuver with one hand.

1. INCORRECT. This is not the first step.

2. CORRECT. This is the recommendation of the American Red Cross and American Heart Association for the treatment of choking in an infant.

> ***TEST-TAKING TIP:*** Always identify the client and the key words before selecting an intervention.

3. INCORRECT. The introductory statement indicates that the coughing is ineffective, since no sound is heard. This client is cyanotic. Effective action needs to be taken immediately.

4. INCORRECT. This is not the age-appropriate recommendation of the American Red Cross and American Heart Association for the treatment of choking in an infant.

STRATEGY: TYPE OF STEM

5. An elderly client is admitted with a broken right arm and contusions to the left wrist following an automobile accident. The nurse is preparing to feed the client. Which of the following nursing actions is least effective in preventing aspiration?

1. Offer small bites of food.
2. Order pureed foods.
3. Have the client use her dentures while eating.
4. Allow enough time for the client to chew the food well before offering more.

1. INCORRECT—this action is effective. Offering small bites of food helps prevent the client from choking caused by too much food in the mouth. Look for the action that is NOT effective.

2. CORRECT. You spotted the action that was least effective. Pureed foods should be used for clients who are not able to chew or do not have teeth. A client who is able to chew should receive foods of normal texture.

3. INCORRECT—this action is effective. Dentures provide the mechanism for the client to chew foods. If dentures are not used, then the client is at risk for choking on unchewed foods that are too large to swallow. You are looking for the action that is least effective.

4. INCORRECT—this action is effective. Choking can occur if the client does not have time to chew food well. Attempts may be made to swallow large boluses of food, or the mouth may become too full if the nurse feeds the client at a fast pace. You are looking for the action that is least effective.

STRATEGY: ISSUE

6. To monitor a client for the most common complication arising from the administration of total parenteral nutrition, the nurse should:

1. Weigh the client at the same time each day using the same scale.
2. Keep accurate records of total intake and total output.
3. Determine the increase or decrease in body weight each day.
4. Take the client's temperature at least every four hours.

1. INCORRECT. The issue in this question is TPN. Weighing the client daily is an appropriate nursing action to assess whether the primary purpose of TPN is being met, but the stem is asking you to select a nursing action that monitors for the most common complication. Poor weight gain can be a problem, but it is not a complication. Note also that the same idea is expressed in option 3; similar distractors generally are wrong and can be eliminated.

2. INCORRECT. The idea in this option is to record intake and output. This is an appropriate nursing action, but it does not monitor for the most common complication. Try again!

3. INCORRECT. Weighing the client daily to assess weight and nutritional status is an appropriate nursing action, but it is not the answer to the question. The issue is TPN, and the stem asks you to select a nursing action that monitors for the most common complication. Note that the same idea is expressed in option 1. Similar distractors generally are wrong and can be eliminated.

4. CORRECT. Catheter-related infections are the most common complication. Taking the client's temperature at least every four hours is the nursing action that monitors for the most common complication.

> ***TEST-TAKING TIP:*** Note that options 1 and 3 are very similar to each other and can be eliminated.

STRATEGY: COMMUNICATION TOOLS AND BLOCKS

7. A hospitalized client has just found out that her mother has died of a heart attack. She is crying and has her face buried in the pillow. The best nursing action is to:

1. Return in 15 minutes to see how the client is doing.
2. Sit with the client for a little while.
3. Tell the client that she will feel better in the morning.
4. Share with the client that you lost your mother within the last year and that you know how she feels.

1. INCORRECT. This response does not promote therapeutic communication for the "here and now" of this question. By leaving, the nurse indicates to the client that she is not willing to offer herself by staying with her during this stressful time. If the client wanted to communicate, there wouldn't be anyone to listen.

2. ***CORRECT. The nurse lets the client know that she is important by providing time for her. Being silent is a communication tool that is appropriate during times of grieving. This response also addresses the "here and now" in this question.***
3. *INCORRECT. This response devalues the client's feelings and puts them on hold. This response does not encourage therapeutic communication. It also offers false assurance, since she may not feel better in the morning.*
4. *INCORRECT. This response focuses on an inappropriate person (the nurse). When the nurse says that she knows how the client feels, it inhibits communication, since this implies that there is no need for the client to express her own feelings. There also is an assumption by the nurse that grieving is the same for everyone. This response is not therapeutic for the client.*

STRATEGY: COMMUNICATION TOOLS AND BLOCKS

8. An elderly client is admitted to the hospital for surgery after finding a lump in his right testicle. He asks the nurse, "Do you think the doctor will find cancer?" The best response by the nurse initially is:

1. "Most lumps found in the testicles are benign."
2. "It must be difficult for you not to know what the doctor will find."
3. "I think that you should discuss this with your doctor."
4. "It might be, but the doctor won't know until the surgery is performed."

1. *INCORRECT. This statement provides some general information (about "most lumps found in the testicles"), but does not allow the client to express his fears concerning cancer. This response blocks communication between the client and the nurse.*

> ***TEST TAKING TIP:*** Identify the key words! The word "initially" is your clue to use the communication theory guideline that the nurse should first address the client's feelings.

2. ***CORRECT. This response promotes communication by allowing the client to express his feelings. The key word is "initially," and communication theory identifies that the nurse should first address the client's feelings.***
3. *INCORRECT. Referring the client's concern to the doctor puts the client's concern "on hold" and is not a therapeutic nursing response. The client's feelings and concerns need to be addressed by the nurse.*
4. *INCORRECT. This response might be a true statement, but it does not help the client to explore his feelings and is not a therapeutic nursing response.*

STRATEGY: COMMUNICATION TOOLS AND BLOCKS

9. An elderly male client was admitted to the hospital for surgery for a fractured hip. The client says to the nurse, "I guess I've lived long enough, and my number's up." How should the nurse respond initially?

1. "You are in really good shape for your age."
2. "This is just a minor setback. You will be on your feet in no time."
3. "You feel that your life is ending?"
4. "The doctors and nurses are going to take good care of you while you are here. There's nothing to worry about."

1. *INCORRECT. This response contradicts the client and fails to address the client's feelings. He has made a statement that implies he is going to die. The nurse needs to explore these feelings further to be able to promote therapeutic communication. This response devalues the client's feelings and is an inhibitor to effective communication.*
2. *INCORRECT. This response devalues the client's feelings about dying, and it also uses the communication blocks of cliché and false assurance, which inhibit communication. The nurse needs to address this client's feelings of doom.*
3. ***CORRECT. The client has made a statement that implies he is going to die. The nurse needs to explore these feelings further to be able to promote therapeutic communication. This response addresses the client's concerns and uses restatement and clarification of the client's feelings to promote therapeutic communication.***
4. *INCORRECT. This response focuses on inappropriate persons (the doctors and nurses) and not on the client. The feelings of the client concern death, but this response devalues his feelings by using the communication blocks of cliché and false assurance.*

STRATEGY: COMMUNICATION TOOLS AND BLOCKS

10. A daughter has come to take her mother home from the hospital after a colostomy. The daughter tells the nurse that she doesn't know how she is going to care for her mother's colostomy. The nurse's most helpful response to the daughter is:

1. "Your mother can take care of her colostomy without difficulty."
2. "What part of your mother's care are you concerned about?"
3. "A home health nurse will be stopping by tomorrow. If you have any questions, you can ask her."
4. "It is quite simple. I'll make sure that her colostomy bag is clean before she leaves."

1. *INCORRECT. This may be a true statement, but it does not allow the client to express her concerns. The daughter is the client in this question, and the nurse's response should always be therapeutic for the client.*

> ***TEST-TAKING TIP:*** Remember that the client in a communication question isn't always the person with the health problem.

2. ***CORRECT. The daughter is the client in this question. This response is therapeutic for the daughter because it uses the communication tool of clarification to allow her to express her concerns.***
3. *INCORRECT. The daughter is the client in this question, and the nurse's response should be therapeutic for the client. This response uses the communication block of putting the client's concerns "on hold," and is not therapeutic for the client. This cannot be the best response.*
4. *INCORRECT. The daughter is the client in this question, and the nurse's response should be therapeutic for the client. This response uses the communication block of false reassurance. It is not therapeutic because it fails to address the client's concerns.*

STRATEGY: CLIENT

11. A client is scheduled for a mastectomy in the morning. Her daughter is visiting her and says to the nurse, "I should call my brother and sister and have them here in the morning, just in case something goes wrong." The most helpful nursing response is to:

1. Ask the mother if she would like her children there in the morning.
2. Suggest to the daughter that she ask her mother how she feels about that.
3. Say to the daughter, "If your brother and sister want to be here, they are welcome."
4. Ask the daughter what she knows about her mother's surgery and diagnosis.

1. *INCORRECT. Although the mother is the person with the health care problem, the client in the question is her daughter. The nursing response should be addressed to the daughter.*
2. *INCORRECT. The daughter is the client in this question. This response is not therapeutic for the daughter because it does not address her concern about her mother's impending surgery.*
3. *INCORRECT. The daughter is the client in this question. This response is not therapeutic because it focuses on the needs of the brothers and sisters, not on the daughter's concerns about her mother's surgery. This response might also appear to the daughter to validate her fears about the surgery. Finally, the mother is in the room, and it is not up to the nurse to say whether the brother and sister are "welcome." This option cannot be the answer.*
4. ***CORRECT. The daughter is the client in this question, and the nurse is addressing the daughter's needs by clarifying the daughter's understanding of her mother's health problems. This response is therapeutic for the daughter.***

STRATEGY: COMMUNICATION: TOOLS AND BLOCKS

12. An 84-year-old married man is admitted from his home to a skilled nursing facility with a diagnosis of Alzheimer's disease. While speaking with the admitting nurse, his wife begins to cry and says, "I never thought it would come to this. I feel so guilty bringing him here." Which nursing response is best?

1. "You have done all you could. We will take good care of him here."
2. "This has been a difficult time for you. Let's find a quiet place where we can talk."
3. "Admitting your husband was the right decision. He requires more care then you can provide at home."
4. "What are you feeling guilty about?"

1. *INCORRECT. This statement is not the best nursing response because it uses a form of false reassurance. The nurse is assuming the wife did all she could, but the nurse does not know that this is true. The nurse is also referring to an inappropriate issue—the quality of care at the skilled nursing facility. The client in this question is the wife, and the issue is her feelings of guilt. The nursing goal is to help the wife deal with her feelings so she will be able to support her husband with his adjustment to the nursing home.*
2. ***CORRECT. The nurse acknowledges the wife's feelings and offers an availability to assist her with them. The nursing goal is to help the wife deal with her feelings so she will be able to support her husband with his adjustment to the nursing home.***

> ***TEST-TAKING TIP:*** This response uses the therapeutic communication tools of empathy and offering self.

3. *INCORRECT. This is not the best option. The nurse is giving advice and approval, instead of helping the wife to deal constructively with her feelings.*

> ***TEST-TAKING TIP:*** Giving advice and giving approval or disapproval are communication blocks. This cannot be the correct answer.

4. INCORRECT. The nurse does not need further clarification. The wife has told the nurse that she feels guilty about admitting her husband to the long-term care facility. Asking this question indicates that the nurse either has not listened or is not sensitive to the wife's feelings.

STRATEGY: CLIENT

13. A client is admitted to the hospital. He has been on bed rest at home and has been incontinent of urine. His wife has been caring for him, and there is a strong odor of urine. The wife says that she is sorry and embarrassed about the unpleasant smell. Which response by the nurse is therapeutic?

1. "It must be difficult to care for someone who is confined to bed. How have you been able to manage?"
2. "Don't worry about it. He will get a bath, and that will take care of the odor."
3. "A lot of clients that are cared for at home have the same problem."
4. "When was the last time that he had a bath?"

1. ***CORRECT. The wife is the client in this question. The nurse's response must be therapeutic for the client. This response addresses the feelings***

of the client by using the communication tool of showing empathy. It also facilitates therapeutic communication because it is nonjudgmental and encourages the client to express her feelings.

2. *INCORRECT. Telling the client not to worry blocks communication by devaluing her feelings and her concern about the odor. The nurse's response must be therapeutic for the client. Look for a response by the nurse that addresses the feelings of the client and uses a therapeutic communication tool.*
3. *INCORRECT. This response implies that caregivers in the home are not able to keep the client odor free. It is a judgmental statement that is not therapeutic. Look for a response by the nurse that addresses the feelings of the client and uses a therapeutic communication tool. .*
4. *INCORRECT. Asking about the last bath implies to the client that the odor of urine indicates that her husband has not been bathed for some time. The wife is the client in this question, and she has expressed her feelings to the nurse. The nurse's response must be therapeutic for the client. Look for a response by the nurse that addresses the feelings of the client and uses a therapeutic communication tool.*

STRATEGY: CLIENT

14. A general anesthesia has been given for multiple tooth extractions on a three-year-old child. He returns crying, but awake, from the recovery room. What approach by the nurse is most likely to be successful?

1. Assess the child, examining the mouth first.
2. Assess the child, leaving the mouth until last.
3. It really makes no difference what is done first.
4. Medicate the child for pain first.

1. *INCORRECT. Since this is the area of discomfort, this is likely to cause more crying and uncooperative behavior.*
2. ***CORRECT! Leave the most distressing part of an exam on a toddler until the end. You must assess the child before pain medication can be administered.***

> ***TEST-TAKING TIP:*** This question focuses on the nursing process and growth and development.

3. *INCORRECT. The issue in this question is postoperative care for a toddler.*
4. *INCORRECT. The issue in this question is postoperative care. An assessment is always performed immediately upon transfer from recovery.*

STRATEGY: NURSING PROCESS

15. The nurse's clinical assessment of a two-year-old child who is poorly nourished is most likely to include:

1. Mother's statement that the child is a "picky eater."
2. Height and weight in the 25th percentile.
3. Observing that the child is slender and active.
4. Dry, colorless hair and pale skin.

1. *INCORRECT. This is a possibility, but it is not the best option. This assessment is not really helpful. Many healthy toddlers are described as picky eaters by their families, because they are too busy to sit for meals. Read all the options before selecting the one that best describes a malnourished child.*
2. *This assessment reflects an adequate amount of growth and does not describe a poorly nourished child. The introductory statement tells you that the child is poorly nourished.*
3. *INCORRECT. Slender and active describes a healthy child. The introductory statement tells you that the child is poorly nourished. .*

> ***TEST-TAKING TIP:*** Options 1 and 3 are similar in that they describe the child's <u>behavior</u>. Similar options can generally be eliminated.

4. ***CORRECT. This is the classic picture of a poorly nourished child. Inadequate nutrients may cause a low hemoglobin, which will cause pale skin, and since the body is poorly nourished the hair is dry, brittle, and lacking in color.***

STRATEGY: COMMUNICATION TOOLS AND BLOCKS

16. A mother expresses concern about her infant's lack of eye muscle control at two days of age because her neighbor's daughter is mentally retarded and her eyes cross the same way. What is the nurse's best reply?

1. "You should probably talk to the doctor about your concerns."
2. "Newborns all lack the ability to control eye movement until they are three to four months of age."
3. "I will take the baby back to the nursery and assess other neuromuscular activity."
4. "It's nothing to worry about."

1. *INCORRECT. This response "passes the buck" and suggests that there could be a problem that the physician needs to know about. The nurse can use knowledge of normal growth and development to respond to this client's concern.*
2. ***CORRECT. Lack of eye muscle control is present in all newborns. This mother needs to know this so she will not think this is abnormal. This response is therapeutic because it addresses the client's concerns and provides correct information.***
3. *INCORRECT. This statement suggests that the lack of eye muscle control warrants further assessment of the newborn. The nurse can use knowledge of normal growth and development to respond to this client's concern.*
4. *INCORRECT. This statement is not therapeutic. It provides no information, does not reassure the client that this finding is normal, ignores the client's fears, and discourages further communication.*

> ***TEST-TAKING TIP:*** This option uses the communication blocks of using cliché and devaluing the client's concern.

STRATEGY: MASLOW

17. A mother watches the nurse in the pediatrics ward place her toddler in a highchair for a meal. After placing the client in the highchair, what nursing action would be most essential initially?

1. Pour a small amount of milk into the glass.
2. Ask the mother to feed the child.
3. Belt the child securely to the chair.
4. Cut the child's food into bite size pieces.

1. *Wrong choice. This is an appropriate action; never fill a glass or cup more than half full. However, this action is not the "most essential initially."*

> ***TEST-TAKING TIP:*** Identify the key words in the stem, and read all the options before selecting the best one.

2. *Wrong choice. This is an appropriate action. Toddlers have severe separation anxiety, and having mother feed the child will decrease their fear and increase their intake of food. However, this action is not the "most essential initially." Remember—always identify the key words in the question.*
3. ***Very good! The key words "most essential initially" make this a prioritizing question, and the priority in this clinical situation is safety. The toddler is at immediate risk of falling. The nurse should assess this potentially unsafe situation and make the appropriate changes to provide a safe environment.***
4. *This is an appropriate action. A toddler should always have small pieces of food that can be picked up with the fingers. However, this is not the "most essential" action "initially."*

STRATEGY: TYPE OF STEM

18. An 82-year-old client is admitted to the hospital for hip replacement surgery. She appears alert and cooperative, although in great pain. While doing an assessment, the nurse learns she is disoriented to time and believes she is in a hotel. The nurse identifies acute confusion as a nursing problem. Of the following, which does the nurse understand would least impact the client's confusion:

1. Her age.
2. Relocation to the hospital.
3. Her physical pain.
4. Bed confinement.

1. ***CORRECT. Although acute confusion commonly occurs in persons over the age of 80, this condition is caused by physical and psychological problems that occur in advanced old age, not by age itself. Acute confusion can be successfully resolved by diagnosing and treating the underlying problem(s).***
2. *INCORRECT. Relocation to a new environment, particularly when the move is sudden or unplanned, can result in a period of acute confusion for an elderly person. You are looking for an option that is NOT a likely cause of this client's confusion. .*
3. *INCORRECT. Pain or discomfort from unmet physical needs is often the cause of acute confusion in persons of any age, including the elderly. You are looking for an option that is NOT a likely cause of this client's confusion.*
4. *INCORRECT. Bed confinement, especially in a horizontal position, is often associated with acute confusion because the individual does not have access to the full range of visual cues needed to maintain good orientation. You are looking for an option that is NOT a likely cause of this client's confusion.*

STRATEGY: KEY WORDS

19. A client has right-sided paralysis following a stroke. He is not able to talk but can make gestures to make himself understood. To effectively communicate with the client, the nurse should:

1. Speak very loudly to the client.
2. Speak quickly to the client, since his attention span may be short.
3. Use gestures while speaking slowly.
4. Wait until the family comes in, so they can interpret his behavior.

1. *INCORRECT. The client is not hard of hearing. What is the issue in the question?*
   This client, with right-sided paralysis, also has impaired mobility. This question identifies several <u>safety</u> risk factors.
2. *INCORRECT. Fast speech is difficult to understand. Also, there is no information that the client has a short attention span.*

> ***TEST-TAKING TIP:*** Identify the key words! The client cannot speak and has difficulty making himself understood.

This client, with right-sided paralysis, also has impaired mobility. This question identifies several <u>safety</u> risk factors.

3. ***CORRECT. This client is at a high safety risk, due to both impaired mobility and impaired ability to communicate. The nurse must use all appropriate means to be sure that the client understands what the nurse is saying, and to enable the client to express his needs.***
4. *INCORRECT. The client may have needs that cannot wait for the family. This option does not respect the client's needs or assure his comfort and safety.*

STRATEGY: TYPE OF STEM

20. A client in a long-term care facility has been given a cane to assist her with ambulation. In caring for this client, which of the following would place the client at risk?

1. Inspect the rubber tip often and replace it if appears to be worn.
2. Place the cane on the side of the weak leg.
3. Position the cane to support and balance the client with decreased strength in one of the lower extremities.
4. Keep the cane within easy reach when sleeping or sitting.

1. *INCORRECT—you are looking for an option that is UNSAFE. A cane that does not have a good rubber*

tip on it places the client at risk for falling, since the wood or metal on the bottom of the cane can cause it to slip on the floor.

2. ***CORRECT. You have identified the unsafe action! The cane should be placed on the strong side of the client. Since weight is placed on the cane at the same time that it is placed on the weakened extremity, the body weight will be divided equally between the cane and the weakened leg.***
3. *INCORRECT—You are looking for an option that is UNSAFE. The client must have some strength in the affected extremity, or a cane will not provide enough support to allow for ambulation.*
4. *INCORRECT—You are looking for an UNSAFE action. If a cane is needed for ambulation, then it should be kept within the client's reach in order to prevent falling while trying to locate the cane.*

STRATEGY: NURSING PROCESS

21. An elderly female client has been in the hospital for a week on bed rest. She complains of elbow pain. The best nursing action is to:

1. Place elbow pads on the client.
2. Examine the elbow.
3. Call the physician for an order for pain medication.
4. Reposition the client so that she is more comfortable.

1. *INCORRECT. This is an implementation action. Since the case scenario does not tell you what is causing the elbow pain, you cannot assume that it is related to pressure or skin breakdown. More information must be obtained by the nurse before implementing any actions.*
2. ***CORRECT. Examining the elbow is an assessment of the client's complaint. The nurse does not know enough about the elbow pain or its probable cause. The elbows can be assessed for redness, swelling, or joint pain. Then, after assessing the problem, the nurse can analyze the situation and develop a plan of care and implement the appropriate nursing interventions.***

> ***TEST-TAKING TIP:*** The other three actions are all implementation actions. This question uses the nursing process as a priority setting guideline.

3. *INCORRECT. This is an implementation action. Calling the physician at this time is not appropriate! The nurse does not know enough about the elbow pain or what is causing it. After obtaining further information, the nurse may not need to notify the physician if nursing interventions will alleviate the problem. If the physician must be notified, the nurse needs to gather the information that the physician will need to analyze the problem and order appropriate medical treatment.*
4. *INCORRECT. This is an implementation action. Repositioning the client provides for the client's comfort. However, the nurse does not know what is causing the pain. Repositioning the client should not precede the nurse's investigation of the client's complaint of pain. The nursing process requires that assessment be performed before planning or implementing any other nursing action, because those actions must be based on information obtained during the assessment.*

STRATEGY: KEY WORDS

22. The nurse is preparing to transfer a client from a bed to a chair. To avoid back injury to the nurse, the safest technique is to:

1. Bend at the waist while maintaining a wide stance, lift the client to a standing position, and then pivot the client toward the chair.
2. Have the client lock his or her hands around the nurse's neck, so that the client will feel more secure during the transfer.
3. Place the bed in an elevated position so that the client's hips are at the same level as the nurse's hip, resulting in the center of gravity being the same for both individuals.
4. Bend at the knees, while maintaining a wide stance and straight back, with the client's hands on the nurse's shoulders and the nurse's hands at the client's axillae.

1. *INCORRECT. Bending at the waist places strain on the small lower back muscles, which are prone to injury.*

> ***TEST-TAKING TIP:*** Be sure to identify and focus on the key words in each option, especially when comparing lengthy options! The key words here are "bend at the waist." This cannot be correct.

2. *INCORRECT. If the client's hands are locked around the nurse's neck and then the client starts to fall, all of the client's weight is placed on the cervical vertebrae of the nurse, which can result in a serious injury. The client's hands should rest on the shoulders of the nurse.*

> ***TEST-TAKING TIP:*** Be sure to identify and focus on the key words in each option, especially when comparing lengthy options! The key words here are "hands around the nurse's neck." This cannot be correct.

3. *INCORRECT. The bed should be in the low position, which provides a place for the client to sit if he is unable to stand. With the bed elevated, once the client attempts to stand, the client cannot sit back down on the bed if he becomes weak or faint. If the client begins to fall, the nurse is at risk for back injury in attempting to prevent the fall.*

> ***TEST-TAKING TIP:*** Be sure to identify and focus on the key words in each option, especially when comparing lengthy options! The key words here are "bed in an elevated position." This cannot be correct.

4. ***CORRECT. Bending at the knees results in the use of the large muscles of the legs. Keeping the back straight avoids using the small, easily injured back muscles. When the client's hands rest on the nurse's shoulders, this provides security for the client. Placing the hands under the axillae of the client avoids placing pressure on the chest, which can be uncomfortable for the client.***

> ***TEST-TAKING TIP:*** Be sure to identify and focus on the key words in each option, especially when comparing lengthy options! In the other three options, the key words are all in the first phrases, and the rest of each option is just a rationale.

STRATEGY: TYPE OF STEM

23. The nurse would demonstrate a good understanding of safe body mechanics by avoiding which of the following actions?

1. Move muscles quickly, using short tugs in order to avoid muscle fatigue.
2. Use the longest and strongest muscles of the body whenever possible.
3. Lean toward objects being pushed, such as a stretcher.
4. Carry objects close to the body without touching your clothing.

1. ***CORRECT. The question is asking you to select an action to AVOID. The key word in this option is "quickly." Jerky movements produce increased strain on muscles and are usually uncomfortable for the client. This question has a false response stem.***

2. INCORRECT. The longest, strongest muscles are less likely to become injured than the small muscles. This is a correct action, but the question is asking you to select an option to AVOID.

> ***TEST-TAKING TIP:*** Did you identify that this question has a false response stem?

3. INCORRECT. Body weight adds force to muscle action when pushing any object. This is a correct action, but the question is asking you to select an option to AVOID.

> ***TEST-TAKING TIP:*** Did you identify that this question has a false response stem?

4. INCORRECT. When objects are close to the body, the line of gravity is within the body's base of support, which improves balance and reduces strain on the arm muscles. This is a correct action, but the question is asking you to select an option to AVOID.

> ***TEST-TAKING TIP:*** Did you identify that this question has a false response stem?

STRATEGY: MASLOW

24. A male client sustained a fracture of the tibia and fibula while playing football. A long leg cast has been applied, and the client is admitted to the orthopedic unit. In providing nursing care for the client, which of the following is a vital consideration?

1. Elevation of the leg in the cast on a pillow will minimize edema.
2. Healing of a fractured bone requires an extended period of time.
3. A long period of immobility may lead to atrophy of the muscle.
4. Analgesics may be needed for pain associated with the fracture.

1. ***CORRECT. When caring for a client with a newly applied cast, it is important to keep the affected extremity elevated to reduce swelling. Note that the words "leg" and "cast" appear in the stem as well as in this option.***

2. INCORRECT. While this is a true statement, it does not answer the question asked in the stem. The issue is a newly applied cast, and the stem asks you to select an option that is a vital consideration.

3. INCORRECT. While this is a true statement, it does not address the question asked in the stem. The issue is a newly applied cast, and the stem asks you to select an option that is a "vital consideration."

> ***TEST-TAKING TIP:*** Note that options 2 and 3 both refer to the long run. This is a prioritizing question. Look for an option that addresses an immediate physiological need.

4. INCORRECT. While this is a true statement, it does not address the question asked in the stem. The issue is a newly applied cast, and the stem asks you to select an option that is a "vital consideration."

> ***TEST-TAKING TIP:*** This is a prioritizing question. Look for an option that addresses an immediate physiological need.

STRATEGY: NURSING PROCESS

25. A client has been incontinent of loose stool and is complaining of a painful perineum. The most appropriate initial nursing action is to:

1. Notify the physician to obtain an order for the loose stools.
2. Check the client's perineum.
3. Turn the client every two hours.
4. Increase the client's fluid intake to prevent dehydration.

1. INCORRECT. Informing the physician is a possibility, but this action does not address the client's concern. The issue in the question is perineal pain. This is the client's concern. Also, note that this option is an implementation action. The key word in this question is "initial." The nurse should always assess first!

2. ***CORRECT. This option addresses the client's concern, which is the painful perineum. This is the issue in the question. This option is also the best because it is an assessment action. The nurse should always assess first!***

3. INCORRECT. Turning an immobilized client every two hours will help prevent skin breakdown, but it does not address the issue in the question, which is the perineal pain. Also, this is an implementation action. What should the nurse do first?

4. INCORRECT. Preventing dehydration is important for the client with loose stools. Although this is the client's medical diagnosis, it is not the issue in this question.

The issue is perineal pain, which is the subject of the client's complaint. Also, this is an implementation action. What should the nurse do first?

STRATEGY: ISSUE

26. A teenage client had an appendectomy. When the nurse offers meperidine (Demerol) for postoperative pain, the client says, "No, I don't want to get hooked." Which is the most appropriate nursing response?

1. "You are right. Why take a chance?"
2. "Tell me what you mean by getting hooked."
3. "You will not get addicted for the short amount of time that you will be in the hospital."
4. "The Demerol will make you more comfortable, not make you an addict."

1. INCORRECT. The client appears to have made an incorrect assumption concerning risks of the medication. This response is not therapeutic because it does not properly address the client's concern about addiction or the issue of the client's physical discomfort. It also blocks communication by using a cliché ("Why take a chance?").

> ***TEST-TAKING TIP:*** Responses that include a communication block cannot be correct.

2. CORRECT. This response enhances therapeutic communication by asking for clarification. The nurse is addressing the client's concern and asking for important information about the client's knowledge and feelings, as well as any history of problems with medications or other substances that may be habit forming or addictive. This teenage client has raised the issue of the risk of chemical dependency.

3. INCORRECT. This statement uses false reassurance and devalues the client's feelings. The nurse should communicate therapeutically by trying to learn more about the client's knowledge and feelings.

> ***TEST-TAKING TIP:*** Responses that include a communication block cannot be correct.

4. INCORRECT. The first part of this response gives the client correct information and addresses the issue of the client's pain. However, the nurse should first ask for clarification of the client's concerns about "getting hooked."

STRATEGY: MASLOW

27. An elderly client has a draining pressure sore. The culture of the drainage reveals staphylococci. The best nursing action is to:

1. Reinforce the pressure dressing with a sterile towel before ambulating the client.
2. Wear gown and gloves when changing the client's bed linen.
3. Use sterile technique when changing the dressing on the pressure sore.
4. Discourage the client's use of his personal effects until they have been sterilized.

1. INCORRECT. Reinforcing the dressing will not prevent the spread of the pathogens.

> ***TEST-TAKING TIP:*** This option and option 3 are similar because they both concern the dressing itself. These similar distractors can be eliminated.

2. CORRECT! The nurse should always wear a gown and gloves when changing the client's bed linen. This is to prevent the spread of pathogens, which may attach to the nurse's clothing during the bed change; then, when the nurse goes to another client's room, there is no threat of contaminating that client with this client's pathogens.

> ***TEST-TAKING TIP:*** This question is a prioritizing question. Since no physiological need is identified, the priority is safety. The nurse will provide the safest environment by this action.

3. INCORRECT. Sterile technique will help prevent secondary pathogens from infecting the wound, but it will not prevent the spread of the pathogens. This is not the best option.

> ***TEST-TAKING TIP:*** This option and option 1 are similar because they both concern the dressing itself. These similar distractors can be eliminated.

4. INCORRECT. Sterilizing the client's linen and personal effects will not prevent the spread of the pathogens.

STRATEGY: KEY WORDS

28. Before administering an injection, the nurse performs aseptic handwashing. This technique includes:

1. Avoiding soap, since it causes drying of the skin.
2. Using paper towels to turn the faucet on and off.
3. The use of lotion to prevent drying.
4. Holding arms and hands upright so that all organisms will drain away from hands while washing.

1. INCORRECT. This is not aseptic! Soap is necessary in handwashing to remove organisms from the skin. After handwashing, lotion should often be used to prevent drying and chapping, which may cause cracks in the skin that provide portals of entry for infectious organisms.

2. CORRECT. Faucets have many bacteria on the handles. To prevent transmission of the bacteria, paper towels are used to turn faucets on and off.

> ***TEST-TAKING TIP:*** The key word in the question is "aseptic," and the issue is aseptic handwashing. The correct option must address the issue.

3. INCORRECT. Using lotion does not clean the hands, so this option does not address the issue in the question and this cannot be the correct answer. After handwashing, however, lotion should be used as necessary to prevent drying and chapping, which may cause cracks in the skin that provide portals of entry for infectious organisms.

> ***TEST-TAKING TIP:*** This option is similar to option 1, since it concerns preventing dryness of the skin. These similar options can be eliminated.

4. *INCORRECT. The water and organisms will run to the elbow instead of off the hand into the sink.*

STRATEGY: ISSUE

29. An infant is in respiratory isolation. The nurse can most effectively prevent the spread of pathogens via droplet infection by:

1. Wearing a gown and mask when feeding the client.
2. Using sterile gloves when changing her diapers.
3. Having the baby wear a mask when in the playroom.
4. Using enteric precautions when caring for the baby.

1. ***CORRECT. This question seeks to identify the main threat to the general population from this client's infection. To prevent the spread of pathogens to others, the nurse must ensure that respiratory secretions are not transmitted. During feeding and burping of the infant, the respiratory secretions will become mixed with the formula. When the baby burps, there is risk of spreading the pathogens via droplet as well as by contact with the nurse's uniform. Wearing a gown and mask will decrease the probability of transmitting the organisms.***
2. *INCORRECT. This will not prevent the transmission of respiratory secretions.*

> ***TEST-TAKING TIP:*** This option does not address the issue in the question.

3. *INCORRECT. An infant in respiratory isolation should not leave the room. Taking the baby to the playroom is inappropriate. It is also inappropriate to put a mask on an infant!*
4. *INCORRECT. Enteric precautions are not appropriate for a baby in respiratory isolation. They will not prevent the transmission of respiratory secretions.*

> ***TEST-TAKING TIP:*** This option is similar to option 2 and does not address the issue in the question.

STRATEGY: TYPE OF STEM

30. An infant with AIDS is being prepared for discharge. The nurse is instructing the grandmother, who will care for the infant, in methods of home care. Which statement made by the grandmother represents the greatest safety hazard?

1. "I know that handwashing is an important preventive measure."
2. "I'll use disposable diapers, discarding them in separate plastic bags."
3. "Blood spills should be washed up immediately with hot soapy water."
4. "Gloves should be worn by whoever changes the baby's diapers."

1. *INCORRECT. This statement by the grandmother indicates a good understanding of transmission of the disease and of the role of handwashing in preventing the spread of infection to the client and to the family. You are looking for an INCORRECT statement.*
2. *INCORRECT. This statement by the grandmother indicates a good understanding of an acceptable method of infection control. Any items that cannot be disposed of in the toilet should be kept in a closed plastic bag until trash disposal. You are looking for an INCORRECT statement.*
3. ***CORRECT. This is an inadequate method of cleaning blood or potentially contaminated body substances. Bleach solution should be used and gloves worn whenever coming in contact with blood products. This INCORRECT statement by the grandmother is the correct answer to this question, which has a false response stem.***
4. *INCORRECT. This statement by the grandmother indicates a good understanding of transmission of the disease and one important action in preventing the spread of infection to the client and to the family. Gloves should be worn by anyone when changing the diaper of a child who has tested HIV positive or has the AIDS virus, because blood and body fluids are a means of disease transmission. You are looking for an INCORRECT statement.*

STRATEGY: TYPE OF STEM

31. A client seen at the clinic is to receive an injection. When preparing to administer a medication for injection from an ampule, which nursing action would place the client at risk?

1. Score the neck of the ampule with a file.
2. Protect the thumb and fingers with a gauze square or alcohol wipe.
3. Snap the neck of the ampule toward the body when breaking the top free from the ampule.
4. Insert the needle into the ampule without touching the needle to the edges of the ampule.

1. *INCORRECT. This is safe! Scoring the neck of the ampule provides a place for the ampule to break easily without jagged edges. You are looking for an UNSAFE action. This question has a false response stem.*
2. *INCORRECT. This action is safe! Using a gauze or alcohol wipe protects the thumb and finger from being cut if contact is made with the hand and edges of the broken ampule. You are looking for an UNSAFE action. This question has a false response stem.*
3. ***CORRECT, you spotted the action that is unsafe! The neck of the ampule should be broken away from the body, to prevent shattering of glass toward the hand or face.***
4. *INCORRECT. This action is safe! The rim of the ampule is considered contaminated. Touching the edges with the needle will contaminate the needle. You are looking for an UNSAFE action. This question has a false response stem.*

STRATEGY: MASLOW

32. A new order is written for ear drops for a three-year-old child. In preparing for the procedure, the nurse knows the lowest priority is to:

1. Anticipate the need for assistance to restrain.
2. Check the child's name bracelet, before administration.
3. Explain the purpose of the medication to the child.
4. Check which ear is to receive the drops prior to administration.

1. *INCORRECT. This is not a low priority. You may very well need help to prevent injury to the child and to correctly instill the medication.*
2. *INCORRECT. This is not a low priority! Checking the name bracelet is always a high priority for drug administration.*
3. ***CORRECT. Even though you want to have an informed client, this isn't the highest priority—especially since this child is three years old and does not have the cognitive ability to understand the reason for the medication. Safety is more important.***

> ***TEST-TAKING TIP:*** Note that this prioritizing question has a false response stem. Remember Maslow's Hierarchy of Needs! This question does not identify a physiological need, and the other three options all identify safety concerns. This option is the lowest priority of those offered.

4. *INCORRECT. This is not a low priority. The client has two ears and the nurse must be certain that the medication is administered in the proper ear!*

STRATEGY: CLIENT

33. The nurse is assessing a young child with asthma in order to determine the usefulness of a metered dose inhaler. The nurse assesses that the use of the inhaler is discouraged by the:

1. The child's inability to follow directions.
2. The family's poor financial situation.
3. The size of the medication particles.
4. The severity of the child's disease.

1. ***CORRECT. In order to effectively use a metered dose inhaler, the child must be able to inhale as the medication is released. Children can use an inhaler as soon as they can follow these directions.***

> ***TEST-TAKING TIP:*** Remember the critical elements—Always identify the client!

2. *INCORRECT. This would not discourage use. The relative costs of oral medications, metered dose inhalers, and nebulizers are the same. In fact, nebulizers may be more costly initially.*
3. *INCORRECT. This would not discourage use. Medication particles are the smallest when delivered by metered dose inhaler. Because children's airways are narrower than adults' airways, a metered dose inhaler is the route of choice. The inhaler cannot be used, however, by children too young to understand how to use the inhaler.*
4. *INCORRECT. When used properly, a metered dose inhaler can deliver a sufficient amount of medication to treat an asthma attack. The inhaler has the advantage of being more transportable and, therefore, more readily available. The severity of the illness, therefore, is a poor factor in determining effectiveness.*

STRATEGY: NURSING PROCESS

34. A client has returned after major surgery and is complaining of pain. The physician ordered morphine sulfate to control her pain. Before administering the medication, the nurse would first:

1. Discuss the side effects with the client.
2. Take the client's vital signs.
3. Provide mouth care.
4. Have the client turn, cough and deep breathe.

1. *INCORRECT. This is not the first nursing action. Clients do need to be informed of possible side effects, but the nurse should save any teaching until the client is more alert.*

> ***TEST-TAKING TIP:*** This is an implementation option. What should the nurse do first?

2. ***CORRECT. Vital signs should be taken before administering morphine to provide a baseline for measuring respiratory depression, which can occur afterwards.***

> ***TEST-TAKING TIP:*** The nursing process is the best prioritizing guideline in this question. Note that this is the only assessment action described for this postoperative client.

3. *INCORRECT. This is not the first nursing action. Mouth care will be needed postoperatively but it is not needed prior to morphine administration.*

> ***TEST-TAKING TIP:*** This is an implementation option. What should the nurse do first?

4. *INCORRECT. The client will be better able to cooperate when she has less pain, after the medication is administered.*

> ***TEST-TAKING TIP:*** This is an implementation option. What should the nurse do first?

STRATEGY: ISSUE

35. A client is to receive eye drops. Which of the following nursing actions best prevents injury to the eye during administration?

1. Apply gentle pressure over the opening to the naso-lacrimal duct.
2. Hold the tip of the container above the conjunctival sac.
3. Instruct the client to look upward.
4. Deposit the drops into the conjunctival sac.

1. *INCORRECT.. Occlusion of the nasal lacrimal ducts prevents systemic absorption, but does not protect the eye from injury. This action is appropriate, but it does not address the specific safety issue in the question.*
2. ***CORRECT. The tip of the container can injure the client's eye and should not come in contact with the eye.***
3. *INCORRECT. Having the client look up decreases the likelihood of a blink reflex but does not protect the eye from injury. This action is appropriate, but it does not address the specific safety issue in the question.*
4. *INCORRECT. Depositing the drop into the conjunctival sac helps to distribute the medication throughout the eye, but it does not protect the eye from injury. This action is appropriate, but it does not address the specific safety issue in the question.*

STRATEGY: COMMUNICATION TOOLS AND BLOCKS

36. The nurse has been assigned to care for a recently diagnosed diabetic client who is resistant to learning self-injection of insulin. The client insists that the nurse administer all the injections. What is the appropriate nursing response in dealing with the client's resistance?

1. "You won't be able to go home unless you learn to give yourself the insulin injection."
2. "I will have to tell your doctor that you refuse to give yourself the insulin injections. I'm sure she will be angry with you."
3. "Don't worry about it. Your daughter can come over to your house every morning to give you the insulin injections."
4. "It is important that you learn to give yourself the insulin injections. What can I do to help you overcome your fear of giving the injections?"

1. *INCORRECT. This is an inappropriate response as well as an untrue statement. It is also a threat to the client, which is uncalled for and unprofessional.*
2. *INCORRECT. This is an inappropriate response that is intended to coerce the client into doing what the nurse wants. Notice that it uses the communication block of referring to an inappropriate person.*

> ***TEST-TAKING TIP:*** Options that include a communication block cannot be correct.

3. *INCORRECT. This response refers to an inappropriate person and uses false reassurance, because the nurse cannot assume that the daughter is able to give her mother daily insulin injections. The nurse needs to help the client become knowledgeable and independent in the care of her diabetes.*

> ***TEST-TAKING TIP:*** Options that include a communication block cannot be correct.

4. ***CORRECT. The nurse shows acceptance of the client's feelings and emphasizes the importance of self-care. The nurse is responsible for assisting the client in overcoming her fear of injections, by offering support and encouragement as well as client education materials. Referral to a home health nurse may be indicated for follow-up.***

STRATEGY: MASLOW

37. While caring for a client 24 hours following surgery, the priority nursing action is to:

1. Monitor his comfort level.
2. Encourage the client to verbalize his fears.
3. Observe safety precautions.
4. Instruct the client in self-care skills.

1. *INCORRECT. Although comfort is important, safety is the priority.*
2. *INNCORRECT. Although fears need to be identified so they can be explored, safety is the priority.*
3. ***CORRECT. Safe nursing care takes precedence over any other nursing interventions.***
4. *INCORRECT. Although learning proper skills to care for IOL is important, safety is the priority.*

STRATEGY: MASLOW

38. An 88-year-old client is admitted to the hospital for surgery. The nurse places the bed in the low position and puts the call light within easy reach. He is scheduled to have surgery in the morning. The most important nursing action during the admission of this client is to:

1. Explain the surgical procedure to the client and family.
2. Explain to the client how to use his call light if he needs the nurse.
3. Tell the client and his family about visiting regulations.
4. Teach the client how to deep breathe and cough.

1. *INCORRECT. It is the physician's responsibility to explain the surgical procedure to the client. This is not a nursing action.*
2. ***CORRECT. Explaining the use of the call light provides for the client's safety.***
3. *INCORRECT. Knowledge of visiting hours is important; however, the key word in the stem is "most." This is not the most important nursing action during admission. Look for an option that represents a higher priority.*
4. *INCORRECT. Deep breathing and coughing should be taught prior to surgery. However, teaching it at the time of admission is inappropriate and overwhelming for an 88-year-old client.*

STRATEGY: ISSUE

39. A client is scheduled for an abdominal hysterectomy. In order to prevent pneumonia from developing postoperatively, the most important nursing action is to:

1. Teach the client how to deep breathe and cough before surgery.
2. Inform the client that even though she will have pain after surgery, she will have to move from side to side in bed.
3. Tell the client that if she does not ambulate soon after surgery that there is a good chance that she may develop complications.
4. Tell the client that it is very important that she deep breathe and cough often after surgery to prevent complications.

1. ***CORRECT. Teaching the client how to cough and deep breathe prior to surgery is the most important nursing action to prevent pneumonia from developing after surgery. Having the client practice before she has incisional pain increases compliance, since she will know how to perform.***
2. *INCORRECT. It is a true statement, but it is not the most important nursing action and does not address preventing pneumonia postoperatively, which is the issue in the question.*
3. *INCORRECT. This is a true statement, but it is not the most important nursing action and does not specifically address prevention of pneumonia postoperatively, which is the issue in the question.*
4. *INCORRECT. This option may appear to be similar to Option 1, but it does not teach the client how to accomplish this task.*

STRATEGY: MASLOW

40. In preparing a client for surgery, the preoperative checklist has been completed, and the nurse has just administered the preoperative injection. What would the nurse do next?

1. Take the client to the bathroom to void.
2. Dim the overhead and bedside lights.
3. Review deep breathing and coughing exercises.
4. Put the side rails up on both sides of the bed.

1. *INCORRECT. The introductory statement tells you that the preoperative checklist has been completed, and the nurse has just administered the preoperative injection. The client should have voided before being given the injection, and there is no information that the client needs to void at this time. If he gets up now, he is at risk for falling. If a client expresses the need to urinate after the preoperative medication has been given, then the urinal or bedpan would be used.*
2. *INCORRECT. This is an appropriate action, but it is not the priority at this time. The client is at risk to fall.*

> ***TEST-TAKING TIP:*** When prioritizing nursing actions, look for an option that provides for the client's safety.

3. *INCORRECT. This action is an important part of preoperative teaching. However, this review is inappropriate at this time, because of the preoperative injection. The client is at risk to fall.*

> ***TEST-TAKING TIP:*** When prioritizing nursing actions, look for an option that provides for the client's safety.

4. ***CORRECT. The client is at risk of falling because of the injection. This action ensures the client's safety.***

> ***TEST-TAKING TIP:*** When prioritizing nursing actions, remember Maslow's Hierarchy of Needs. If no physiological need is identified, look for an action that provides for the client's safety.

STRATEGY: KEY WORDS

41. In assessing postoperative clients for manifestations of early hypovolemic shock, the nurse notes that an initial observation would most likely be:

1. Thirst.
2. Warm, flushed skin.
3. Irritability.
4. Bradycardia.

1. *INCORRECT. The key words in the stem are "early" and "initial." Thirst is not an early sign of hypovolemic shock. True thirst is caused by fluid volume deficits, but it comes after other diagnostic signs and symptoms.*
2. *INCORRECT. Warm, flushed skin is seen in early septic shock, which is usually caused by gram-negative bacteria. It is not an early sign of hypovolemic shock.*
3. ***CORRECT. Early in hypovolemic shock, hyperactivity of the sympathetic nervous system with increased secretion of epinephrine usually causes the client to feel anxious, nervous, and irritable.***
4. *INCORRECT. Bradycardia is not seen in shock conditions. The pulse is rapid and becomes weaker, thready and irregular as shock progresses.*

STRATEGY: CLIENT

42. A 15-year-old client has had an appendectomy. As the nurse prepares to give discharge instructions, the best approach is to:

1. Instruct both parents.
2. Explain to the client and one parent.
3. Explain to only one parent.
4. Instruct any family member.

1. *INCORRECT. Not the best choice. Look at the age of the client.*
2. ***CORRECT. When the client is an adolescent, the nurse needs to include him in the teaching, or compliance will probably not be achieved.***
3. *INCORRECT. This is not optimal. Look at the age of the client!*
4. *INCORRECT. You are missing an important element in the question.*

> ***TEST-TAKING TIP:*** Identify the client!

STRATEGY: NURSING PROCESS

43. While taking vital signs, the nurse notices an irregularity in the heart rate. Which nursing action is best?

1. Request the assistance of another staff member and take an apical/radial pulse.
2. Count the apical pulse rate for one full minute and describe the irregularity in the chart.
3. Call the doctor and request an order for a Holter monitor recording for the next day.
4. Take the pulse at each peripheral site and count the rate for 30 seconds.

1. *INCORRECT. An apical/radial pulse is used to identify a deficit between the apical and radial rates. It is not used to assess irregularity in the pulse, which is the issue in this question. This option doesn't describe the most appropriate nursing action when assessing a cardiac irregularity.*
2. ***CORRECT. When the pulse is regular, it may be counted for 15 seconds and multiplied by four, or counted for 30 seconds and multiplied by two. However, if the pulse is irregular, it must be counted for a full minute to obtain an accurate rate. The irregularity should be described in the chart.***

> ***TEST-TAKING TIP:*** Note that the word "irregularity" appears in the stem of the question and in this option. Although this test-taking strategy is not foolproof, in this question these similar words are a good clue!

3. *INCORRECT. An irregular pulse rate must be accurately counted and described and should be followed up immediately, generally by continuously monitoring the cardiac rhythm by telemetry. A Holter monitor recording the next day may be too late!*
4. *INCORRECT. Assessment of all peripheral pulses is appropriate for a client with a cardiovascular problem. That assessment, however, is related to the adequacy of circulation to each extremity rather than to regularity of the heart rate. This option does not address the issue in this question. The stem asks you to select the best nursing action when assessing a cardiac irregularity.*

STRATEGY: NURSING PROCESS

44. A confused elderly client is found wandering around the ward wearing a bathrobe and cotton socks. He also is bumping into walls as he walks. What is the priority nursing action?

1. Take the client's shoes to him and assist him in putting them on.
2. Accompany the client to his room and obtain a baseline assessment.
3. Ask the client to return to his room and rest until he feels better.
4. Tell the client to be careful of any wet spots on the floor.

1. *INCORRECT. In this option, the nurse fails to ensure the client's immediate safety. He is at risk of falling because of ambulating in stocking feet and bumping into walls. This option does not address the issue of the client's bumping into walls at all.*
2. ***CORRECT. The nurse ensures the client's safety by accompanying him to his room. Assessment is also essential because the client's bumping into walls suggests that oxygenation problems may be interfering with the client's balance and level of consciousness.***
3. *INCORRECT. In this option, the nurse fails to ensure the client's immediate safety. Also, the nurse does not know that the client feels ill or will feel better later. The nurse needs more information to determine the cause of the client's behavior.*
4. *INCORRECT. The question does not tell you anything about wet spots on the floor, and this option does not address the issue of the client's bumping into walls. The nurse must act to provide for the client's immediate safety, and the nurse needs more information to determine the cause of the client's behavior.*

STRATEGY: NURSING PROCESS

45. The day after abdominal surgery, a 10-year-old girl is lying quietly in bed when the nurse makes rounds. The last rounds were made four hours ago, and she was last medicated six hours ago. At this time, the nurse should first:

1. Encourage her to turn, cough, and deep breathe.
2. Assess the need for pain medication.
3. Ambulate her to the door.
4. Ask her if she is hungry, and provide fluids.

1. *INCORRECT. Although this is part of thorough postoperative care, you have missed an important piece of assessment data in the question.*
2. ***CORRECT. A child lying quietly, medicated six hours ago, who is one day postoperative, is very probably in pain. Children at this age are apt to lie motionless to prevent pain. They may not request pain medication for fear of needles. Before any other nursing care is provided, the nurse should complete an assessment of pain and medicate the child. Ambulating and deep breathing will be better tolerated with pain relief.***
3. *INCORRECT. Ambulating is not the priority, given the information in the question.*
4. *INCORRECT. Although fluids are important to the postoperative client, this is not the priority of care. You do not have enough information to know if oral intake is appropriate on the first day.*

STRATEGY: TYPE OF STEM

46. A client is ordered to have a hypothermic or cooling blanket applied because of a very high body temperature. When caring for this client, which of the following is the least appropriate nursing action?

1. Check the client's body temperature frequently.
2. Place a layer of cloth, such as a bath blanket, between the client and the cooling blanket if the cooling blanket does not have a protective covering.
3. Keep the cooling blanket in place until the client's body temperature is a couple of degrees below the desired level recommended by the physician.
4. Remove the cooling blanket when the client's body temperature is a couple of degrees above the desired level recommended by the physician.

1. INCORRECT—this action is appropriate. The client's temperature needs to be checked frequently in order to determine the body's response to the therapy and to prevent hypothermia.

> ***TEST-TAKING TIP:*** This question has a false response stem. Look for something the nurse should NOT do.

2. INCORRECT—this action is appropriate. The client's skin should never come in direct contact with any method used for cooling purposes since tissue damage can occur.

> ***TEST-TAKING TIP:*** This question has a false response stem. Look for something the nurse should NOT do.

3. CORRECT. This action would be inappropriate. The client's body temperature will continue to cool after the blanket is removed. The client will become too cold if the blanket is not taken off until the temperature is below the desired level.

4. INCORRECT—this action is appropriate. The cooling blanket should be removed when the client's temperature is a couple of degrees higher than the desired level indicated by the physician, since the body will continue to cool after the blanket is removed.

> ***TEST-TAKING TIP:*** This question has a false response stem. Look for something the nurse should NOT do.

STRATEGY: NURSING PROCESS

47. An elderly client is admitted to the hospital with chest pain. His daughter tells the nurse that he has certain routines for his personal hygiene and for taking his medicine. The best nursing response is to:

1. Assure the daughter that everything possible will be done to accommodate her father's needs.
2. Ask the daughter what routines and medicines her father uses at home.
3. Inform the daughter that the hospital has policies that have to be followed, and that you will provide the best care for her father.
4. Tell the daughter that she should inform the doctor about her father's routines so that orders can be written to meet the client's needs.

1. INCORRECT. The daughter is the client in this question. She will interpret this response as a cliché and false reassurance. The nurse has not clarified exactly what the father's needs are! This option does not address the daughter's concerns or encourage further communication.

2. CORRECT. This option promotes communication and encourages the daughter to tell the nurse more about her concerns. This response also focuses on the nurse's responsibility to assess the client's needs.

> ***TEST-TAKING TIP:*** This question prioritizes assessment and uses the communication tool of clarification.

3. INCORRECT. This response devalues the daughter's concerns about her father. This is a block to therapeutic communication and therefore not the best nursing response.

4. INCORRECT. This response "passes the buck" to the doctor and puts the client's feelings and concerns on hold. This response inhibits communication.

STRATEGY: MASLOW

48. The nurse is preparing the staffing assignment. An infant on the unit has AIDS and cytomegalovirus (CMV). Which staff person should the nurse assign as the primary care giver for this child?

1. An experienced practical nurse who is six months pregnant.
2. A male graduate nurse, recently oriented to pediatrics.
3. An experienced nurse's aide who is healthy.
4. A licensed practical nurse with eczema.

1. INCORRECT. You probably selected this nurse due to her experience. This would place the nurse's fetus at undue risk, since pregnant women should avoid exposure to CMV. What prioritizing guideline should be applied in this question?

2. CORRECT. A graduate nurse should be able to carry out the care, maintaining appropriate technique based on the principles of communicable disease transmission.

> ***TEST-TAKING TIP:*** Note the safety reasons why the other options are incorrect: Option 1 would place the nurse's fetus at undue risk. Option 3 is not correct because this client should have a licensed caregiver above the level of nurse's aide. And Option 4 is incorrect because the eczema puts this nurse at risk for infection. When you make a decision about an option, know the reason WHY it is correct or incorrect.

3. INCORRECT. Although the aide is "healthy" and experienced, this client should have a licensed caregiver. The implied level of care is above that of the aide. What prioritizing guideline should be applied in this question?

4. INCORRECT. This nurse is at risk for injury from this assignment. She has open areas on her skin, which is the body's first line of defense from communicable disease. What prioritizing guideline should be applied in this question?

STRATEGY: ISSUE

49. The nurse tells the client that she is going to be catheterized for a urine specimen. The client pulls the covers to her neck. She glances at the open door and says, "Someone might see me out there!" At this time, the best nursing action is to:

1. Explain the procedure to the client.
2. Obtain some assistance, since the client does not appear to be comfortable and may be resistant to the procedure.
3. Close the door and assure the client that you will cover her as much as possible during the procedure.
4. Gather all of the needed equipment before starting the procedure.

1. *INCORRECT. Explaining the procedure is an appropriate nursing action, but it doesn't address the client's concern. The issue in this question is the client's privacy.*
2. *INCORRECT. Although the client exhibits concern about privacy, the introductory statement does not indicate that she will be uncooperative. Do not "read into" the question! The client is communicating both verbally and nonverbally to the nurse to indicate her concern for privacy. The nurse should respond therapeutically and address the client's concern.*
3. ***CORRECT. The client has expressed her concern for privacy. The nurse uses both verbal and nonverbal communication to respond therapeutically, addressing the client's concern.***
4. *INCORRECT. This is an appropriate nursing action, but it does not address the client's concern. The issue in this question is the client's privacy.*

STRATEGY: TEACHING/LEARNING THEORY

50. Following a colostomy, a client and his wife have been taught to perform a colostomy irrigation. Which behavior by the client would best indicate readiness for discharge?

1. The client's wife verbalizes all steps in the irrigation procedure.
2. The client performs the irrigation following written instructions.
3. The client and his wife attend all classes given about colostomy care.
4. The client asks appropriate questions about irrigations.

1. *INCORRECT. The question specifically asks for a behavior by the client himself.*
2. ***CORRECT. The client has demonstrated ability to perform the skill using the instructions that he will have when he is at home.***
3. *INCORRECT. This may sound good, and it demonstrates involvement and effort—but it doesn't prove competence in the skill. Consider teaching/learning theory and how learning is best evaluated.*
4. *INCORRECT. This demonstrates involvement and effort, but not skill in performing the procedure. Consider teaching/learning theory and how learning is best evaluated.*

Chapter 11

DRILL QUESTIONS ON FUNDAMENTAL NURSING CONCEPTS

The following questions on fundamental nursing topics are designed to provide additional practice in using your test-taking techniques and strategies. You may also wish to use these drill questions as part of your review for exams covering these specific topics.

When practicing your test-taking skills, *be sure to time yourself and practice using the pacing strategy* explained in Chapter Eight. Determine the total number of questions you will answer in a practice session, and allow yourself one minute per question.

Don't forget to keep a score-card! Be sure to record your answers, calculate your score, and record the results. *You will be impressed with your progress* as you polish and improve your test-taking skills!

Finally, be sure to turn to Chapter Twelve and read the rationales for each section when you have finished it. Be sure you know *why* you missed any questions you got wrong—and be sure you answered the others correctly *using the correct rationales.*

MEDS Publishing congratulates you on your determination to improve your test-taking skills. We believe that good test-takers are better problem-solvers.

We also believe that nothing succeeds like success. Your new and improved test-taking skills will not only increase your test scores—they will also increase your confidence. We encourage you to continue practicing these skills as you complete your nursing education.

Section 1: The Role of the Nurse

The role of the nurse in providing safe and effective client care is critical and complex. The nurse assesses, analyzes, plans, implements and evaluates nursing care, using the nursing process to identify and solve clinical problems and prioritize care. In all phases of the nursing process, the nurse has the important responsibility of documenting client care. The nurse works with physicians, physical therapists, nutritionists and other members of the health care team, supervises the work of licensed practical nurses and nursing assistants, and utilizes community resources to meet client needs and provide continuity of care. The nurse also teaches clients to care for their own health needs.

The nurse/client relationship is critical to the practice of nursing. The nurse is responsible for establishing and maintaining a therapeutic relationship with the client and protecting client rights, including privacy and the right to receive—or refuse—care. The nurse also has varying other legal responsibilities.

1. The nursing assistant says to the nurse, "This client is incontinent of stool three or four times a day. I get angry when I think that he is doing it just to get attention. I think adult diapers should be used for him." How should the nurse initially respond to the nursing assistant?

1. "You probably are right. Soiling the bed is one way of getting attention from the nursing staff."
2. "Changing his bed and cleaning him must be tiresome for you. Next time it happens, I'll help you."
3. "It's upsetting to see an adult regress."
4. "Why don't you spend more time with him if you think that he is behaving this way to get more attention?"

2. A client is to have a perineal examination, which requires the dorsal recumbent position. Which of the following nursing actions provides the client with the most privacy?

1. Place a bath blanket on the client with one corner at the chest, two corners wrapped around the feet and legs, and the fourth corner draped between the client's legs.
2. Drape a draw sheet over the client's knees covering the abdomen and legs.
3. Place a bath blanket on the client, with the top at the chest and the bottom draped over the knees to cover the legs and feet.
4. Close the examination room door.

3. While administering a bed bath it is important for the nurse to maintain privacy. Which is the best method for maintaining the client's privacy?

1. Allow the client to wear a gown, and reach under the gown with the washcloth and towel to bathe the client.
2. Use towels to protect the bed linen.
3. Cover the client with a bath blanket and expose only the portion of the body that is being bathed.
4. Use the bed sheet to cover the client during the bath.

4. In protecting the privacy of a client, the nurse should avoid reporting which of the following to a government agency?

1. Child abuse.
2. Deaths.
3. Client's change of employment.
4. Elder abuse.

5. The nurse knows that it is not necessary to report which of the following events to a government agency?

1. Births.
2. Child abuse.
3. Marital quarrels.
4. Typhoid fever.

6. The nurse understands that which action is inconsistent with a client's right of privacy:

1. Refusing to have a gunshot wound reported, upon timely request.
2. Refusing to receive visitors.
3. Generally being able to wear one's own clothing.
4. Requesting the presence of a member of the same sex during a physical examination.

7. The home health nurse notes several suspicious bruises and old burns on a 10-month-old child while making an initial home visit. The priority nursing action to provide for the child's safety is to:

1. Call the child protection hotline and report possible abuse.
2. Discuss the family with the physician and social worker at the next team meeting.
3. Tell the mother that child protection will be notified if injuries are noted on the next visit.
4. Carefully record the visit for follow-up.

8. An elderly male client is to have Foley urinary catheter care daily. Which of the following is the best action to provide for the client's privacy during this treatment?

1. Pull the curtain around the client's bed.
2. Cover the penis with a towel while performing catheter care.
3. Close the door to the client's room.
4. Ask the client's roommate to leave until the treatment is finished.

9. The nurse knows which action is the most common cause of violation of a client's privacy?

1. Over-exposing a client during a treatment or examination.
2. Failing to pull the curtain while performing a treatment or examination.
3. Talking about the client to other staff members who are not involved with the care of the client, or within hearing of the public.
4. Helping a client with a tub bath.

10. An elderly client is confused. The charge nurse says that the client is constipated and is to have a soap suds enema. As the nurse is explaining the procedure, the client states that she doesn't think that she is supposed to have an enema. At this time, the nurse should:

1. Tell the client that her doctor must have ordered the procedure.
2. Assure the client that although the procedure sounds unpleasant, she will feel better afterwards.
3. Check the client's chart for the doctor's order to help clarify the situation.
4. Record on the chart that the client refused the enema.

11. An elderly client is admitted to a long-term care facility. Which of the following nursing measures would be most important in planning his care?

1. An explanation of the roles of the registered nurse, practical nurse and the nursing assistant.
2. Obtaining information about his routine for his own care at home.
3. An assessment of his mobility.
4. An introduction to his health care team members.

12. Of the following information, which should the admitting nurse record first in the client's record?

1. The client's vital signs.
2. The plan that was developed for the care of the client while in the hospital.
3. Nursing actions performed for the client.
4. Assessment of the client.

13. A female client with a history of severe multiple sclerosis has requested a living will and has asked the nurse to witness it. The nurse's appropriate response is:

1. "I would be honored to witness the will."
2. "I think your physician should witness the will."
3. "It would be a conflict of interest for me to witness the will, since I do not believe in living wills."
4. "I am unable to witness the will because of my professional relationship with you. Is there someone else you know who could do so?"

14. Which of the following is the most effective nursing action to maintain maximum privacy for the client during a medical procedure?

1. Closing the door of the client's room.
2. Pulling the curtains around the client's bed.
3. Asking family members to leave the room.
4. Using sterile drapes to cover the client.

15. The nurse is caring for an elderly client who will soon be discharged to a long-term care facility. What nursing action is most important to promote her continued recovery?

1. Reviewing the client's nursing care plan with the client's daughter.
2. Discussing the client's nursing care needs with her physician.
3. Telephoning the charge nurse at the long-term care facility to explain the client's nursing care needs.
4. Sending a written summary of the nursing care plan for the client to the long-term care facility.

16. In preparing a client to be discharged, the nurse teaches him to position himself for postural drainage. To achieve success in this teaching program, which information about the client does the nurse recognize to be most important?

1. The type of bed the client will be using at home for the procedure.
2. The amount of time required for the client to change positions.
3. The client's goal concerning his ability to be self-sufficient.
4. The client's ability to move about without assistance from others.

17. A client tells the nurse that he is feeling short of breath and requests that the nurse assist him in changing position. In addition to repositioning the client, which nursing action should be given the highest priority?

1. Put the client on 15 minute checks.
2. Call the charge nurse to report the shortness of breath.
3. Observe the rate, depth, and character of the client's respirations.
4. Give a back rub to help the client to relax.

Section 2: Safety, Body Mechanics and Mobility

Safety first! Safety is the essence of nursing care. The nurse ensures that nursing care is always provided in a safe manner.

The use of proper body mechanics is essential to the safety of the nurse and the client. The nurse uses proper body mechanics at all times in providing nursing care, especially in assisting the client with transfers and ambulation and in maintaining alignment and positioning.

To provide for the client's safety and well being, the nurse also ensures a safe environment for the client. The nurse assists the client in the event of an emergency, including choking, poisoning, electrical hazards and fire. The nurse assesses and addresses such client safety factors as sensory and intellectual deficits, limited mobility, and safe care of the confused client, and the client who requires the use of restraints.

1. A client is confused and disoriented when admitted to the hospital. The doctor has ordered bed rest. Before leaving the client's room, the most important nursing action to provide for the client's safety is to:

1. Put all of the client's belongings in a safe place.
2. Place the bed in the highest position with the side rails up.
3. Place the bed in the lowest position with the side rails up.
4. Explain where everything is in the room.

2. A client is admitted to the hospital and the physician orders stat blood work. The laboratory technician says to the nurse, "I can't do the stat blood work because the client doesn't have an identification bracelet on." The best nursing action is to:

1. Draw the blood for the laboratory technician, since the nurse can identify the client.
2. Assure the laboratory technician that you will verify that he has the correct client.
3. Obtain an identification bracelet for the client as quickly as possible.
4. Ask the client to identify himself to the laboratory technician.

3. A confused elderly client is on strict bedrest. Which nursing intervention will provide for this client's safety?

1. Place the client in a room away from the noise and confusion of the nurses' station.
2. Avoid the use of nightlights, since they tend to distort images and confuse clients.
3. Discuss with the client the need for restraints if she continues to get out of bed.
4. Provide opportunities for regular toileting, and include this information in the client's care plan.

4. An elderly, confused client is on bed rest. Which nursing intervention will be ineffective in providing for this client's safety?

1. Provide regular toileting.
2. Explain to the client that she should use the call light if she needs to get up.
3. Place the side rails in the up position and check on the client often.
4. Initiate the proper use of restraints.

5. A middle-aged client is hospitalized following myocardial infarction. He is to be transferred from a cart to a bed in a room on a unit. When transferring the client from a cart to his bed, the priority nursing action is to:

1. Have the client place his arms on his chest.
2. Lock the wheels on the cart and the bed.
3. Have at least four people to help with the transfer.
4. Use a draw sheet to move the client.

6. A client has left-sided weakness secondary to a stroke. In assisting him out of bed, which nursing action is safest?

1. Allow the client to do as much of the transfer as possible.
2. Lock the wheels of the bed and wheelchair.
3. Place the client's hands around the nurse's neck for support.
4. Place the front of the wheelchair at a right angle to the bed.

7. The doctor has ordered restraints for a very agitated client. When applying restraints to the client, which nursing action is least appropriate?

1. Using the least restrictive type of restraint that will effectively protect the client from injury.
2. Fastening the restraints to the bed frame.
3. Tying the restraint with a knot that cannot be undone easily, in order to prevent the client from untying it.
4. Explaining to the client and family the type of restraint and the reason for applying the restraint.

8. A postoperative client is ambulatory and wishes to go to the day room. While the nurse is walking down the hall with the client, the client says that she feels faint and starts to fall. The nurse should:

1. Grasp the client around the waist and hold her up so she doesn't fall and injure herself.
2. Hold the client up against the wall to keep her from falling.
3. Ease the client gently to the floor.
4. Ask another client to get some help while supporting the client to prevent her from falling.

9. The first, most important nursing action when a nurse discovers a fire in a client's room is to:

1. Pull the fire alarm and notify the hospital operator.
2. Close fire doors and client room doors.
3. Remove the client from the room.
4. Place moist towels or blankets at the threshold of the door of the room with the fire.

10. The nurse finds an elderly client standing in a puddle of water in the hallway of the unit. The nurse does not know this client. What is the nurse's initial action?

1. Ask the client for her name and room number.
2. Wipe up the water until the floor is completely dry.
3. Call the supervisor for assistance in identifying the client.
4. Have the client wait in the lounge until security arrives.

11. A client is paralyzed from the waist down. He is to be up in a chair three times a day. What is the best nursing approach when transferring the client from a bed into a wheelchair?

1. Place the wheelchair close to the foot of the bed.
2. Utilize the principles of body mechanics while providing a safe transfer for the client.
3. Slide the client to the edge of the bed, keeping the nurse's back straight and using a rocking motion to pull the client.
4. Place the nurse's arms under the client's axillae from the back of the client.

12. When transporting a client, the nurse should:

1. Always use a stretcher.
2. Push the stretcher quickly so the client does not become chilled during the transport.
3. Never cover a client with a blanket, since it can get caught in the wheels.
4. Use the safety rails or straps that are available on the equipment.

13. The nurse finds an elderly client with her IV pulled out, standing next to her bed, with the side rails in the up position. The client is confused, does not have an identification bracelet on, and cannot remember her name. What action should the nurse take first?

1. Help the client into bed, and remind her to call the nurse when she wants to get out of bed.
2. Help the client into bed, and then restart the IV.
3. Place a restraining vest on the client.
4. Put an identification bracelet on the client and help her back to bed.

14. A client tells the nurse that his name is not spelled right on his identification bracelet. The best nursing action is to:

1. Tell the client that as long as his medical record numbers are correct, the mistake is not a problem.
2. Ask the client for the correct spelling and change his medical records.
3. Notify the admitting office of the spelling error and obtain a correct identification bracelet for the client.
4. Notify the physician.

15. A client is admitted to the hospital for evaluation of inadequate circulation to her lower extremities. The doctor orders a tub bath at the client's request. In assisting the client with her bath, which nursing action would place the client at risk?

1. Place a rubber mat on the bottom of the tub.
2. Fill the tub approximately half full.
3. When the client steps into the tub, ask her if the water is the right temperature for her.
4. Obtain all of the supplies necessary for the bath and place them within easy reach of the client.

16. The client is very confused and combative. The physician orders the client to be placed in a jacket restraint and wrist restraints. In order to prevent injury to the client with restraints, the best nursing action is to:

1. Explain the procedure and reason for the restraints to the client and the family.
2. Remove the restraints and observe the extremities for circulation at least every four hours.
3. Tell the client that if he is more cooperative the restraints will not be necessary.
4. Document the use of restraints in the chart.

17. Restraints may be used to immobilize a client, or the client's extremity. The nurse understands that an appropriate use of restraints is to:

1. Prevent a client from pulling out an IV or other type of therapy.
2. Reduce the risk to all elderly clients from falling out of bed or off a chair.
3. Prevent removal of life support equipment.
4. Prevent injury to health care personnel by combative clients.

18. A client has just been admitted to the hospital. In showing the client how to use the call system, the nurse understands which of the following statements should be avoided?

1. The call system allows the client to signal for help.
2. The call system should be limited to use in emergencies.
3. The client should be able to reach the call button easily.
4. The client should be taught how to use the call system.

19. A client has just returned to her room after abdominal surgery. She has a nasogastric tube in place and a drain attached to a Hemovac. The Foley catheter is draining clear yellow urine. The nurse understands the reason for maintaining the side rails in the raised position is to:

1. Prevent the urine collection bag and tubing from getting tangled up in the side rails when the client is turned in bed.
2. Prevent the client from falling out of bed after receiving an anesthetic.
3. Provide a place to attach the nasogastric tubing to prevent it from being dislodged.
4. Attach the call light so it is within easy reach.

20. A client is ambulating down the tile hallway in her stocking-covered feet. How should the nurse ensure the client's safety?

1. Remind the client to avoid any wet spots on the floor.
2. Tell the client that she should always wear slippers or shoes when ambulating.
3. Get the client's slippers and have her put them on.
4. No action is necessary, since the client has her feet covered.

21. A client is very irritable at breakfast. When asked if there is a problem, the client states that he was unable to sleep because of noise made by the staff on the night shift. The best initial response by the nurse is:

1. "It must be very distressing to be unable to sleep at night. Would you like to take a nap this morning?"
2. "I'll report that to the supervisor."
3. "Maybe we can move you to a room further from the nurses' station when one of those rooms becomes available."
4. "Why don't you close your door at night? Sometimes the nurses make noise and don't realize it."

22. The physician has determined that a client is extremely dehydrated and in need of intravenous fluids. The client is confused, and she has pulled out one intravenous catheter and caused another intravenous site to become infiltrated. The nurse restarts the IV in the client's left arm. An order for restraints is given. The best nursing action is to:

1. Apply a vest restraint and extremity restraints to ensure that the intravenous site will be protected.
2. Apply a restraint to the left arm.
3. Apply a restraint to the right arm.
4. Apply restraints to the right and left arms.

23. The physician has ordered extremity restraints for safety reasons for a confused elderly client. After placing the client in extremity restraints, the priority nursing action is to:

1. Release each extremity every two hours for range of motion exercises.
2. Discuss the rationale for the restraints with the family members.
3. Reduce the client's distress by dimming the lights and closing the door.
4. Tie the restraints to the side rails using a half bow knot.

24. An elderly client requires extremity restraints for safety reasons. After applying restraints to the client's extremities, the nurse should consider which of the following as a priority action concerned with the client's safety?

1. Documenting the type of restraints applied to the client.
2. Explaining to family members the reason for the restraints.
3. Checking the restraints for circulatory adequacy once during each shift.
4. Observing the restrained extremities for color and pulses at least every hour.

25. While caring for a client receiving fluids using an IV pump that is plugged into an electrical outlet, which of the following is the least appropriate nursing action?

1. Palpate the client's IV site while resetting the pump for the next bag of IV solution.
2. Assess the IV site.
3. Change the tubing according to hospital protocol.
4. Observe the pump for correct operation.

26. The nurse notices a fire in the linen room. Which type of extinguisher should the nurse use?

1. Dry powder.
2. Water.
3. Dry chemical.
4. Carbon dioxide.

27. A confused elderly client has wrist restraints for safety reasons. Which nursing action is the safest?

1. Checking the pulse, color, and temperature of extremities every shift and reporting these findings.
2. Making sure the call light is within the client's reach.
3. Notifying the client's family of the restraints and explaining the rationale for their use.
4. Removing the restraints at night while the client is sleeping.

28. A client complains that he is unable to rest because of the noise from his roommate's TV. The best action by the nurse is to:

1. Have the client moved to a private room.
2. Provide ear phones for the client who is watching television.
3. Explain that the roommate is hard of hearing, so the television is louder than usual.
4. Ask the roommate to shut off the television so the client can rest.

29. While bathing a preschooler in a tub, which would be the least appropriate nursing action?

1. Check the temperature of the water with a thermometer.
2. Never leave the child unattended.
3. Make sure the temperature in the room is warm.
4. Allow the child to determine if the water temperature is comfortable by placing the child's feet in the water.

30. The nurse is caring for an elderly client in a long-term care facility. When applying a hot water bottle to the client, it would place the client at risk if the nurse:

1. Wrapped the hot water bottle in a cloth before placing it next to the client's skin.
2. Filled the hot water bottle with as much hot water as it will hold.
3. Eliminated as much air as possible from the hot water bottle.
4. Checked the temperature of the water with a thermometer.

31. The nurse is about to instruct parents of young children about poison control in the home. The nurse should:

1. Instruct the parents to induce vomiting with syrup of ipecac.
2. Instruct the parents to immediately bring the child to the emergency room.
3. Provide labels for the parent's telephone with the Poison Control Center's telephone number, and give instructions to call that number after an accidental ingestion.
4. Notify social services to investigate the home situation for safety.

32. An adolescent client is to have a water system heating device ("K-Pad"), applied to a pulled muscle. The client tells the nurse that the device does not feel very warm. The safest nursing action is to:

1. Tell the client these heating devices never feel hot.
2. Check the temperature setting on the heating unit and feel the pad for warmth.
3. Call the appropriate repair department and have them fix the unit.
4. Turn the temperature up on the unit if it doesn't feel warm enough to the client.

33. While working the night shift, the nurse notices a mouse running down the hallway of the clinical unit. The best nursing action is to:

1. Place rat poison in the vicinity where the mouse was seen.
2. Set some mouse traps to catch the mouse, and then dispose of it in a plastic bag labeled as contaminated.
3. Notify the supervisor of the problem.
4. Call the environmental health department of the hospital, and report the incident.

34. A vest restraint is placed on a confused elderly client who is at high risk for falling. Which nursing action is the least appropriate?

1. Provide an opportunity for the client to use the bedpan, toilet, or other toilet facilities at regular intervals.
2. Assess the respiratory status of the client frequently.
3. Utilizing help from other nurses, approach the client and apply the vest as quickly as possible, in order to avoid any resistance from the client.
4. Change the client's position at least every two hours.

35. The nurse discovers a fire in the hospital. Which of the following nursing actions would place the client at risk?

1. Sound the nearest fire alarm.
2. Move clients who are in the immediate area of the fire.
3. Turn off any oxygen or electrical equipment.
4. Open the doors and windows to let the smoke out.

36. A client is in the bathroom after taking a shower. The nurse hears a loud thud. The nurse opens the bathroom door to find the client on the floor and a hair dryer in the sink with the basin full of water. The first nursing action is to:

1. Assess the client to determine if she is breathing.
2. Assess the client for a heart rate.
3. Unplug the hair dryer, while taking care not to touch the client or any water or wet surface.
4. Perform a neurological assessment.

37. A young client is paralyzed from the waist down. He has a TV, radio, video tape player, stereo, and video game unit, which are all used throughout the day. The nurse notices that there are not enough

electrical outlets, and that extension cords with multiple outlets are in use to accommodate this equipment. The best nursing action is to:

1. Have the client's family take some of the equipment home.
2. Unplug as much of the client's equipment as necessary, after informing the client that an overloaded circuit can cause an electrical fire and that extension cords are not allowed.
3. Tell the client that only single-outlet cords can be used, and that you will check often to see if he wants to use anything not currently connected.
4. Call the maintenance department and have more wall outlets installed in the client's room.

38. While caring for a client, the nurse notices that the call light cord is frayed. The nurse should:

1. Tell the client not to use the call light until it is fixed.
2. Remove the call light, and report the problem to the supervising nurse immediately.
3. Tape up the cord until the maintenance people can fix it, so the client will have a call light.
4. Tell the client to call out if he needs help, and to use the call light only in an emergency.

39. An elderly client is scheduled for surgery tomorrow. The nurse enters the client's room and finds that flames are coming out of the waste basket. The nurse would demonstrate an understanding of safety priorities by first:

1. Placing the folded blanket from the client's bed over the entire opening of the waste basket.
2. Finding nearest fire extinguisher to put the fire out.
3. Telling the client he is not supposed to be smoking.
4. Pulling the nearest fire alarm.

40. A client spills hot coffee on himself during breakfast. The first action by the nurse is to:

1. Remove the clothing from the burn area and apply cold water to the area.
2. Call the physician.
3. Make out an incident report.
4. Cover the area with sterile towels.

41. An elderly client has an IV with an infusion pump. While examining the infusion pump, the nurse experiences a slight tingling sensation in the hand as the plug is checked. What is the safest nursing action?

1. Shut the pump off immediately.
2. Inform the repair department to immediately shut off the pump.
3. Recheck the equipment in one hour.
4. Use a different electrical outlet site.

42. While caring for an infant, the nurse notices that one of the infant's stuffed animals in the crib has eyes that can easily be pulled off. The safe nursing action is to:

1. Take the toy out of the crib immediately.
2. Remove the eyes from the stuffed animal and return it to the crib.
3. When the mother comes to visit, show her the eyes and explain that the infant could pull them off and choke on them.
4. Send the toy home with the mother.

43. A client is to have an electrical heating device applied to his lower back area. The plug on the heating device has three prongs, and the electrical wall outlet available only has two-pronged openings. The client's radio is plugged into a three-pronged outlet. The best action by the nurse at this time is to:

1. Unplug the client's radio, which is plugged into a three-pronged outlet, and use that outlet for the heating device.
2. Obtain an extension cord with a three-pronged outlet on it.
3. Use a 2-pronged adapter to plug into the wall outlet; then plug the heating device into the adapter.
4. Call central supply to see if you can get a heating device with a two-pronged plug on it.

44. A client is confused and confined to bed. He has attempted to crawl over the side rails. The safe nursing action is to:

1. Apply restraints to the client immediately.
2. Stay with the client and notify the supervising nurse.
3. Remind the client to stay in bed.
4. Tell the client to stay in bed, or else the nursing staff will have to restrain him.

45. In a hospital pediatric unit, which action by the nurse is best for preventing accidental poisoning to a toddler?

1. Place cleaning supplies on a counter out of reach of the toddler.
2. Do not allow any plant life on the pediatric unit.
3. Place cleaning supplies in a locked cabinet.
4. Place all toddlers in specific rooms where they are supervised frequently.

46. The nurse, walking by a client's room, notices that the top sheet on the client's bed is on fire and the client is in the bed. What is the first action by the nurse?

1. Get a fire extinguisher and spray the entire bed, including the client, who is at risk for burns.
2. Grab a towel and beat the flames out by hitting the burning sheet.
3. Take the blanket at the foot of the bed, place the blanket over the burning sheets to smother the flames, and smooth the blanket to remove any pockets of oxygen.
4. Use the nearest fire hose to extinguish the flames.

47. The nurse notices a crack in an electrical outlet. The IV pump that is plugged into the outlet appears to be working without any problems. Which is the safest nursing action?

1. Use another outlet; then call the maintenance department to have the outlet changed.
2. Since the pump is working, no action is necessary.
3. Test the outlet by moving the plug a bit in the outlet, and observing if this affects the pump.
4. Since the outlet works, continue to use it until maintenance can replace it.

48. The nurse is caring for a client who is scheduled for surgery. When the transporter arrives to take the client to the operating room, the client is sitting in a chair. To achieve the client's safe transfer onto the stretcher, the best nursing action is to:

1. Assist the client to get back into bed, and then move her across to the stretcher with the help of a drawsheet.
2. Have the client use the chair to step up onto the stretcher.
3. Assist the client to climb up onto the stretcher.
4. Together with the transporter, lift the client from the chair onto the stretcher, keeping a wide stance and a straight back.

49. While mixing a solution o[illegible] used as a disinfectant spray, th[illegible] there is more solution than will fit [illegible] Which of the following actions by th[illegible] place the client at risk?

1. Pour the excess solution into an empty co[illegible] label the container as to contents, and place it in [illegible] cleaning supply closet.
2. Discard the excess solution.
3. Use the excess solution for the immediate cleaning job, then discard what is left.
4. Pour the excess into another cleaning solution container that has only a small amount of an ammonia solution left in the bottom.

50. During an electrical storm, the lights go out for a few seconds. Some of the lights come back on, but the ventilator is not working. What is the first nursing action?

1. Remove the client from the ventilator and ventilate with a bag and mask.
2. Quickly check the electrical outlets to determine if the ventilator is plugged into an emergency power outlet.
3. Call a code.
4. Ventilate the client with oxygen using a positive pressure bag attached to the endotracheal tube, until full power is restored.

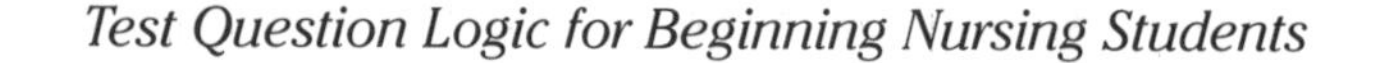

on 3: Infection Control

r preventing the spread of infection in all aspects of nursing care. tion and implements measures to ensure medical asepsis, proper iques, and prevention of postoperative infection. Handwashing is ve measure in client care. The nurse also knows the routes by which sis, and other infectious diseases are spread, and implements mea- ssion. The nurse is also responsible for client teaching to prevent the

1. An ... tted to the hospital with a lung ... f the following isolation categories should be implemented in order to prevent transmission of the HIV virus?

1. Strict isolation.
2. Respiratory isolation.
3. Universal precautions.
4. Enteric precautions.

2. While changing the linen on a client's bed, how should the nurse handle the linen?

1. Hold it close to the body to avoid dropping it.
2. Place soiled linen on the chair until done making the bed.
3. Hold the linen away from the body and uniform.
4. Shake clean linen to unfold it and provide ease in making the bed.

3. A client is recovering from surgery. While changing the linens on the client's bed, the nurse notes that drainage from an infected wound has soiled the bed sheet. What is the best method for changing this linen?

1. Carefully place the soiled sheet in the cloth linen bag and label it as contaminated.
2. Spray the soiled area with a bleach solution prior to placing it in the linen bag.
3. Carefully place the soiled sheet in a moisture-resistant plastic linen bag designated for soiled articles.
4. Discard the sheet into a plastic trash bag.

4. The best nursing action to prevent the spread of infection among hospitalized clients is:

1. Using sterile technique when performing any procedure.
2. Hand washing before coming in contact with each client.
3. Wearing gloves to perform any procedure.
4. Wearing a mask and gown while performing any procedure.

5. A client is admitted to the hospital with a diagnosis of active pulmonary tuberculosis. An immediate nursing goal is to control the spread of infection. To control the spread of active tuberculosis, the nurse would:

1. Wear a gown and mask when caring for the client.
2. Recommend that the client wear a mask when she has visitors.
3. Teach the client how to cover her nose and mouth when she coughs or sneezes.
4. Use blood and needle precautions.

6. When changing dressings for an HIV positive client, the nurse should remember to wash her hands and to:

1. Wear a mask.
2. Wear gloves.
3. Maintain strict isolation.
4. Wear a gown and gloves.

7. While starting an intravenous infusion, the nurse's gloved hands get spotted with blood. The client has not been diagnosed with any organisms that are transmitted by way of the blood stream. The first action the nurse should take upon completion of the task is to:

1. Remove the gloves carefully and follow with handwashing.
2. Wash the gloved hands, and then throw the gloves away.
3. Prepare an incident report so that this occurrence will be documented, in case a health care problem develops at a later date.
4. Ask the client to have a blood test to determine if a bloodborne pathogen is present in the client's blood.

8. While the nurse is caring for a client, the intravenous tubing becomes disconnected from the intravenous catheter, resulting in the client's blood spilling onto the side of the bed and floor. The nurse knows that which solution is recommended for disinfection of blood spills?

1. Betadine solution.
2. Alcohol.
3. Soap and water.
4. Sodium hypochlorite or chlorine bleach solution.

9. The nurse would select which infection control precautions as appropriate in caring for an AIDS client?

1. Strict isolation.
2. Respiratory isolation.
3. Contact isolation.
4. Universal blood and body fluid precautions.

10. The nurse caring for an AIDS client accidentally pierces her hand with a needle used to give the client his pain medication. The priority nursing action is to:

1. Report the incident to the charge nurse.
2. Cover the wound with a sterile gauze dressing and report the incident to employee health.
3. Complete an incident report.
4. "Bleed" the site and rinse under water, apply an antibiotic ointment, and cover the area with a dry dressing.

11. Which exposure would place the nurse at greatest risk for contracting AIDS?

1. Vaginal secretions and semen.
2. Blood.
3. Cerebrospinal fluid.
4. Sputum.

12. A postoperative client has an infected surgical incision. The area is red and swollen with a small amount of thick, yellow drainage. The correct term for the nurse to use in describing this drainage is:

1. Purulent.
2. Sanguineous.
3. Serous.
4. Serosanguineous.

13. In planning to teach a client who has the human immunodeficiency virus (HIV), the nurse should remember to alert the client that the virus can be transmitted:

1. As soon as the client develops symptoms.
2. To anyone having contact with the client's blood.
3. Via the respiratory route, like tuberculosis.
4. Only during the active phase of the virus, but not while it is inactive.

14. Universal precautions requires that a nurse wear which protective equipment when performing a nasogastric tube irrigation on a client with acquired immunodeficiency syndrome (AIDS)?

1. Sterile gloves.
2. Goggles and nonsterile gloves.
3. Nonsterile gown, sterile gloves.
4. Nonsterile gloves.

Section 4: Client Hygiene and Comfort Needs

To ensure the highest possible level of client well being, the nurse provides care to promote client hygiene and comfort needs. The nurse's responsibilities in this area range from bed making to bathing the client and care of the skin, hair, mouth, perineum, and feet and nails. The nurse assesses for pain, implements pain relief measures, provides backrubs, and promotes rest and sleep.

1. The nurse is caring for a client who is paralyzed on his right side following a stroke. In preparing to give a bed bath to this client, which of the following nursing actions is the most appropriate?

1. Adjust the bed to the lowest position, in case the client falls.
2. Raise the bed to the high horizontal position.
3. Put the bed in low semi-Fowler's position.
4. Unplug the bed.

2. A client is in the intensive care unit and is in a coma as a result of a head injury. The most important nursing action in performing mouth care on this client is to:

1. Turn the client to her side before starting mouth care.
2. Use a soft toothbrush.
3. Use a mouth bite to keep her mouth open.
4. Wear gloves.

3. When giving a partial bath, which nursing action is the least appropriate?

1. Arrange equipment and linen for easy access.
2. Open the window to let fresh air in.
3. Pull the curtain for privacy.
4. Rinse off all of the soap.

4. A client with osteoarthritis complains of discomfort when performing exercises prescribed by the physical therapist. Which response by the nurse is most appropriate?

1. "The exercises will prevent pain."
2. "The exercises will prevent worsening of the disease."
3. "The exercises will help to maintain as near normal joint function as possible, as well as range of motion."
4. "The exercises will make you feel better."

5. An elderly client is to receive a bath. In preparing the bath, which action would place the client at risk?

1. Check the temperature of the tub room.
2. Gather and take all of the necessary equipment to the tub room prior to the bath.
3. Test the temperature of the bath water by having the client place his hand in the water.
4. Place a mat or towel in the bottom of the tub.

6. The nurse caring for a client who is unconscious would place the unconscious client in which position?

1. Semi-Fowler's.
2. Trendelenburg.
3. Prone.

Section 5: Physical Assessment of the Client and Basic Nursing Skills

Before planning or implementing nursing care, the nurse must always *assess first.* The nurse assesses vital signs and is responsible for other measures of client health and well being, including level of consciousness, weight and edema. The nurse collects specimens, including blood, urine, stool and sputum, and is skilled in such basic procedures as the insertion and removal of nasogastric tubes and the use of cooling blankets.

1. A female client returns to the postoperative unit following abdominal surgery. She has a nasogastric tube to low continuous suction and complains of a sore throat. She asks the nurse when the nasogastric tube will be taken out. Which response by the nurse is most appropriate at this time?

1. "The doctor will discontinue the tube when your bowel sounds return."
2. "The tube probably will be removed tomorrow, but you'll remain NPO for three to five more days."
3. "The tube will be removed when peristalsis returns through the entire GI tract, usually in three to five days."
4. "You'll have to ask that question of your doctor. He's the one who has to give the order to discontinue the tube."

2. The physician orders a stool specimen to be collected for ova and parasites. What is the proper procedure for collection of this specimen by the nurse?

1. Send the entire stool immediately to the lab.
2. Use a sterile container.
3. Take feces from several areas of the bowel movement.
4. Refrigerate the specimen until it can be delivered to the lab.

3. A client is admitted to the hospital, and a urine specimen is ordered. When obtaining a urine specimen from the client, which action should be avoided?

1. Place the urine cup in the client's bathroom.
2. Take the full specimen cup to the lab pick up area and then place it in a clean plastic bag.
3. Attach the client's name to the specimen cup.
4. Explain to the client the procedure for obtaining a urine specimen.

4. A child weighing 1800 gm is admitted. The nurse knows that the infant's weight in pounds is:

1. 3.9 lbs.
2. 8.1 lbs.
3. 18 lbs.
4. 36 lbs.

5. Which approach by the nurse is best when taking the blood pressure of a client with hypertension?

1. Measure the blood pressure under the same conditions each time.
2. Take the blood pressure with the client sitting on the side of the bed.
3. Place the blood pressure cuff on the right arm above the elbow.
4. Measure the blood pressure with the client in supine position.

6. The nurse has just collected a liquid stool specimen for ova and parasites. The test results may not be accurate if the nurse:

1. Places the specimen into a clean container.
2. Puts the collected specimen in the refrigerator.
3. Instructs the client to defecate into a bedpan.
4. Sends only the bloody and mucoid portions of the stool.

7. The physician has ordered a sputum specimen to be collected for culture and sensitivity. The nurse is aware that the preferable time to collect this specimen is:

1. In the morning.
2. In the evening, after forcing fluids all day.
3. After antibiotics have been started.
4. After the client has taken an expectorant.

8. To assess for correct placement of a nasogastric tube, the nurse should:

1. Instill 30 ml of saline to assess client tolerance.
2. Instill 10 ml of air into the tube and listen for gurgling sounds with a stethoscope over the gastric area.
3. Aspirate stomach contents with a syringe.
4. Place the end of the tube in water to assess for bubbling.

9. When obtaining a urine specimen from an indwelling catheter for culture and sensitivity, the nurse should:

1. Empty the drainage bag from the urometer port.
2. Wear sterile gloves.
3 Cleanse the entry site on the catheter prior to inserting the needle.
4. Drain the bag and wait for a fresh urine sample to send from the drainage bag.

10. When collecting a urine specimen for a routine urinalysis, which of the following nursing actions is the most important?

1. Label the container with the client's room number.
2. Check the identification of the client.
3. Avoid using gloves when handling a urine specimen.
4. Instruct the client to put the specimen on the counter at the nurses' station for pick up.

11. In obtaining a blood pressure measurement, the most appropriate nursing action is to:

1. Obtain the proper equipment, place the client in a comfortable position, and record the appropriate information in the client's chart.
2. Measure the client's arm, if you are uncertain of the size of cuff to use.
3. Have the client recline or sit comfortably in a chair with the forearm at the level of the heart.
4. Document the measurement, which extremity was used, and the position that the client was in during the measurement.

12. The physician requests a stool specimen for culture, for an alert and ambulatory client. The nurse would give which directions to the client for proper stool collection?

1. Restrict food and liquids the night before the collection.
2. Maintain a sterile procedure.
3. Require the collection of specimens on three consecutive days.
4. Retrieve from the toilet with sterile gloves and then place in the container.

13. Assisting the doctor in examining a two-year-old who has otitis media, the nurse should have the child:

1. Lie down on the examining table while his throat and ears are examined, and then allow him to sit up for the rest of the exam.
2. Lie down on the examining table, while the physician starts with examining the head and proceeds downward with the exam.
3. Sit in his mother's lap while the heart and lungs are auscultated, and then examine the rest of his body, doing the throat and ears last.
4. Allow him to sit in his mother's lap while his ears are examined with an otoscope, and then take his BP and vital signs.

14. A postoperative client has an electronic blood pressure machine automatically measuring her blood pressure every 15 minutes. The nurse notes that the blood pressure machine is reading the client's blood pressure at more frequent intervals, and that the readings are not similar. The nurse checks the machine settings and observes additional readings, but the problem continues. At this time, the best nursing action is to:

1. Record only those blood pressures that are needed for the 15-minute intervals.
2. Disconnect the machine and measure the blood pressure with a sphygmomanometer and stethoscope.
3. Turn on the machine every 15 minutes to obtain the client's blood pressure.
4. Measure the blood pressure manually and compare readings obtained by the machine with readings obtained manually.

15. Six hours into the collection of a 24-hour urine specimen, one voided specimen is accidentally discarded by the client. The nurse should:

1. Continue the collection, noting the loss on the lab slip.
2. Notify the nurse in charge.
3. Discard the previously collected urine and start the collection again.
4. Notify the lab so that the collection can be reduced to six hours.

16. The physician orders a urine test. The nurse understands that specific gravity of urine is used to determine the amount of:

1. Proteins in the urine.
2. Uric acid crystals in the urine.
3. Solutes in the urine.
4. Epithelial cells in the urine.

Section 6: Growth and Development

In the course of providing nursing care, the nurse encounters clients in all stages of growth and development. To properly assess and assist the client, the nurse must know not only the normal vital signs and lab values for different ages, but also the developmental tasks, behaviors, and problems common to each developmental stage, and the measures to be used to adapt care to their needs.

1. The nurse is preparing a seven-year-old female for hospitalization. The child had a previous hospital experience. To best prepare this child, the nurse would:

1. Suggest a role play and provide materials.
2. Remind the child of the experience of her past hospitalization.
3 Read her a story about another child having a similar operation.
4. Tell her she is only going in to have her throat checked.

2. A nephrectomy (removal of the kidney) is scheduled for the next day on a three-year-old client. How would the nurse best prepare this child for this procedure?

1. On the evening before the procedure, demonstrate by pointing on the child's body where the incision will be made.
2. Give the preoperative sedation as ordered with a small needle so that a Band-Aid will not be needed.
3. Ask the child's parents to leave the room while the preoperative medication is administered.
4. Explain the procedure to the child in simple sentences just before giving the preoperative sedation.

3. During a well-child visit, the mother of a five-year-old expresses concern that her son refuses to wear his helmet while riding his bicycle. What is the best nursing response?

1. "Tell him the bike doesn't leave the garage without the helmet."
2. "It isn't that important, since he won't be riding in the road."
3. "Gradually encourage the wearing of the helmet with small rewards."
4. "I'll explain to him the potential for injury without a helmet."

4. On the tenth day of hospitalization, an 11-month-old child is quiet and sad when his mother leaves. The nurse knows this behavior indicates:

1. An understanding of his mother's need to leave.
2. Despair at his mother's absence.
3. Protest that his source of emotional support is gone.
4. Developing autonomy.

5. A 30-month-old male is admitted with asthma. To decrease the stress of hospitalization for the toddler, the nurse should:

1. Explain procedures and routines.
2. Encourage contact with children of the same age.
3. Provide for privacy.
4. Encourage rooming-in.

6. A disruptive 10-year-old child is having difficulty interacting with other children on the unit. Which nursing action would be best initially?

1. Have a unit conference with other staff members and discuss strategies to solve the problem.
2. Talk to the child about the behavior that is causing the problem and identify possible solutions.
3. Tell the other children to stop teasing the client and to observe for changes in the client's behavior.
4. Tell the client's mother that she needs to talk to her son about his disruptive behavior.

7. In caring for a preschooler who is being admitted the evening before surgery, the nurse knows that which activity is least appropriate for reducing the stress of hospitalization?

1. Explaining the surgical procedure.
2. Playing "surgery" with cap and masks.
3. Showing her the call light and bathroom.
4. Having her mother undress her.

8. A four-year-old is visiting his brother who is critically ill and may be dying. In talking with this young visitor, the nurse is aware that he would be least likely to believe that death is:

1. Like going to sleep.
2. The result of magic.
3. Permanent and lasting.
4. The result of a wish.

9 Anticipatory guidance is given to the parents of a 10-year-old girl. The nurse knows the parents

understand this information if they say they will reinforce:

1. Sex education and self breast exam.
2. The need for increased caloric intake.
3. The child's increasing need for sleep.
4. The need for fewer dental visits.

10. The nurse knows that which of the following behaviors would indicate regression in a hospitalized five-year-old?

1. Bedwetting several times a day.
2. Crying when mother leaves.
3. Eating only food from home.
4. Wanting his teddy bear for bedtime.

11. A nine-year-old girl is admitted with asthma. In planning her care, the nurse should anticipate that the child will prefer to:

1. Play with another girl her age.
2. Be with older girls.
3. Associate with small groups of boys and girls.
4. Have male companions.

12. In caring for elderly clients, the nurse understands that the aging process generally results in:

1. A decline in physiological and sensory systems of the body.
2. A decreased skin resilience.
3. A diminished hearing acuity.
4. An absence of sexual interest and activity.

13. A four-year-old is admitted to the hospital with croup. When the mother comes to visit the next day, she finds the nurse changing the bedding after the client has wet the bed. The mother says, "He never wets the bed at home. I am so embarrassed." Which nursing response is most helpful to the mother?

1. "I know this can really be embarrassing, but I have kids myself, so I understand and it doesn't bother me."
2. "It is not uncommon for children to regress during a hospitalization. His toileting skills will return when he is feeling better."
3. "It's probably due to the medication we are giving him for his infection."
4. "I plan to discuss your child's incontinence with the physician, as this may require further investigation."

14. In developing a plan to improve the self-image of an eight-year-old client with asthma, the nurse should consider that:

1. The client is not able to understand the causes or limitations of chronic illness.
2. The client's peers, parents, and teachers should be instructed in strategies for encouraging her.
3. Teaching the client self-care skills will increase her sense of control.
4. The client should be told about all potential long-term complications.

15. The mother of a two-year-old who is hospitalized asks how she should handle her son's temper tantrums. The nurse should advise the mother to:

1. Restrain the child physically.
2. Ignore the behavior.
3. Let the child know his temper tantrums are not acceptable.
4. Play a game with him, or rock him quietly.

16. A hospitalized eight-year-old is losing a game of checkers. He stands up and says, "I quit." The nurse understands that this behavior probably is:

1. A personality change due to hospitalization.
2. Immaturity for his age.
3. A sign that this game is too hard for him.
4. Normal for his social development.

17. The nurse is evaluating the effectiveness of teaching performed for the mother of a six-month-old who is teething. The nurse would consider the teaching to be successful if the mother:

1. Provides the infant with a hard rubber toy to bite.
2. Places aspirin against the erupting tooth.
3. Rubs a topical anesthetic on the sensitive area.
4. Places sherry and water mixture on gums at bedtime.

18. At nine months of age, an infant has been in the hospital four times for a total of 42 days. The nurse notices that the infant does not seem upset when her parents leave. The nurse would evaluate this behavior as:

1. An infant with an easy temperament.
2. A mature infant who is very secure.
3. A strong attachment to the nurse.
4. Experiencing detachment.

19. The father of a four-year-old son tells the nurse that his child believes there are monsters in his closet at bedtime. The nurse's best suggestion for dealing with this problem is:

1. Letting the child sleep with his parents.
2. Keeping a night light on in the child's bedroom.
3. Tell the child that these fears are not real.
4. Staying with the child until he falls asleep.

20. A three-year-old is brought to the clinic for evaluation because he is thin and his mother is concerned

about his appetite. The best response the nurse can give his mom is:

1. "His appetite should be increasing, so he needs to be fed."
2. "You should discourage food rituals."
3. "His growth is slow, and so his appetite is, too."
4. "If this continues, he will need testing."

21. In caring for a confused elderly client, which statement by the nurse indicates the best understanding of the principles of reality orientation?

1. "Good morning, Mr. Jones. Did you sleep well? It's time to get dressed."
2. "Good morning. This is your second day in Shady Pines and I am your nurse for the day."
3. "Do you remember who I am? We met yesterday when you were admitted."
4. "Good morning, how are you today? I am your nurse for the day. My name is Ms. Smith."

22. The nurse caring for clients in a long-term care facility understands that remotivation therapy is used to:

1. Stimulate and encourage social participation.
2. Reorient clients with cognitive problems.
3. Encourage clients to share memories of past experiences and events.
4. Resolve emotional problems.

23. An elderly client is able to walk with a cane and enjoys ambulating in the hall. Since he has memory problems, he has great difficulty remembering which room is his. What nursing action would best alleviate this problem?

1. Assign him a room close to the nursing station so staff members will be available to help him.
2. Assign him to a room with a roommate who can watch out for him.
3. Do not allow him to leave his room unaccompanied.
4. Put his picture and his name written in large letters on the door to his room.

24. While working in a pediatric unit, the nurse encounters all ages of children. The nurse knows that a child's social interactions with peers are very important. During which periods of a child's life is this need greatest?

1. Preschool and school age.
2. Toddler and preschool.
3. School age and adolescence.
4. Late adolescence and early adulthood.

25. The nurse knows that it is characteristic of the development of a 30-month-old child to:

1. Tell tall tales.
2. Have a command vocabulary of about 10 words.
3. Weigh double his birth weight.
4. Have achieved complete primary dentition.

26. In developing a plan for perioperative teaching for an adolescent, the nurse should be guided by the knowledge that:

1. He may act as if he knows much more than he actually does.
2 He will only be interested in reassurance that things will go well.
3. The major part of the teaching should be delayed until after the surgery.
4. His parents should be the major focus of the teaching.

27. The nurse would best describe the most important aspect of planning the discipline of a hospitalized toddler as:

1. Consistency in enforcing the rules.
2. Delaying punishment for wrongdoing until parents are present.
3. Eliminating discipline while the child is ill.
4. Giving several warnings before actually disciplining.

28. In caring for the elderly, the nurse is guided by Erikson's observation that the elderly need to resolve conflicts between:

1. Ego, integrity, and despair.
2. Intimacy and isolation.
3. Generativity and stagnation.
4. Identity and isolation.

29. The nurse has been caring for an elderly client who was admitted for hip replacement and is disoriented to time and place. The nurse requests to be assigned to stay with the client when she returns to the unit after her surgery. The rationale for this request is:

1. The elderly client requires close postoperative supervision because of her unpredictable preoperative behavior.
2. The elderly client will most likely be agitated when she regains consciousness after surgery.
3. The many stresses associated with surgery could lead to further cognitive impairment in this elderly client.
4. Elderly clients are particularly vulnerable to the development of postoperative complications.

30. The nurse working with elderly clients knows that organic mental disorders:

1. Are the most prevalent type of psychiatric problem in this age group.

2. Are almost always chronic.
3. Need careful evaluation as they may be caused by a medical problem that could be treated effectively.
4. Can be controlled with supportive and behavioral approaches, but eventually will lead to further deterioration and death.

31. The nurse working with elderly clients should remember that dementia in the elderly:

1. Is easy to distinguish from depression.
2. May coexist with depression.
3. Is not affected by medications.
4. Cannot be concealed by the client.

32. At what age would the nurse expect that the anterior fontanel would be closed?

1. Three weeks.
2. Three months.
3. Eighteen months.
4. Four years.

33. When working with three-year-olds, which speech patterns does the nurse expect?

1. Speech that is not understood by strangers.
2. Sentences average four to five words.
3. Only direct commands are understood.
4. Practices speech by talking constantly.

34. The mother of a four-year-old says that she is worried about her son's fine motor development. The nurse expects the child to be able to:

1. Tie shoelaces.
2. Copy a square and circle.
3. Draw a stick man with seven to nine parts.
4. Print name without errors.

35. The nurse observes that, in the first few days of hospitalization, an 18-month-old client sits quietly sucking her thumb in the corner of her crib. When the nurse approaches the crib, the client shyly turns her head away from the nurse. The nurse understands that the toddler's behavior:

1. Indicates a pathological reaction to being hospitalized.
2. Indicates that the relationship between parents and child should be assessed.
3. Demonstrates an anxiety reaction to the stress of hospitalization.
4. Is an example of negative behavior and a beginning attempt at autonomy.

36. A client is in the hospital, and he is dying. He is very weak, tired, and short of breath. The nursing plan of care for the client and his family should emphasize:

1. Limiting visiting hours to help conserve his energy.
2. Having the client do as much as he can for himself to increase his self-esteem and independence.
3. Encouraging the family to spend as much time as possible with him and do whatever they feel comfortable with in caring for him.
4. Planning to perform as much of his care as possible at one time, so he can rest for long intervals.

Section 7: Meeting Basic Needs of Fluids, Nutrition, Elimination and Oxygenation

This area includes the nurse's thorough knowledge of problems and procedures relating to fluid and electrolyte balance, therapeutic diets and enteral feeding, TPN, intestinal intubation, intake and output, incontinence, constipation, fecal impaction diarrhea, bowel training, enema, and urinary catheters. The nurse also addresses the client's needs for oxygenation, measures to prevent aspiration, emergency measures like the Heimlich maneuver and CPR as used with clients of different ages, and devices used to increase respiratory function.

1. An elderly male client is admitted to the hospital with complaints of abdominal pain and distention. He has a history of no bowel movement for the past 10 days. After a diagnostic evaluation, it is determined that the client has a fecal impaction. Which treatment can the nurse anticipate will be ordered initially?

1. Soap suds enemas until clear.
2. Bisacodyl (Dulcolax) suppository.
3. Oil retention enema.
4. Tap water enema.

2. Following a stroke that affected the left side of the brain, an elderly client had the tube feeding removed and is ready to begin oral feedings. Which of the following nursing actions would be best?

1. Feed from right side of mouth; upright position; mouth care before feeding.
2. Verbal encouragement; check gag reflex; feed thinned foods and liquids.
3. Check gag reflex; feed on left side of mouth; upright position.
4. Sensory stimulation; verbal encouragement; favorite foods.

3. A client is recovering from surgery. The nurse is preparing to irrigate his urinary catheter. To prevent injury to the mucosa of the bladder when irrigating the catheter, the nurse should:

1. Gently compress the ball of the syringe to instill the irrigating solution.
2. Quickly instill the irrigating solution, using some pressure to loosen any clots or mucous.
3. After instilling the solution, apply gentle pressure to remove the irrigating solution from the bladder.
4. Place a sterile cap on the end of the drainage tubing to protect it from contamination.

4. Postural drainage with percussion is ordered for a client with pneumonia. What would the nurse include in the plan for this procedure?

1. Perform this procedure before meals.
2. Cup and clap lightly, to avoid causing redness to the client's skin.
3. Administer bronchodilators after percussion and before postural drainage.
4. Provide analgesia prior to each treatment.

5. At a boy scout camp the nurse encounters a child who exhibits a high-pitched inspiratory sound, and cyanosis. Describe the procedure that the nurse should perform.

1. Stand behind the child and apply an upward thrust below the xiphoid.
2. Monitor the child, and if respirations cease, use the Heimlich maneuver.
3. Bend the child forward and deliver back blows to dislodge the object.
4. Begin cardiopulmonary resuscitation.

6. The nurse takes precautions to prevent constipation and fecal impaction in an immobilized client. The nurse is aware that, if a client develops a fecal impaction, which of the following serious complications could result?

1. Intestinal obstruction.
2. Bowel perforation.
3. Peritonitis.
4. Rectal bleeding.

7. A person in a restaurant puts his hand to his throat. A nurse who sees this happen begins to administer the Heimlich maneuver. After the client falls to the floor, the nurse should take the following initial action:

1. Check for the pulse.
2. Sweep the mouth.
3. Attempt to ventilate.
4. Administer five abdominal thrusts.

8. The physician has ordered an indwelling urinary catheter for a male client. Where should the nurse tape the catheter to prevent pressure on the urethra at the penoscrotal junction?

1. Medial thigh.
2. Upper abdomen.
3. Mid-abdominal region.
4. Lateral thigh.

9. During a home visit, the wife of your client collapses. There is neither a pulse nor respirations. Which of the following accurately describes the CPR the nurse would provide?

1. 5 to 1 ratio of compressions to ventilations, at a rate of 100 beats/min.
2. 15 to 2 ratio of compressions to ventilations, at a rate of 80 beats/min.
3. 15 to 2 ratio of compressions to ventilations, at a rate of 100 beats/min.
4. 5 to 1 ratio of compressions to ventilations, at a rate of 80 beats/min.

10. A client has just been catheterized and has an indwelling Foley catheter in her bladder. If all of the following actions were taken, improper technique was used when the nurse:

1. Cleansed the client's urinary meatus with soap and water prior to inserting the catheter.
2. Placed the client in the lithotomy position.
3. Inserted the catheter one to two inches further into the urinary meatus when urine was observed in the catheter tubing.
4. Used sterile normal saline to inflate the retention balloon on the catheter.

11. When inserting a nasogastric tube in a comatose client for internal tube feedings, it is least appropriate for the nurse to:

1. Measure the amount of the tube to be inserted.
2. Lubricate the distal portion of the tube.
3. Tilt the client's head back when inserting the tube.
4. Check placement of the tube.

12. A client is in the hospital and has weakness on her left side because of a stroke. She becomes upset when eating because liquids drool out of her mouth on her weak side. What is the best nursing intervention?

1. Provide only pureed and solid foods to prevent drooling, so the client will not become upset.
2. Have a member of the family assist with the client's feedings.
3. Teach the client how to drink fluids on the unaffected side to prevent drooling.
4. Have the client use a syringe to squirt liquids into the back of her mouth.

13. Which nursing action is contraindicated for a client with an indwelling Foley catheter?

1. Instill sterile distilled water in the catheter.
2. Use minimal pressure to clear the catheter of clots or mucous plugs.
3. Use sterile equipment for irrigation.
4. Use the flow of gravity for return of the irrigant.

14. A client has a nasogastric tube in place following abdominal surgery. Which nursing action would the nurse avoid when planning the care for a client with a nasogastric tube?

1. Attach the nasogastric tube to high suction.
2. Provide frequent oral hygiene.
3. Measure the amount of drainage from the nasogastric tube.
4. Attach the nasogastric tube to the client's gown in order to prevent pulling at the insertion site.

15. The nurse is assisting a frail elderly client to eat. The client begins to choke and indicates to the nurse that she cannot talk. The first nursing action is to:

1. Perform the Heimlich maneuver to obtain a patent airway.
2. Begin mouth to mouth resuscitation.
3. Place an oxygen mask on the client.
4. Go to the nurses' station to get some help.

16. CPR has been initiated on a client in the emergency room. Which finding by the nurse would indicate effective cardiac compressions?

1. An EKG pattern with each compression.
2. Compression depth of 1 1/2 to 2 inches.
3. A palpable femoral pulse during each compression.
4. Pupils changing from pinpoint to dilated.

17. A client who is incontinent of stool has been placed on a bowel training program. The nurse understands that the goal of bowel training is to:

1. Prevent soiling of the bed.
2. Prevent cancer of the colon.
3. Prevent loose stools.
4. Provide the client with control over his bowels.

18. A client is scheduled for surgery on his bowel. The doctor orders a cleansing enema for the morning of surgery. The best nursing approach is to:

1. Wear gloves to insert the tubing.
2. Use universal precautions and provide comfort measures to help the client relax during the procedure.
3. Lubricate the tubing well prior to insertion.
4. Position the client on his side and drape the client for warmth and privacy.

19. The client is admitted with anorexia nervosa. A nasogastric tube is to be inserted. In preparing the client for this procedure, what would be the initial nursing action?

1. Assist the client to a sitting position.
2. Explain the procedure to the client.
3. If the client has dentures, make sure that they are in place in the client's mouth.
4. Have a stethoscope available to listen for proper placement.

20. A 10-year-old is overweight. He has no dietary restrictions. The nurse is helping him make out his menu. Which diet should the nurse encourage?

1. A glass of whole milk, hot dog on a roll with pickles, and a candy bar.
2. A glass of skim milk, baked fish sandwich on whole wheat roll with lettuce, and a medium apple.
3. A glass of diet lemonade, hamburger and roll, medium orange and mashed potatoes.
4. A salad plate of low fat cottage cheese, potato salad, and macaroni salad with a croissant and a glass of water.

21. A client develops a fecal impaction. Before digital removal of the mass, what type of enema is usually given by the nurse to loosen the feces?

1. Fleets.
2. Oil retention.
3. Soap suds.
4. Tap water.

22. During the resuscitation of a client, the physician orders the client to be defibrillated by receiving a controlled electrical shock. The nurse knows that it would place the client at risk to:

1. Move away from the bed while the client is defibrillated.
2. Observe the other nurses to be sure they are not in contact with the client or the bed during defibrillation.
3. Hold the IV pole out of the way while the client is defibrillated.
4. Make sure the client's chest is dry, except where the electrode paste or pads are applied for placement of the defibrillator paddles.

23. A trauma client, admitted through the Emergency Room, has a urinary catheter inserted to monitor kidney function and assess for early signs of shock. The nurse would report which urinary output measurements as suggestive of cardiac failure or hypovolemia?

1. 20 ml/hour.
2. 35 ml/hour.
3. 40 ml/hour.
4. 50 ml/hour.

24. The nurse is assessing an immobilized client for symptoms of a fecal impaction. The most definitive symptom is:

1. The absence of bowel sounds.
2. Diarrhea stools with abdominal cramping.
3. A rigid board-like abdomen.
4. Constipation with liquid fecal seepage.

25. The physician has ordered a urine specimen to be sent to the lab for analysis of specific gravity. How should the nurse collect the specimen?

1. Clean-catch midstream urine.
2. Catheterized urine specimen.
3. Random urine sample.
4. 24-hour urine collection.

26. The nurse is instructing the client regarding good food sources for potassium. Which menu choice by the client indicates to the nurse that the client has understood the instruction?

1. Baked chicken, boiled potato, pudding.
2. Boiled chicken, rice, cranberry juice.
3. Broiled meat, baked potato, citrus fruit salad.
4. Beef stew, bread and butter, jello.

27. A client in an extended care facility is in the dining room, having dinner with the other clients. The client has stopped eating, is grasping his throat with his hands, and cannot talk. The first and most effective action by the nurse is to:

1. Call a code and obtain assistance, before taking further action.
2. Perform the Heimlich maneuver.
3. Place the client on the floor and begin mouth-to-mouth resuscitation.
4. Slap the client on the back several times.

28. The nurse is assisting an elderly client to eat. The client suddenly coughs a few times, then appears to be attempting to cough, making a whistling sound as he inhales. When using the Heimlich maneuver on a conscious client, which of the following nursing actions is most effective?

1. Ask the client what he is choking on.
2. Place your arms around the client and position your fist in the abdomen, between the bottom of the breast bone and the navel.
3. Slap the client on the back until the object is expelled or until the client becomes unconscious.
4. Stand in front of the person.

29. The nurse is caring for a client who is on a moderate sodium diet. Which of the following lunch selections by the client would signify an understanding of the diet?

1. Grilled cheese sandwich and tomato soup.
2. Bologna sandwich and dill pickles.
3. Chinese vegetables with soy sauce.
4. Chicken salad sandwich with tossed salad.

30. During cardiopulmonary resuscitation (CPR), the nurse should assess the adult's pulse by feeling the:

1. Carotid pulse in the neck.
2. Brachial pulse in the arm.
3. Femoral pulse in the groin.
4. Radial pulse in the wrist.

31. In the initiation of cardiopulmonary resuscitation (CPR), which assessment must be made by the nurse PRIOR to beginning chest compressions?

1. Absence of respirations.
2. Dilated pupils.
3. Absence of pulse.
4. Unresponsiveness.

32. When an infant is choking and turning blue, but still is conscious, the best initial action by the nurse is to:

1. Turn the child on his back and attempt mouth-to-mouth ventilation.
2. Support the child in a prone position with the head down and give four back blows.
3. Perform the Heimlich maneuver.
4. Call an ambulance.

33. During cardiopulmonary resuscitation (CPR), the preferred method that the nurse should use for opening the airway is to:

1. Turn the head and open the mouth.
2. Perform a finger sweep of the mouth.
3. Use the jaw thrust and head tilt method.
4. Tilt the head and lift the chin.

34. The nurse is to insert a Levin nasogastric tube. The nurse understands that an inappropriate use of the NG tube is:

1. Maintaining NPO status.
2. Decompression.
3. Lavage.
4. Gavage.

Section 8: Administration of Medications

The safe administration of medications is a primary nursing responsibility. In addition to checking the time and identifying and assessing the client prior to giving a medication, the nurse must practice medical asepsis, know the proper safety precautions for different drugs and different methods of administration, and ensure the proper dosage and proper route. Remember the "Five Rights!"

1. A 12-year-old child is being discharged from the hospital with a diagnosis of asthma. She is to be maintained on metered dose inhalers at home. The nurse is preparing a care plan on the use of cromolyn (Intal). Which of the following nursing instructions to the parents should the nurse avoid including in the client's care plan?

1. Intal will decrease the inflammation in your child's bronchioles.
2. Do not rely on Intal for relief of an acute attack.
3. Have your child rinse her mouth after using the puffer.
4. Your child should breathe more easily after a dose of Intal.

2. The nurse is to apply topical ointment to the client's skin for a dermatological condition. Which action should the nurse avoid?

1. Massaging the ointment into the skin.
2. Removing excess ointment.
3. Applying ointment with ungloved fingertips.
4. Documenting a description of the skin prior to application of the ointment.

3. During the administration of a medication, a 19-year-old client asks the nurse if this is a "new pill" and tells the nurse that he has never had that particular pill before. The safest nursing action is to:

1. Check the client's identification bracelet again.
2. Review the physician's orders to see if this is a new medication.
3. Assure the client that the medication package has his name on it.
4. Ask the client to take the medication, since the identification bracelet and medication administration record indicate the client is to receive the medication.

4. A child with a rectal temperature of 39° C has an order for acetaminophen (Tylenol) 280 mg by mouth. The label on the bottle reads 160 mg/5 cc. How many cc's should the nurse give to the child?

1. 8.8 cc.
2. 1.8 cc.
3. 7.0 cc.
4. 12.7 cc.

5. A concerned mother calls the physician's office. Her child has a respiratory infection and a temperature of 39° C orally. She needs to give her son 240 mg of acetaminophen (Tylenol). The label on her bottle at home reads 160 mg/5 cc. The nurse's accurate response is:

1. Give 1/2 teaspoon.
2. Give 1 1/2 teaspoons.
3. Give 1 1/2 cc.
4. Give 15 cc.

6. During administration of medications to a client, the priority nursing action is to:

1. Help the client swallow medications without aspirating by keeping the head in a neutral position.
2. Identify the client by checking the client's identification bracelet and asking for his name.
3. Keep all prepared medications in sight.
4. Check the client for desired or undesired drug effects within an hour after administration of the medication.

7. A 10-month-old client is scheduled for OR. The preoperative medication is ordered IM, and the volume will amount to 1.5 cc. The nurse should give the injection in the:

1. Deltoid muscle.
2. Gluteus maximus.
3. Rectus femoris.
4. Vastus lateralis.

8. The nurse discovers that the wrong medication was given to a confused client who answered to the name stated when the nurse entered the room. The physician is notified and states that the medication that the client received will not harm him and nothing needs to be done. The priority nursing action after notifying the physician is:

1. Apologize to the client involved.
2. Make out an incident report documenting the occurrence.
3. Try to avoid being responsible for administering medications again, since this could have been terrible situation.
4. Realize that everyone makes mistakes, and continue to administer the rest of the medications to the other clients.

9. The nurse is preparing medications for administration in a pediatric unit. Of the following nursing actions, which would be inappropriate?

1. Prepare medications for one client at a time.
2. Calculate correct drug dosage.
3. Open unit dose tablets and place medications in medication cup.
4. Avoid touching tablets or capsules with the hands.

10. The nurse is preparing to administer medication to a client who is scheduled to receive his insulin at 8:00 a.m. The best nursing approach is to:

1. Read the label three times.
2. Check the client's identification bracelet.
3. Administer the correct medication to the right client.
4. Check the dosage prescribed.

11. While caring for the client with an IV, it is most important for the nurse to:

1. Report any signs of infection to the charge nurse.
2. Record the condition of the IV site and the rate of infusion, and report any unusual findings.
3. Record intravenous intake.
4. Ask the client if the IV site is painful or tender.

12. When administering ear drops with a dropper, which nursing action best prevents contamination of the bottle of medication?

1. Thorough handwashing prior to preparing the medication.
2. Hold the dropper with the tip above the ear canal.
3. Wash the client's ear prior to instilling the medication.
4. Fill the dropper with only the prescribed number of drops.

13. The nurse is to administer an intramuscular injection. The most important action by the nurse to prevent introduction of the medication into the venous system is to:

1. Inject the medication slowly to allow for slow absorption.
2. Insert the needle at a 45-degree angle where there are fewer blood vessels.
3. Use the Z track method of injection.
4. Aspirate the drug after insertion of needle.

14. While preparing to give a morning medication, the first nursing action is to:

1. Read the label.
2. Check for the right dose.
3. Wash hands.
4. Check for the right time.

15. A client is admitted to the hospital for cataract surgery of the left eye. The physician has ordered eye drops to be administered to both eyes at frequent intervals prior to surgery. Which nursing action is most appropriate?

1. Use aseptic technique and avoid dropping the medication onto the cornea.
2. Gently wash away any crust along the eyelid margin with warm water.
3. Have the client look up toward the ceiling prior to instillation of drops.
4. Drop prescribed number of drops into the conjunctival sac.

16. A client has left her used insulin syringe on the bedside table. What is the best action by the nurse to help prevent spread of infection by way of the contaminated needle?

1. Explain to the client that the syringe should be disposed of in the garbage can, to avoid a potential needle stick by someone providing care for the client.
2. Cap the syringe and take it to the needle disposal container.
3. Place the uncapped syringe in the needle disposal container.
4. Have the nurse administer the injection next time, since the client is not responsible enough to follow through with the correct procedure.

17. An elderly female client is admitted to the hospital. She brings all of her medicines, including a bottle with no label. She says this is her cough medicine, which she put in a small bottle so it would fit in her purse. At this time, the safest nursing action is to:

1. Pour the liquid down the drain, since it has no label.
2. Instruct the client concerning safety issues related to this practice, and suggest that she have the pharmacy put the medication in smaller containers that will fit in her purse.
3. Send the bottle home with a family member.
4. Tell the client that this is a dangerous practice, which could result in the death of one of her small grandchildren.

18. A 16-year-old male is to receive an intramuscular injection. To gain cooperation with this procedure, the nurse's first intervention is to:

1. Tell him what he will feel.
2. Explain the purpose of the medication.
3. Offer him a choice of injection sites.
4. Describe the steps in the procedure.

19. A client is seen in the health clinic and is diagnosed with conjunctivitis of the right eye. An antibiotic ophthalmic ointment has been ordered. Which instruction would be appropriate for the nurse to give to this client?

1. Use a sterile glove and applicator to apply the antibiotic ointment.
2. When washing your face, wash the infected eye first.
3. Other family members may share your washcloth as long as you rinse it out first.
4. Apply the ointment in a thin line, beginning at the inner corner and proceeding outward.

20. A client is admitted to the hospital with a compound fracture. While making the client's bed, the nurse finds a capsule of medication in the sheets. The nurse knows that it would be least appropriate to:

1. Administer the medication to the client.
2. Notify the physician of the missed dose.
3. Determine what medication the capsule contains.
4. Document the incident in the nurse's notes.

21. Acetaminophen (Tylenol) is ordered for a nine-year-old child with a temperature of 102° F. The nurse preparing to administer the medication to the client realizes that he looks very thin for his age. What action would the nurse take first?

1. Give him one-half the ordered dose.
2. Give the prescribed dose.
3. Measure his weight and calculate the dosage range.
4. Call the doctor and question the dosage.

Section 9: Perioperative Nursing Responsibilities

Pre- and postoperative nursing care includes specific responsibilities in preparing the client for surgery and preventing and monitoring for postoperative complications. The nurse must use a wide range of assessment, analysis, planning, implementation and evaluation skills in providing postoperative care. Prioritizing is especially critical for the client's safety. The nurse also provides preoperative and discharge client teaching and has specific responsibilities with regard to informed consent.

1. **A client is recuperating from abdominal surgery performed under general anesthesia. The nurse should encourage the client to use the incentive spirometry a minimum of how many times per hour?**

    1. Two.
    2. Five to 10.
    3. 10 to 15.
    4. 20 to 25.

2. **An adolescent client had surgery on his foot and has just been returned to his room from the recovery room. The initial assessment indicates that he is stable. An hour later, his roommate turns on the call light and tells the nurse that the client has gotten up and hopped on one foot to the bathroom, using his IV pole for support. What is the priority nursing action?**

    1. Open the bathroom door to assess if the client is okay.
    2. Help the client back to bed and get him a urinal.
    3. Explain to the client that it is not safe for him to be hopping around on one foot.
    4. Get a wheelchair and help the client back to bed when he is done in the bathroom.

3. **A male client was admitted to the hospital for possible abdominal surgery. Following x-ray and diagnostic procedures, the doctor decided that the surgery was necessary. The nurse's preoperative teaching should include which information?**

    1. Most clients are admitted to the intensive care unit after abdominal surgery.
    2. Minor discomfort is expected in the operative site during the first few postoperative days.
    3. Moving as little as possible will decrease the discomfort following this procedure.
    4. Learning to cough and deep breathe will help prevent postoperative respiratory breathing complications.

4. **A postoperative client is to ambulate for the first time after surgery. The nurse understands that which of the following would place the client at risk?**

    1. Have the client get up and sit in the chair next to the bed.
    2. Have the client sit on the edge of the bed with his feet down for a few minutes before he starts to ambulate.
    3. Have the client stand at the side of the bed for a few minutes before taking his first steps.
    4. Encourage the client to try to walk straight ahead while you assist him with his walking.

5. **A client is scheduled for left below-the-knee amputation in the morning. Before surgery, the preoperative teaching plan included deep breathing and coughing. In evaluating the effectiveness of preoperative teaching, the nurse should ask the client:**

    1. "Do you understand what we have just discussed about deep breathing and coughing?"
    2. "Do you think that you will need to have a sedative to help you sleep tonight?"
    3. "Will you demonstrate for me the correct method of deep breathing and coughing?"
    4. "Do you have any questions concerning your scheduled surgical procedure?"

6. **A client is seen in the emergency room for abdominal pain and is scheduled for emergency surgery. In preparing to do the client's preoperative teaching, the nurse knows that it is most important to:**

    1. Explain the hospital billing process for clients receiving surgery.
    2. Teach deep breathing and coughing with abdominal splinting.
    3. Obtain the surgical consent.
    4. Explain where the incision will be and how much drainage to expect on the dressing after surgery.

7. **While changing a surgical dressing, the nurse notes green, foul-smelling drainage at the incision site. Another postoperative client is sharing the same room with this client. The most appropriate nursing action is to:**

    1. Place the client with the drainage in a private room.
    2. Institute drainage and secretion precautions.
    3. Move the other client to another room.
    4. Place the client in strict isolation until the organism has been cultured and identified.

8. **The nurse is planning discharge teaching for a client following abdominal surgery. Which of the follow-**

ing instructions about changing dressings in the home would the nurse consider most appropriate?

1. The appropriate opening of bandages to maintain their sterility.
2. Proper aseptic technique.
3. Proper gloving technique.
4. Good handwashing technique.

9. The nurse is caring for a client who had abdominal surgery two days ago. The nurse should be most concerned about which finding?

1. A urinary drainage bag with 100 ccs of straw colored urine.
2. A wound dressing with thick, light green drainage.
3. A blood pressure reading of 98/66.
4. Shallow respirations, with a rate of 30.

10. A client fell at home and fractured her hip. She is to have surgery in the morning. In preparing the client for surgery, which option is outside the scope of the nurse's responsibilities?

1. Assessing the health status of the client.
2. Explaining the operative procedure and any risks that may be involved with the procedure.
3. Determining that the history, physical, and specific laboratory tests have been ordered or completed according to hospital protocol.
4. Determining that a signed surgical consent form is completed.

11. A client is scheduled for a colostomy after being diagnosed with cancer of the large intestine. The nurse should begin client teaching about the ostomy:

1. Postoperatively, after the pain has subsided, when the client will be better able to concentrate.
2. Postoperatively, after meeting with the ostomy nurse.
3. When the client demonstrates an interest in learning about the ostomy.
4. Preoperatively, to involve the client in his care and give him a sense of control over his life.

12. In planning preoperative care for a client, the nurse is aware that obtaining legal, informed consent to perform surgery is the responsibility of:

1. The nurse.
2. The surgeon.
3. The client's family physician.
4. The client.

13. Before giving preoperative medication to a client going to surgery, the nurse must make sure that:

1. The client has an empty bladder.
2. Vital signs are documented on the preoperative check list.
3. Dentures are removed.
4. The consent form has been signed.

14. A postoperative client should be assessed frequently for any manifestation of hemorrhage, which can lead to hypovolemic shock. In hypovolemic shock, which assessment would most likely be made by the nurse?

1. Rising blood pressure.
2. Hyperthermia.
3. Bradycardia.
4. Tachypnea.

15. A postoperative client's knee dressing becomes completely saturated with blood one hour after returning to the clinical unit. Initially, the nurse should:

1. Reinforce the knee dressing.
2. Apply a tourniquet around the closest artery.
3. Apply direct pressure to the knee.
4. Apply ice to the knee.

16. A client who had surgery 24 hours ago is experiencing dyspnea and tachycardia, and has developed a fever. The nurse suspects atelectasis. If this complication is present, the nurse's auscultation of the client's lung sounds would reveal:

1. Diminished breath sounds.
2. Rhonchi.
3. A pleural friction rub.
4. Absent breath sounds.

17. The nurse is planning to reinforce the doctor's preoperative teaching. The child is seven years old and is scheduled for abdominal surgery. The best nursing approach is to:

1. Explain the procedure to the child by pointing to the child's abdomen.
2. Discuss the procedure only with the child's parents.
3. Tell the child about the procedure using an age-appropriate explanation.
4. Demonstrate the procedure to the child using a drawing or doll.

Section 10: Therapeutic Communication

We have saved communication until last—but therapeutic communication is **absolutely essential** to the safe and effective practice of nursing.

The nurse must always be in a therapeutic role. Without top-notch communication skills, you cannot establish and maintain a therapeutic nurse/client relationship or achieve effective cooperation with other members of the health care team. As you will see in the following drill questions, therapeutic communication is an integral part of the *assessment, implementation* and *evaluation* phases of the nursing process.

Chapter Five in *TQLogic for Beginning Nursing Students* reviews communication tools and blocks, and provides useful guidelines for prioritizing nursing responses; you may wish to review Chapter Five before proceeding with the drill questions.

1. A client is sitting by his food tray, pushing the food around on his plate. He says to the nurse, "I hate hospital food. Is this the only thing that I can get to eat?" The nurse's best response is:

1. "What is it about the food that you dislike?"
2. "Well, the other clients haven't complained about the food. Is something else bothering you?"
3. "I'll call the kitchen and order something else for you."
4. "Is there something special you would like to eat?"

2. When the nurse is making morning rounds, a client says, "I almost died last night." The most therapeutic nursing response is:

1. "You made it through the night."
2. "Patients do have dreams that they die when they are hospitalized."
3. "Are you feeling okay now?"
4. "That must have been frightening for you. Tell me more about it."

3. A client is told by her doctor that he has found a lump in her breast and that a biopsy would have to be done. The client states to the nurse, "Do you think it is cancer?" The best initial response by the nurse is:

1. "You seem to be worried about what the doctor may find."
2. "Do you have a family history of breast cancer?"
3. "We won't know anything until the biopsy is done."
4. "Most lumps are not cancerous, so you really shouldn't worry."

4. An elderly client is constantly putting her call light on. When the nurse answers the light, the client does not appear to need anything. Which action by the nurse is least appropriate?

1. Ask the members of the family if they can spend more time with the client.
2. Remove the call light from easy reach of the client.
3. Make frequent visits to the client's room.
4. Spend more time in the client's room while charting.

5. A client is taught to do colostomy care for herself prior to discharge. She says to the nurse, "I don't think that I will be able to take care of this colostomy myself." Which of the following is the most helpful response by the nurse?

1. "Don't worry about it. Most clients feel like that at first."
2. "What part of the colostomy care are you having trouble with?"
3. "In time, you will become better at this than I am."
4. "A home health nurse will be visiting you, so if you have any problems, she can help you."

6. A client is in the hospital because of severe weight loss and refusal to eat. The physician ordered the insertion of a nasogastric tube for feeding. The nurse finds the client with the tube removed. The client tells that nurse that he "doesn't need that thing." The most appropriate response by the nurse is:

1. "You shouldn't have done that! Now I have to put it down again."
2. "Why did you pull that tube out? Do you want to die?"
3. "Tell me what you don't like about the tube."
4. "Your doctor is going to be very upset with you for doing this."

7. The nurse is caring for a client who is mourning a recent loss. The nurse understands that it is important to avoid saying that mourning:

1. Is a normal response to loss.
2. Functions to free the individual from an attachment to the lost object so that future relationships can be

established.
3. Is accompanied by a growing realization that the loss has occurred.
4. Occurs only in humans.

8. The wife of an alcoholic client says to the nurse, "I told my husband I would leave him if he did not get into treatment. Now that he is here, I feel differently. What can I do to help him?" The most therapeutic nursing response is:

1. "You should attend an Al-Anon meeting. The group can teach you how best to help him stay sober."
2. "You have already done a great deal by getting him to come into treatment. Now it is up to him to make the best use of his time here."
3. "Are you feeling some responsibility for his drinking?"
4. "Tell me more about the kind of help you feel you are able to provide at this time."

9. An elderly client asks the nurse to telephone her husband and ask him if he remembered to pick up his suit at the cleaners. The nurse knows that her husband died five years before. The best nursing response initially is:

1. "It may seem like your husband is still here, but he died five years ago."
2. "You miss your husband a lot, don't you? It must seem like he's almost here with you."
3. "You've forgotten that your husband is dead, haven't you?"
4. "Don't worry. Your husband will remember to pick up his cleaning."

10. The nurse enters a client's room. The client's son tells the nurse, "You people can't do anything right. Ever since my father was admitted to this hospital, it has been one mistake after another. I am taking him out of here before you kill him." The appropriate response by the nurse to the son is:

1. "You feel that your father is not being well taken care of?"
2. "We have the best intentions for the clients."
3. "I'll get the supervisor for you."
4. "Your father hasn't complained about the care. What specifically is the problem?"

11. A client has been told by the doctor that he has cancer and that it has advanced so far that treatment will not help. When the nurse comes to help him with his bath, he says to the nurse, "I'm not an invalid, you know! I can take care of myself. Get out and leave me alone." How should the nurse respond?

1. "I know that you are not an invalid. However, I was trying to help you."
2. "It sounds to me like you are angry about something. Did somebody do something wrong?"
3. "You are pretty upset. Let's talk about it."
4. "I'll just set up this equipment for you to bathe and come back later when you're not so angry."

12. The nurse tells a client that the doctor has ordered an intravenous line to be started. The client appears to be upset but says nothing. What should the nurse say?

1. "Do you have any questions about the procedure?"
2. "The doctor wants you to have antibiotics, and this method eliminates getting frequent injections."
3. "What is there about this procedure that concerns you?"
4. "It only hurts a little bit. It'll be over before you know it."

13. An elderly client is admitted to the hospital. His daughter, who takes care of him at home, says to the nurse, "I'm so glad he is here. You can take much better care of him than I can." What is the best nursing response to the daughter?

1. "We do have the equipment and people to take care of sick clients."
2. "It is not easy to care for the elderly. How do you manage?"
3. "Sir, your daughter takes good care of you at home, doesn't she?"
4. "Are you feeling guilty because your father has pneumonia?"

14. A client is to have a nasogastric tube inserted. The nurse explains the procedure to him and is about to begin the insertion, when the client says, "No way! You are not putting that hose down my throat. Get away from me." Which is the most appropriate nursing response?

1. "You have the right to refuse treatment. Why don't you talk to your doctor about it?"
2. "Something is upsetting you. Can you tell me what it is?"
3. "What do you feel about this hose?"
4. "I would just get it over with, because you won't get better without this tube."

15. The nurse observes an elderly client trying to climb over the side rails of the bed. When the nurse begins to place a vest restraint on the client, the client's daughter says to the nurse, "My mother does not need to be tied down in bed. I've been caring for her for years, and she hasn't fallen out of bed yet." Which response is therapeutic for the daughter?

1. "I just saw your mother trying to climb over the side rails. Since I am concerned about her falling and hurting herself, I think this is best for her safety."
2. "Tell me how you managed to care for her at home."
3. "Hospital policy requires restraint vests on clients who are at risk for falling. I just saw your mother trying to climb over the rails. You don't want her to get hurt, do you?"
4. "The elderly may become confused in an unfamiliar place and do things they wouldn't do at home. It is difficult to see her restrained. While you are with her, the restraints can be off. Let me know when you are ready to leave."

16. The nurse is preparing to give an elderly client a bath. The client says to the nurse, "I don't think that I need a bath today. I just had one yesterday. My skin is going to get too dry. I bathe completely every other day at home." Which response by the nurse is best?

1. "My head nurse wants all of the clients bathed daily. She believes that it decreases the number of germs on your skin that cause infection. Would you like to talk to her?"
2. "A bath can make you feel refreshed and make the day seem brighter. Don't you agree?"
3. "Would you like to compromise and just wash your face and hands today?"
4. "I heard you say that you didn't want a bath today."

17. A visitor asks the nurse about the client in the next room, who cries out frequently. "That person must have a terrible disease. What is the matter with him?" The most appropriate response by the nurse is:

1. "That client has cancer and is quite uncomfortable."
2. "Mr. Jones is being kept as comfortable as possible."
3. "That person is quite uncomfortable. Does his crying out bother you?"
4. "I cannot reveal anything about his diagnosis. Why don't you ask his family when they visit? I'm sure they would appreciate your concern."

18. A young client has been admitted to the acute diseases unit. She has recently been diagnosed with AIDS. When the nurse enters her room, the nurse finds the client is crying. What is the most appropriate response demonstrated by the nurse?

1. Ignore the crying and proceed to take the client's vital signs.
2. Acknowledge her feelings and offer to help.
3. Consult with the charge nurse immediately.
4. Notify her physician and suggest an antidepressant medication.

19. The nurse learns that an elderly client's sleeping problems began six months ago, when his physician diagnosed prostatic cancer. Prior to that time, he had enjoyed good physical health. The nurse also knows that his wife of 50 years died one year ago. One day the client tells the nurse, "I'd be better off dead because I am totally worthless." The nurse's most therapeutic response is:

1. "I have seen some very valuable things about you."
2. You feel worthless now because you are so depressed. You will feel differently when you depression begins to improve."
3. "You really have a great deal to live for."
4. "You have been feeling very sad and alone for some time now."

20. A client who has just been diagnosed with cancer tells the nurse that he would rather be dead than go through the treatment for cancer. The most appropriate nursing response is:

1. "What is it about the cancer treatment that concerns you?"
2. "If you don't receive the treatment, you will get your wish."
3. "Why don't you talk to your doctor about your feelings?"
4. "That wouldn't be fair to your family, would it?"

21. The client tells the nurse that he does not know how he is ever going to stay on the low cholesterol diet that his doctor ordered after his heart attack. The best response by the nurse is:

1. "If you don't follow the diet, you will probably have another heart attack, which could kill you."
2. "What is it about the low cholesterol diet that seems to be a problem for you?"
3. "I've been on that same diet for the last five years, and I'm sure you will learn how to change your eating habits after a while."
4. "I will have the dietitian talk to you before you are discharged. She's the expert, and she can be really helpful."

22. A client has advanced cancer of the lung with metastasis. His wife says to the nurse, "I know my husband is in severe pain. I wish I could do something to make him feel better." Which of the following responses by the nurse would be most helpful to the wife?

1. "It must be very difficult for you to see your husband suffering."
2. "I wish there was more that I could do to relieve his pain, too."
3. "I'm sure he will begin to feel better after his next pain medication."
4. "Your husband tries hard not to show the pain when you are with him."

23. A 29-year-old diabetic is admitted to the hospital for dialysis because of poor renal function. He says to the nurse, "I don't even know why I'm doing this. There is no cure." Which of the following is the most appropriate nursing response?

1. "There is always a chance that through research a cure will be found."
2. "Dialysis will help you live longer."
3. "You shouldn't complain! You are fortunate to be in this good a shape, considering the type of diabetes you have."
4. "It sounds as though you have given up on life."

24. A couple is in the hospital because of a fetal death at 37 weeks gestation. The husband is trying to comfort the wife, who is crying. The husband says to the nurse, "We wanted this baby so much." Which of the following is an appropriate response by the nurse?

1. "You are both young and you can have other children."
2. "It is God's will, and it must be accepted."
3. "It must be very difficult for you both. I will be available if you need anything."
4. "I think you should call your minister. He can help comfort you."

25. A woman is crying continuously after the death of her husband. The son is distressed over his mother's crying and reports to the nurse that she has said that she wants to die. He asks the nurse to help "calm her down." The nurse's best response to the son's request is:

1. "All right, I'll talk with her and see if I can comfort her."
2. "If you just sit quietly with her, I'm sure she will calm down when she gets these feelings out."
3. "It's hard to see her so upset, but she needs to let these feelings out; we can both stay with her for a while."
4. "This seems to bother you more than it does her."

26. A woman is distressed over the death of her husband. The son remarks to the nurse, "My father has been dead for six months now. I think my mother needs to get on with her life." What is the most helpful response by the nurse to the son?

1. "A death is usually a crisis for the whole family. How has your father's death affected you?"
2. "I agree. How can you help her find more pleasure in her life?"
3. "I think it would be helpful if you could give her more support."
4. "Perhaps she needs more time. Grieving often takes a year or more to complete."

27. The nurse observes an elderly depressed client in the day room. The client is shivering. Which response by the nurse would be most helpful to this client?

1. "Come with me to your room, and we will get a sweater for you."
2. "Why do you sit here without a sweater when you are cold?"
3. "What color sweater do you want me to get from your room for you?"
4. "When you are in the day room, you should dress so that you are not cold."

28. Soon after being admitted to a rehabilitation unit, a chronic alcoholic says to the nurse, "I don't really need to be here. My wife and family make me drink. My wife spends all my money. My kid just had an accident with his car that will cost me a fortune in repairs." The therapeutic nursing response is:

1. "Tell me more about how your wife is spending all your money."
2. "Could you tell me more about why your child's car accident cost you money?"
3. "It sounds like you are having a great deal of financial difficulty."
4. "Tell me more about your feelings about being here in the hospital."

29. An elderly male client is admitted to the hospital for an exploratory laparotomy. The client's daughter says to the nurse, "I wish I could stay with my father, but I need to go home to see how my children are doing. I really hate to leave my father alone at this time." The most helpful response by the nurse to the daughter is:

1. "Your father needs opportunities to be independent. This will help him become self-sufficient."
2. "Your father is capable of taking care of himself. Try to allow him more independence."
3. "Stress is not good for your father at this time. Perhaps you could call your children."
4. "You are feeling concern for both your dad and your children. Let me know when you are leaving, and I'll stay with him."

30. A 20-day-old infant is recovering from surgery for pyloric stenosis. The client's mother asked the nurse, "Now that my son has had this surgery, is it likely that pyloric stenosis will cause trouble later?" An appropriate nursing response to the mother would be:

1. "Why don't you talk to the doctor about your uncertainties regarding your son's future?"
2. "He might develop obstructive symptoms later. If so, take him immediately to an emergency room."
3. "He will not have symptoms again in childhood, but may have digestive difficulties in his adult life."
4. "Recurrence of the obstruction or repetition of the surgical procedure would be unlikely."

31. A chronic alcoholic has been hospitalized following a drinking binge. During a lengthy conversation with the nurse about his long history of alcoholism, the client becomes tense and uncomfortable. Which of the following is the initial response by the nurse?

1. "What did I say to make you feel so uncomfortable?"
2. "Drinking for a long time can make anyone feel uncomfortable."
3. "At what point did you begin to feel uncomfortable?"
4. "Talking about your drinking will help you to recover."

32. A female client has been diagnosed with breast cancer. She has become quiet and thoughtful and says to the nurse, "What do you think people will say about me when I'm gone?" Which response by the nurse is the most helpful to the client?

1. "You will be remembered as a very nice person."
2. "Do you feel that people will be talking about you after your death?"
3. "At this time, a positive attitude can influence your recovery."
4. "The thought of your breast cancer must seem hopeless."

33. A woman is admitted to the ICU on a ventilator after attempting suicide. As the husband is talking with the nurse, he begins to cry. He says, "It's all my fault. I should have been home more often to keep an eye on her." Which response to the husband by the nurse would be most helpful initially?

1. "You seem to regret not being there for your wife. How can you feel that way when you have to earn a living?"
2. "At this time you need your privacy. I will return later, and we can talk then."
3. "This is an important issue that you need to bring up at your family therapy session."
4. "It must have been hard to be away when your wife was so sick."

34. A hospitalized client says to the nurse, "I'm a terrible person, and I should be dead." Which response by the nurse would be appropriate initially?

1. "That is why you are here. We are trying to help you with your bad feelings."
2. "Feeling that way must be awful. What makes you feel so terrible?"
3. "Feeling like a terrible person is part of your illness. As you get better, those feelings will lessen."
4. "You are not terrible. You are not a bad person."

35. An elderly client with Alzheimer's disease is admitted to the hospital. His daughter says to the nurse, "I really feel guilty about leaving my father, but I need to go home." The most helpful response by the nurse to the daughter is:

1. "Your father is well cared for here."
2. "Your worried feelings are normal."
3. "When you are getting ready to leave, tell me. I will sit with your father."
4. "Can I call another family member to stay with him?"

Chapter 12

DRILL QUESTIONS ON FUNDAMENTAL NURSING CONCEPTS: ANSWERS AND ANALYSIS

Section 1: The Role of the Nurse

1. The nursing assistant says to the nurse, "This client is incontinent of stool three or four times a day. I get angry when I think that he is doing it just to get attention. I think adult diapers should be used for him." How should the nurse initially respond to the nursing assistant?

1. "You probably are right. Soiling the bed is one way of getting attention from the nursing staff."
2. "Changing his bed and cleaning him must be tiresome for you. Next time it happens, I'll help you."
3. "It's upsetting to see an adult regress."
4. "Why don't you spend more time with him if you think that he is behaving this way to get more attention?"

1. *INCORRECT. The nursing assistant is the client in this question! This response is not therapeutic because it does not address the nursing assistant's feelings and does not encourage expression of feelings. The communication block of showing approval can be identified by the phrase, "You probably are right."*
2. *INCORRECT. This response correctly identifies the nursing assistant as the client in the question and uses the communication tool of empathy. However, this is not the best option. This response does not encourage any further expression of feelings, seek any additional information about the client's soiling the bed purposely, or provide any information. Read all the choices before selecting your answer.*
3. ***CORRECT. The nursing assistant is the client in this question. This response encourages further communication because it is empathetic and offers a possible explanation of the client's behavior. This response is therapeutic.***
4. *INCORRECT. The nursing assistant is the client in this question. This response begins with a non-therapeutic "why" question and does not address the feelings of the client. It also gives advice, which blocks communication. Finally, it fails to address the client's feelings.*

2. A client is to have a perineal examination, which requires the dorsal recumbent position. Which of the following nursing actions provides the client with the most privacy?

1. Place a bath blanket on the client with one corner at the chest, two corners wrapped around the feet and legs, and the fourth corner draped between the client's legs.
2. Drape a draw sheet over the client's knees covering the abdomen and legs.
3. Place a bath blanket on the client, with the top at the chest and the bottom draped over the knees to cover the legs and feet.
4. Close the examination room door.

1. ***CORRECT. This option provides the most privacy for the client by keeping the client completely covered until the examination is performed. The examiner can lift the corner of the blanket that is between the client's legs and expose only the perineal area.***

TEST-TAKING TIP: The phrase "draped between the client's legs" in this option is similar to "perineal" in the question. This is a clue that this may be the correct answer.

2. *INCORRECT. This option does not provide much privacy since the legs are not wrapped and the sheet must be pushed up to expose the perineum, which exposes the legs and thighs.*
3. *INCORRECT. Since the blanket must be pushed up to examine the perineum, the client's legs and thighs are completely exposed.*
4. *INCORRECT. Closing the door is appropriate but draping the client properly provides more privacy, since anyone can open the examination room door.*

3. While administering a bed bath it is important for the nurse to maintain privacy. Which is the best method for maintaining the client's privacy?

1. Allow the client to wear a gown, and reach under the gown with the washcloth and towel to bathe the client.
2. Use towels to protect the bed linen.
3. Cover the client with a bath blanket and expose only the portion of the body that is being bathed.
4. Use the bed sheet to cover the client during the bath.

1. *INCORRECT. The gown should be removed when performing a bed bath. It does not absorb water well and may cause the client to become chilled. Note also that the gown is not clean and may be soiled, which defeats one of the purposes of the bath, which is to cleanse the skin.*
2. *INCORRECT. Using towels to protect the bed linen is appropriate during a bed bath; however, the stem of the question asks about maintaining the client's privacy. This option does not address the issue in the question.*
3. ***CORRECT. The nurse should provide privacy by exposing only the portion of the body that is being bathed. A bath blanket should be used because it provides a covering for the client that absorbs water and avoids chilling of the client.***
4. *INCORRECT. While the bed sheet may provide privacy for the client, it does not absorb water well and will result in the client's being chilled.*

4. In protecting the privacy of a client, the nurse should avoid reporting which of the following to a government agency?

1. Child abuse.
2. Deaths.
3. Client's change of employment.
4. Elder abuse.

1. *INCORRECT. Child abuse must be reported. The nurse should follow the institution's procedures.*
2. *INCORRECT. Deaths must always be reported. The nurse should follow the institution's procedures.*
3. ***CORRECT. Changing employment is a private concern of the client. The client has the right to withhold this information, and it is NOT to be reported.***
4. *INCORRCT. Elder abuse is client data that must be reported. The nurse should follow the institution's procedures.*

TEST-TAKING TIP: This question has a false response stem.

5. The nurse knows that it is not necessary to report which of the following events to a government agency?

1. Births.
2. Child abuse.
3. Marital quarrels.
4. Typhoid fever.

1. *INCORRECT. Births are required to be reported. The nurse should follow the institution's procedures.*
2. *INCORRECT. Child abuse must be reported, and the nurse should follow the institution's procedures.*
3. ***CORRECT. Marital quarrels are not subject to reporting requirements. This client data is protected by the client's right to privacy.***
4. *INCORRECT. Typhoid fever, a communicable disease, must be reported.*

TEST-TAKING TIP: This question has a false response stem.

6. The nurse understands that which action is inconsistent with a client's right of privacy:

1. Refusing to have a gunshot wound reported, upon timely request.
2. Refusing to receive visitors.
3. Generally being able to wear one's own clothing.
4. Requesting the presence of a member of the same sex during a physical examination.

1. ***CORRECT. Gunshot wounds must be reported. The nurse should follow the institution's procedures.***

TEST-TAKING TIP: This question has a false response stem. You are looking for something that is NOT a privacy right of the client.

2. *INCORRECT. Clients have the right to maintain privacy by choosing their company, and they may choose not to receive visitors.*
3. *INCORRECT. The client has the right to wear personal clothing unless it interferes with medical procedures. An example of a situation where personal clothing would interfere is surgery.*

TEST-TAKING TIP: Note that words like "generally" tend to make a statement true. However, this question has a false response stem. You are looking for something that is NOT a privacy right of the client.

4. *INCORRECT. The client does have this right, and such a request should be respected by the nurse.*

> **TEST-TAKING TIP:** This question has a false response stem. You are looking for something that is NOT a privacy right of the client.

7. The home health nurse notes several suspicious bruises and old burns on a 10-month-old child while making an initial home visit. The priority nursing action to provide for the child's safety is to:

1. Call the child protection hotline and report possible abuse.
2. Discuss the family with the physician and social worker at the next team meeting.
3. Tell the mother that child protection will be notified if injuries are noted on the next visit.
4. Carefully record the visit for follow-up.

1. ***CORRECT. This is the necessary first action to take in providing for the child's safety. As a "mandated reporter," the nurse is legally obligated to report any cases of suspected abuse. The reporter does not need to prove the case, just report the facts known. This is the law.***

> **TEST-TAKING TIP:** The issue in this question is suspicion of child abuse. Note the use of the words "child" and "possible abuse" in this option. Also, since this action is legally required and "provides for the child's safety," as asked in the stem of the question, you know it is a correct nursing action. Go with what you know!

2. *INCORRECT. The nurse could be considered negligent according to the laws of the state within which the nurse practices. Waiting "until the next team meeting" is too long a delay before acting to protect the child.*
3. *INCORRECT. This action will drive the family underground and will not help you develop a therapeutic relationship with the mother. She is likely not to be at home the next time you visit. What is the nurse's legal responsibility?*
4. *INCORRECT. You didn't do anything that will either stop the abuse or initiate an immediate investigation. Hint: What does mandated reporter mean?*

8. An elderly male client is to have Foley urinary catheter care daily. Which of the following is the best action to provide for the client's privacy during this treatment?

1. Pull the curtain around the client's bed.
2. Cover the penis with a towel while performing catheter care.
3. Close the door to the client's room.
4. Ask the client's roommate to leave until the treatment is finished.

1. ***CORRECT. Pulling the curtain provides the most privacy for the client. With the curtain pulled, neither the roommate nor anyone entering the room will have visual access to the client or the treatment being performed.***
2. *INCORRECT. Performing catheter care includes cleansing and inspection of the urinary meatus. This cannot be accomplished if the penis is covered.*
3. *INCORRECT. While closing the door provides some privacy for the client, anyone can open the door and unnecessarily expose the client to the person entering the room and others in the hallway.*
4. *INCORRECT. It is not necessary for the client's roommate to leave the room while catheter care is performed. Also, anyone can open the door and unnecessarily expose the client to the person entering the room and others in the hallway.*

9. The nurse knows which action is the most common cause of violation of a client's privacy?

1. Over-exposing a client during a treatment or examination.
2. Failing to pull the curtain while performing a treatment or examination.
3. Talking about the client to other staff members who are not involved with the care of the client, or within hearing of the public.
4. Helping a client with a tub bath.

1. *INCORRECT. It is true that only the body part that is involved in an examination or treatment should be exposed, in order to provide as much privacy as possible for the client. This is not, however, the most common violation of privacy. Read all the options before selecting the best one.*
2. *INCORRECT. It is true that the curtain should be closed whenever a client is to have a treatment or examination that may expose body parts. However, this is not the most common violation of privacy.*
3. ***CORRECT. Talking about the client is the most common cause of invasion of privacy in the health care setting. No information about the client, including personal concerns, diagnosis, and treatment, should be discussed with anyone who is not involved in the care of the client. The nurse should take special care not to compromise the client's privacy by discussing client care in such places as elevators, restaurants, or other areas that are accessible to the public and where the discussion might be overheard.***
4. *INCORRECT. Although there is loss of privacy for the client when assisting with a tub bath, this nursing intervention is performed when necessary to provide for the safety of the client.*

10. An elderly client is confused. The charge nurse says that the client is constipated and is to have a soap suds enema. As the nurse is explaining the procedure, the client states that she doesn't think that she is supposed to have an enema. At this time, the nurse should:

1. Tell the client that her doctor must have ordered the procedure.
2. Assure the client that although the procedure sounds unpleasant, she will feel better afterwards.
3. Check the client's chart for the doctor's order to help clarify the situation.
4. Record on the chart that the client refused the enema.

1. *INCORRECT. This option ignores the client's concern about whether or not she is really supposed to have an enema. The nurse cannot just ignore her concern because she is confused. Ignoring the client's concern is not therapeutic communication! Also, a confused client may be correct about this information. The nurse must address the client's concern and provide for the client's safety.*
2. *INCORRECT. The fact that the client doesn't think she is supposed to have an enema needs to be addressed. This option blocks communication by using a cliché and does not give any credibility to the client's concerns. Also, a confused client may be correct about this information. The nurse must address the client's concern and provide for the client's safety.*
3. ***CORRECT. Looking at the doctor's orders will help to clarify the situation and will reassure the client that the procedure was ordered for her. Even with a confused client, the nurse must address the client's concern and take action to provide for the client's safety.***
4. *INCORRECT. The client didn't refuse the enema.*

11. An elderly client is admitted to a long-term care facility. Which of the following nursing measures would be most important in planning his care?

1. An explanation of the roles of the registered nurse, practical nurse and the nursing assistant.
2. Obtaining information about his routine for his own care at home.
3. An assessment of his mobility.
4. An introduction to his health care team members.

1. *INCORRECT. Although explanations to the client are necessary to help him feel comfortable in the new surroundings, this is not the most important nursing action in planning his care.*

> ***TEST-TAKING TIP:*** Options 1 and 4 involve giving information to the client about the staff and are implementation actions. These similar distractors can be eliminated.

2. ***CORRECT. It is most important that the nurse understand the client's routines at home so that these routines may be integrated in his present care. The goal of the nurse is to create a safe environment for the client and provide for his well-being. Following pre-existing routines will help the client feel more secure and less threatened. This question requires the ability to plan nursing care for an elderly client.***

> ***TEST-TAKING TIP:*** This option is an assessment action, and it is more global than option 3.

3. *CORRECT. The ability of the client to move and care for himself is important in planning his care. However, this is not the most important measure.*

> ***TEST-TAKING TIP:*** Look for an option that is more comprehensive or global.

4. *INCORRECT. The stem asks you to select the most important nursing measure in planning this client's care. Although introducing the client to members of the health care team is important to help the client feel safe and comfortable in his new surroundings, it is not the most important action.*

> ***TEST-TAKING TIP:*** Options 1 and 4 involve giving information to the client about the staff and are implementation actions. These similar distractors can be eliminated.

12. Of the following information, which should the admitting nurse record first in the client's record?

1. The client's vital signs.
2. The plan that was developed for the care of the client while in the hospital.
3. Nursing actions performed for the client.
4. Assessment of the client.

1. *INCORRECT. The client's vital signs should be recorded in the client's record in order to document that the nurse assessed the client's condition on admission. This is an appropriate nursing action and a possible answer, but it is not the best option. Look for one that's more global.*
2. *INCORRECT. The plan of care should be documented. A plan cannot be developed, however, until the nurse finds out more about the client.*
3. *INCORRECT. Nursing actions are documented as the plan of care is implemented. Since the case scenario tells you that the client is being admitted, the nursing process requires that the nurse gather data and develop a plan before implementing actions.*
4. ***CORRECT. The nurse should document the findings on assessment in order to provide information concerning the status of the client on admission.***

> ***TEST-TAKING TIP:*** This prioritizing question uses the nursing process. The nurse must assess first, before planning or implementing care. Also, note that this option is more global than option 1.

13. A female client with a history of severe multiple sclerosis has requested a living will and has asked the nurse to witness it. The nurse's appropriate response is:

1. "I would be honored to witness the will."
2. "I think your physician should witness the will."
3. "It would be a conflict of interest for me to witness the will, since I do not believe in living wills."
4. "I am unable to witness the will because of my professional relationship with you. Is there someone else you know who could do so?"

1. *INCORRECT. A nurse is not permitted to witness the living will of her/his client. Such a witness would be invalid because of the nurse's professional relationship with the client.*
2. *INCORRECT. A physician is not permitted to witness the living will of his/her client. Such a witness would be invalid because of the physician's professional relationship with the client. Also, this response*

by the nurse does not address the issue in the question because it does not identify why the nurse cannot sign the living will.

3. *INCORRECT. There is a conflict of interest here, but it is because of the nurse's professional relationship with the client, not the nurse's beliefs. A nurse is prohibited from witnessing the living will of his/her client, and such a witness would be invalid. Note that this response also uses the communication block of referring to an inappropriate issue: the nurse's beliefs are not important.*

> ***TEST-TAKING TIP:*** There is no information in the introductory statement that the nurse objects to living wills. This cannot be the best option.

4. ***CORRECT. The nurse is prohibited from witnessing the living will because of his/her professional relationship with the client. Such a witness would be invalid. This response also promotes communication by encouraging the client to think of others who could witness the will.***

14. Which of the following is the most effective nursing action to maintain maximum privacy for the client during a medical procedure?

1. Closing the door of the client's room.
2. Pulling the curtains around the client's bed.
3. Asking family members to leave the room.
4. Using sterile drapes to cover the client.

1. *INCORRECT. This action may be appropriate and will help maintain a secure environment, but it is not the best action to maintain privacy for the client. If someone opens the door or enters the room, the client's privacy may be violated.*
2. ***CORRECT. This is the best action for providing maximum privacy for the client. In each of the other options, the client's privacy will not be protected if someone enters the room.***
3. *INCORRECT. This is appropriate, bu not the best action to maintain privacy for the client. After family members leave, someone else may enter the room.*
4. *INCORRECT. During a procedure, the body part that is involved will be exposed to provide access for the nurse or physician. The client's privacy will not be protected if someone enters the room.*

15. The nurse is caring for an elderly client who will soon be discharged to a long-term care facility. What nursing action is most important to promote her continued recovery?

1. Reviewing the client's nursing care plan with the client's daughter.
2. Discussing the client's nursing care needs with her physician.
3. Telephoning the charge nurse at the long-term care facility to explain the client's nursing care needs.
4. Sending a written summary of the nursing care plan for the client to the long-term care facility.

1. *INCORRECT. This is not the most important action. The family should know about the client's needs for care, but there is a better way to promote continuity of care.*
2. *INCORRECT. This action is not sufficient to ensure continuity of nursing care when the client is admitted to the long-term care facility, even for clients who will continue to use the same physician. Look for a nursing action that will promote continuity of the client's nursing care.*
3. *INCORRECT. This action might be a possibility, since it will promote continuity of care, but it is not adequate to accurately communicate complete information of the client's nursing care needs.*
4. ***CORRECT. A written summary of the nursing care plan for the client is the best way of conveying the client's nursing care needs to the nurses who will actually work with her in the long-term care facility.***

> ***TEST-TAKING TIP:*** Note that options 1, 2 and 3 all involve talking with the family or other health care providers. This option is different: it provides written documentation of the client's care and needs, which is an important nursing responsibility.

16. In preparing a client to be discharged, the nurse teaches him to position himself for postural drainage. To achieve success in this teaching program, which information about the client does the nurse recognize to be most important?

1. The type of bed the client will be using at home for the procedure.
2. The amount of time required for the client to change positions.
3. The client's goal concerning his ability to be self-sufficient.
4. The client's ability to move about without assistance from others.

1. *INCORRECT. The type of bed the client will be using at home is important information, since a mechanical bed greatly facilitates the procedure. However, postural drainage can be done without a mechanical bed, using things normally found in the home such as pillows and a straight-back chair. The key word in the stem of this question is "most."*

> ***TEST-TAKING TIP:*** Which of the priority-setting guidelines should be applied in answering this teaching/learning question?

2. *INCORRECT. The amount of time required for the client to change positions is important, but it is not "most important."*

> ***TEST-TAKING TIP:*** Which of the priority-setting guidelines should be applied in answering this teaching/learning question?

3. ***CORRECT. The client's motivation and goals are essential for success, and they are a primary concern in any teaching program. Teaching/Learning theory tells us that if the client is not motivated or goal directed, the discharge teaching program is unlikely to be effective.***

TEST-TAKING TIP: This option is different from all the others, which refer to physical considerations (the type of bed and the client's mobility).

4. *INCORRECT. The client's ability to move about without assistance from others is important, but it is not the "most important" consideration.*

TEST-TAKING TIP: Which of the priority- setting guidelines should be used in answering this teaching/learning question?

17. A client tells the nurse that he is feeling short of breath and requests that the nurse assist him in changing position. In addition to repositioning the client, which nursing action should be given the highest nursing priority?

1. Put the client on 15 minute checks.
2. Call the charge nurse to report the shortness of breath.
3. Observe the rate, depth, and character of the client's respirations.
4. Give a back rub to help the client to relax.

1. *INCORRECT. Any client with a breathing problem must be monitored closely, because a medical emergency may develop. The nurse's decision to check the client every fifteen minutes is an implementation action, and it implies that the shortness of breath does not represent a medical emergency at this time. There is not enough information to support this as the correct answer.*
2. *INCORRECT. This is an implementation action. Additional data should be collected before the charge nurse is notified. The nurse needs to complete collecting data by further monitoring the respirations.*
3. ***CORRECT. This is an assessment activity and should be done first. Before initiating 15 minute checks, calling the doctor, or giving a back rub, an assessment should be made. Following the assessment, one or more of the actions in the other options may be done, as appropriate.***

TEST-TAKING TIP: The nursing process identifies that the nurse must assess before planning or implementing care. When prioritizing, consider whether more data is required by the nurse.

4. *INCORRECT. Giving a back rub is an implementation action that implies that the shortness of breath does not represent a medical emergency. What is the nursing priority at this time?*

Section 2: Safety, Body Mechanics and Mobility

1. A client is confused and disoriented when admitted to the hospital. The doctor has ordered bed rest. Before leaving the client's room, the most important nursing action to provide for the client's safety is to:

1. Put all of the client's belongings in a safe place.
2. Place the bed in the highest position with the side rails up.
3. Place the bed in the lowest position with the side rails up.
4. Explain where everything is in the room.

1. *INCORRECT. This action is appropriate, but it is not the most important action in providing for the client's safety.*
2. *INCORRECT. Placing the bed in the highest position puts the client at risk for falling.*
3. ***CORRECT. This option provides for the client's safety by reducing the risk of falling.***
4. *INCORRECT. The client is confused and disoriented, and may not understand explanations.*

2. A client is admitted to the hospital and the physician orders stat blood work. The laboratory technician says to the nurse, "I can't do the stat blood work because the client doesn't have an identification bracelet on." The best nursing action is to:

1. Draw the blood for the laboratory technician, since the nurse can identify the client.
2. Assure the laboratory technician that you will verify that he has the correct client.
3. Obtain an identification bracelet for the client as quickly as possible.
4. Ask the client to identify himself to the laboratory technician.

1. *INCORRECT. Even though the nurse knows the client, the client must have an identification band to ensure that the name and hospital numbers match the laboratory requisitions. This is necessary to prevent errors in reporting results.*

TEST-TAKING TIP: Options 1 and 2 both include the nurse's identifying the client—and neither resolves the issue of the client's lack of an identification bracelet. These similar options can be eliminated.

2. *INCORRECT. This will not adequately provide for the client's safety. In order to prevent erroneous reporting of lab results, the laboratory technician needs to match the client's name and number from the identification bracelet with those on the laboratory requisition.*

TEST-TAKING TIP: Options 1 and 2 both include the nurse's identifying the client — and neither resolves the issue of the client's lack of an identification bracelet. These similar options can be eliminated.

3. ***CORRECT. The client needs an identification bracelet to provide for his safety in all aspects of hospitalization.***

> **TEST-TAKING TIP:** This option is the only option that addresses the issue of the client's lack of an identification bracelet — and the only one that uses those words. If you weren't sure of the answer, these similar words would be a clue. Note also that options 1 and 2 are similar to each other and can be eliminated.

4. *INCORRECT. The client's name alone is not sufficient identification to ensure the safety of the client. Clients with the same name can be hospitalized in the same health care facility.*

3. A confused elderly client is on strict bedrest. Which nursing intervention will provide for this client's safety?

1. Place the client in a room away from the noise and confusion of the nurses' station.
2. Avoid the use of nightlights, since they tend to distort images and confuse clients.
3. Discuss with the client the need for restraints if she continues to get out of bed.
4. Provide opportunities for regular toileting, and include this information in the client's care plan.

1. *INCORRECT. Any client who is confused should be placed in a room near the nursing station —not away from it.*
2. *INCORRECT. A nightlight is generally used for confused clients, because it decreases image distortion and enhances reality. Also, the use of a nightlight helps orient clients to the hospital environment.*
3. *INCORRECT. This option is a good distractor, because it implies that by talking to the client, the nurse may be able to lessen her confusion. Wrong! If the client is confused, then the issue of safety requires that the nurse should focus on how to adapt the client's environment to decrease the risk of accidents.*
4. ***CORRECT. This client is confused, which means there is a high safety risk due to decreased ability to perceive danger. Providing opportunities for regular toileting helps ensure that the client's basic needs for elimination will be met, and will greatly reduce the risk of the client's falling while trying to get up and go to the bathroom without the assistance of the nurse. This nursing action provides for the comfort and safety of the client, and it should be recorded in the plan of care.***

4. An elderly, confused client is on bed rest. Which nursing intervention will be ineffective in providing for this client's safety?

1. Provide regular toileting.
2. Explain to the client that she should use the call light if she needs to get up.
3. Place the side rails in the up position and check on the client often.
4. Initiate the proper use of restraints.

1. *INCORRECT—this is an important and necessary nursing action. When a confused, elderly client has the physiological need to void or have a bowel movement, an attempt is usually made to find a bathroom. This attempt may result in a fall for the confused client.*

> **TEST-TAKING TIP:** Since this question has a false response stem, the correct answer is something that will NOT help prevent a fall.

2. ***CORRECT. This client is confused, and thus may not be able to perceive danger. A confused client is also unlikely to remember instructions concerning the use of the call light. This action will not effectively provide for the client's safety.***
3. *INCORRECT. This is an important and necessary nursing action. The side rails should be in the up position to prevent the client from falling out of bed, and to serve as a reminder to the client to remain in bed.*
4. *INCORRECT. This nursing action would be effective in preventing a fall. If the client is assessed and it is determined that she needs to be restrained in order to avoid injury, then restraints may be applied, and the physician notified of the situation. Note that the option provides for the PROPER use of restraints.*

> **TEST-TAKING TIP:** Since this question has a false response stem, the correct answer is something that will NOT help prevent a fall.

5. A middle-aged client is hospitalized following myocardial infarction. He is to be transferred from a cart to a bed in a room on a unit. When transferring the client from a cart to his bed, the priority nursing action is to:

1. Have the client place his arms on his chest.
2. Lock the wheels on the cart and the bed.
3. Have at least four people help with the transfer.
4. Use a draw sheet to move the client.

1. *INCORRECT. Although placing the arms across the chest helps protect the client's arms from injury, this option is not the priority.*

> **TEST-TAKING TIP:** In this prioritizing question, see if you can identify something else that the nurse should do FIRST.

2. ***CORRECT. Locking the wheels stabilizes the cart and bed, preventing the client from falling between them during the transfer. This is the priority action for transferring a client.***
3. *INCORRECT. Four people may or may not be the number needed for a transfer. The number will depend on the size of the client and the size of the persons performing the transfer.*

> **TEST-TAKING TIP:** In this prioritizing question, see if you can identify something else that the nurse should do FIRST.

4. *INCORRECT. Although a draw sheet is often used to transfer clients between two level horizontal surfaces, this is neither a requirement nor a priority action.*

6. A client has left-sided weakness secondary to a stroke. In assisting him out of bed, which nursing action is safest?

1. Allow the client to do as much of the transfer as possible.
2. Lock the wheels of the bed and wheelchair.
3. Place the client's hands around the nurse's neck for support.
4. Place the front of the wheelchair at a right angle to the bed.

1. *INCORRECT. While it is important to encourage self care to the extent that is appropriate, this client has left-sided weakness and is at risk for falling. The nurse needs to prioritize so that the client's safety is the most important factor.*
2. ***CORRECT. The bed and wheelchair must both be stabilized to prevent the client from falling and being injured.***
3. *INCORRECT. Holding onto the nurse's neck places undue stress on the neck and back. If the client loses his balance and falls, the nurse, as well as the client, is at risk for injury. The client should place his hands on the nurse's shoulders.*
4. *INCORRECT. With this option, the client would have to turn almost 180 degrees to get into the chair. The wheelchair should be placed parallel to the bed.*

7. The doctor has ordered restraints for a very agitated client. When applying restraints to the client, which nursing action is least appropriate?

1. Using the least restrictive type of restraint that will effectively protect the client from injury.
2. Fastening the restraints to the bed frame.
3. Tying the restraint with a knot that cannot be undone easily, in order to prevent the client from untying it.
4. Explaining to the client and family the type of restraint and the reason for applying the restraint.

1. *INCORRECT. This action is appropriate. Over-restraining a client can intensify the problems caused by immobility. The question asks you to identify an action that is INAPPROPRIATE.*
2. *INCORRECT. This is an appropriate nursing action. The bed frame, rather than the side rails should be used to attach the restraints because the bed frame is more stable. Lowering side rails that have restraints attached can result in injury to the client. The question asks you to identify an INAPPROPRIATE action.*
3. ***CORRECT. This is something that the nurse should NOT do! Restraints should be tied with knots that can be undone easily, in case the client's well being necessitates removal of the restraints. To protect the client from releasing the restraints, the knot should be placed where the client cannot reach it.***
4. *INCORRECT. Restraints can increase the client's confusion and cause anger and hostility in the client and family. An explanation concerning the client's safety can help to promote understanding and cooperation. The question asks you to identify an INAPPROPRIATE action.*

8. A postoperative client is ambulatory and wishes to go to the day room. While the nurse is walking down the hall with the client, the client says that she feels faint and starts to fall. The nurse should:

1. Grasp the client around the waist and hold her up so she doesn't fall and injure herself.
2. Hold the client up against the wall to keep her from falling.
3. Ease the client gently to the floor.
4. Ask another client to get some help while supporting the client to prevent her from falling.

1. *INCORRECT. Preventing injury to the client is the most important action. This option may result in both the client and the nurse falling, putting both individuals at risk for injury.*
2. *INCORRECT. Holding the client against the wall will not prevent the fall and may cause injury to the client from the impact against the wall.*
3. ***CORRECT. Easing the client gently to the floor is the best action, since it protects both the client and the nurse from injury.***
4. *INCORRECT. Attempting to hold a client who is fainting upright places the nurse at risk for injury. If the client becomes too heavy, then the client may be injured if the nurse becomes fatigued and can no longer support her.*

9. The first, most important nursing action when a nurse discovers a fire in a client's room is to:

1. Pull the fire alarm and notify the hospital operator.
2. Close fire doors and client room doors.
3. Remove the client from the room.
4. Place moist towels or blankets at the threshold of the door of the room with the fire.

1. *INCORRECT. Pulling the fire alarm and alerting the hospital operator notifies the appropriate individuals who are needed to fight a fire. But this is not the first nursing action! The immediate safety of the client in the room with the fire takes priority.*
2. *INCORRECT. This action does not address the immediate safety of the client in the room with the fire! After providing for the safety of this client, closing fire doors and other clients' room doors will help prevent the spread of a fire to other areas of the hospital and help prevent smoke and fumes from entering their rooms. What should the nurse do first?*
3. ***CORRECT. The client in the room with the fire is at highest risk for injury. The smoke from a fire can deprive a client of adequate oxygenation, and the fire poses a direct threat to the safety of the client. Moving this client to safety receives first priority.***
4. *INCORRECT. Placing moist towels or blankets at the threshold of the door where the smoke is coming from helps prevent the smoke and fumes from entering other areas. This is an inappropriate action in this situation because the fire is in the client's*

room! The client is at risk for injury and oxygen deprivation. The immediate safety of the client in the room with the fire takes priority.

10. The nurse finds an elderly client standing in a puddle of water in the hallway of the unit. The nurse does not know this client. What is the nurse's initial action?

1. Ask the client for her name and room number.
2. Wipe up the water until the floor is completely dry.
3. Call the supervisor for assistance in identifying the client.
4. Have the client wait in the lounge until security arrives.

1. *INCORRECT. The issue in this question is the puddle of water on the floor. The water on the floor threatens the immediate safety of the client and others on the unit. After the nurse assures safety, she can identify the client and assist with getting her back to where she belongs.*
2. ***CORRECT. The issue in this question is the puddle of water on the floor. The water on the floor threatens the immediate safety of the client and others on the unit. The nurse's first action should be to alleviate the safety hazard by wiping up the water.***

> ***TEST-TAKING TIP:*** Maslow's Hierarchy of Needs indicates that when no physiological need exists, safety needs should receive priority. Note that the word "water" in the question is repeated in this option. The test-taking strategy of looking for similar words in the question would identify this option as a possible answer.

3. *INCORRECT. The issue in this question is the puddle of water on the floor which threatens the immediate safety of the client and others on the unit. After the nurse assures safety, she can identify the client and assist with getting her back to where she belongs.*
4. *INCORRECT. The issue in this question is the puddle of water on the floor which threatens the immediate safety of the client and others on the unit. Asking the client to wait in the lounge until security arrives does not assure safety. Someone may still slip on the puddle of water and injure themselves.*

11. A client is paralyzed from the waist down. He is to be up in a chair three times a day. What is the best nursing approach when transferring the client from a bed into a wheelchair?

1. Place the wheelchair close to the foot of the bed.
2. Utilize the principles of body mechanics while providing a safe transfer for the client.
3. Slide the client to the edge of the bed, keeping the nurse's back straight and using a rocking motion to pull the client.
4. Place the nurse's arms under the client's axillae from the back of the client.

1. *INCORRECT. The wheelchair should be placed as close to the position of the client's buttocks as possible for a safe and easy transfer. The wheelchair should not be placed at the foot of the bed.*
2. ***CORRECT. The nurse is in control of his or her own body and the client's movement during the transfer. Providing for the safety of the client, and utilizing the principles of body mechanics to provide safety for the nurse and the client, is the best nursing approach.***

> ***TEST-TAKING TIP:*** Options 3 and 4 describe specific actions that are correct in transferring a client, but Option 2 is the best option because it is the most comprehensive or global statement of the correct nursing approach.

3. *INCORRECT. This is an appropriate nursing action, which addresses the safety of the nurse and client. Positioning the client near the edge of the bed will reduce the energy required to move the client to the wheelchair, and the nurse's back will be protected by using leg and arm muscles to move the client to the edge of the bed. There is another option, however, that better describes the best nursing approach in transferring this client.*
4. *INCORRECT. This is a correct action, which helps provide for the nurse's and the client's safety. Supporting the upper portion of the client's body helps to place the weight of the client over the nurse's center of gravity. There is another option, however, that better describes the best nursing approach in transferring this client.*

12. When transporting a client, the nurse should:

1. Always use a stretcher.
2. Push the stretcher quickly so the client does not become chilled during the transport.
3. Never cover a client with a blanket, since it can get caught in the wheels.
4. Use the safety rails or straps that are available on the equipment.

1. *INCORRECT. A stretcher is not always necessary for transport; a wheelchair may be used safely in many cases.*

> ***TEST-TAKING TIP:*** The absolute word "always" does not take all circumstances into account and is a clue that this option may be incorrect.

2. *INCORRECT. The stretcher should not be pushed quickly. This may increase the client's anxiety and does not provide for safe transport. It doesn't prevent the client's becoming chilled, either!*

> ***TEST-TAKING TIP:*** When no physiological need is identified, try to find an option that addresses a safety issue.

3. *INCORRECT. The client should be covered to provide warmth and privacy. Tucking in the edges of the blanket will prevent the blanket from getting caught in the wheels of the stretcher.*

4. ***CORRECT. Straps and belts are provided for the client's safety and should be used to prevent falls. This is the best option because it is the only correct option that provides for the client's safety.***

> ***TEST-TAKING TIP:*** When no physiological need is identified, try to find an option that addresses a safety issue.

13. The nurse finds an elderly client with her IV pulled out, standing next to her bed, with the side rails in the up position. The client is confused, does not have an identification bracelet on, and cannot remember her name. What action should the nurse take first?

1. Help the client into bed, and remind her to call the nurse when she wants to get out of bed.
2. Help the client into bed, and then restart the IV.
3. Place a restraining vest on the client.
4. Put an identification bracelet on the client and help her back to bed.

1. *INCORRECT. Reminding a confused client to use a call light is not an appropriate nursing action. The introductory statement tells you that the client cannot remember her name, so she will probably not remember to use a call light. Since a physiological need is not identified in this question, the safety of the client is the most important nursing consideration at this time. Which priority setting guideline will you use in this question? .*
2. *INCORRECT. The introductory statement does not tell you whether the IV has life saving medications or fluids infusing, so you cannot assume that the IV is a physiological need. Do not "read into" the question!*
3. ***CORRECT. The introductory statement tells you that the client got out of a bed that had the side rails up. This is an unsafe situation, since the client is at risk of falling. Such an injury can be life-threatening. Placing a restraining vest on the client will provide for her safety.***

> ***TEST-TAKING TIP:*** This prioritizing question uses Maslow's Hierarchy of Needs. Since no physiological need is identified, look for an option that provides for the client's immediate safety.

4. *INCORRECT. The client's lack of an identification bracelet is an important safety concern. The introductory statement, however, tells you that the client got out of a bed that had the side rails up. This is an unsafe situation, since the client is at risk for falling. Such an injury can be life-threatening. After the immediate physical safety of the client is assured, an identification bracelet can be obtained. Which priority setting guideline will you use in this question?*

14. A client tells the nurse that his name is not spelled correctly on his identification bracelet. The best nursing action is to:

1. Tell the client that as long as his medical record numbers are correct, the mistake is not a problem.
2. Ask the client for the correct spelling and change his medical records.
3. Notify the admitting office of the spelling error and obtain a correct identification bracelet for the client.
4. Notify the physician.

1. *INCORRECT. The client's identification bracelet should be corrected. It is possible that his name also appears incorrectly in his medical chart and other hospital records as well, and these records will have to be checked.*
2. *INCORRECT. The client's records will have to be corrected. However, this is not the correct procedure, since the hospital has other records in addition to the chart. The client's identification bracelet should also be corrected.*
3. ***CORRECT. The admitting office must be informed of the error, and the client's identification bracelet should show his name correctly.***

> ***TEST-TAKING TIP:*** This option includes the words "spelling" and "identification bracelet," like the introductory statement. This is a clue that this may be the correct answer.

4. *INCORRECT. The spelling of the client's name is not a medical problem. This in an inappropriate nursing action. The stem asks for a true statement.*

15. A client is admitted to the hospital for evaluation of inadequate circulation to her lower extremities. The doctor orders a tub bath at the client's request. In assisting the client with her bath, which nursing action would place the client at risk?

1. Place a rubber mat on the bottom of the tub.
2. Fill the tub approximately half full.
3. When the client steps into the tub, ask her if the water is the right temperature for her.
4. Obtain all of the supplies necessary for the bath and place them within easy reach of the client.

1. *INCORRECT. A rubber mat helps prevent slipping on a slippery tub bottom. This is an appropriate intervention. This question has a false response stem, however, so you are looking for an option that represents an action the nurse should NOT do.*
2. *INCORRECT. Since water is displaced when the client sits in the tub, filling the tub about half full will prevent the water from running over, which could result in a fall from water on the floor. This is an appropriate nursing action. This question has a false response stem, however, so you are looking for an option that represents an action the nurse should NOT do.*
3. ***CORRECT. This question has a false response stem, and this correct answer is something the nurse should NOT do. A client with poor circulation in the lower extremities will not be able to accurately detect feelings of hot and cold when stepping into a tub. For the safety and comfort of the client, the nurse should regulate the water temperature to between 105-110° F.***

4. *INCORRECT. The equipment should be available to the client, within easy reach. Safety is a concern here, as the client may slip and fall trying to reach the equipment. This question has a false response stem, however, so you are looking for an option that represents an action the nurse should NOT do.*

16. The client is very confused and combative. The physician orders the client to be placed in a jacket restraint and wrist restraints. In order to prevent injury to the client with restraints, the best nursing action is to:

1. Explain the procedure and reason for the restraints to the client and the family.
2. Remove the restraints and observe the extremities for circulation at least every four hours.
3. Tell the client that if he is more cooperative the restraints will not be necessary.
4. Document the use of restraints in the chart.

1. *INCORRECT. This is an important part of nursing care. However, this action will not prevent injury to the client.*
2. ***CORRECT. This nursing action will help prevent nerve and musculoskeletal injuries to the client as a result of poor circulation caused by the restraints.***
3. *INCORRECT. The introductory statement tells you that the client is confused. Giving him this choice is inappropriate.*
4. *INCORRECT. Documentation of the use of restraints and the client's behavior that warranted their use for the client's safety is very important. However, this action will not prevent injury to the client.*

17. Restraints may be used to immobilize a client, or the client's extremity. The nurse understands that an inappropriate use of restraints is to:

1. Prevent a client from pulling out an IV or other type of therapy.
2. Reduce the risk to all elderly clients from falling out of bed or off a chair.
3. Prevent removal of life support equipment.
4. Prevent injury to health care personnel by combative clients.

1. *INCORRECT—this is an appropriate use of restraints. A confused client may pull out an IV or nasogastric tube because of discomfort or inability to understand the purpose of the therapy.*

> ***TEST-TAKING TIP:*** Always identify the type of stem! You are looking for an INAPPROPRIATE rationale for the use of restraints.

2. ***CORRECT— you identified the inappropriate option. This option implies that ALL elderly clients should be restrained in order to reduce the risk of falls. Many elderly clients can care for themselves without falling. Each individual should be assessed for risk to fall.***

> ***TEST-TAKING TIP:*** Absolute words like "all," "every," and "always," or "none" or "never," are hints that a statement may be false. This question has a false response stem, so this false statement is the answer.

3. *INCORRECT — this is an appropriate use of restraints. Some clients may become combative or confused while on life support systems and may cause life support systems to become dislodged.*

> ***TEST-TAKING TIP:*** Always identify the type of stem! You are looking for an INAPPROPRIATE rationale for the use of restraints.

4. *INCORRECT — this is an appropriate use of restraints. Occasionally a client can become combative, and restraints can be the only means of protecting the health care worker while providing care.*

> ***TEST-TAKING TIP:*** Always identify the type of stem! You are looking for an INAPPROPRIATE rationale for the use of restraints.

18. A client has just been admitted to the hospital. In showing the client how to use the call system, the nurse understands which of the following statements should be avoided?

1. The call system allows the client to signal for help.
2. The call system should be limited to use in emergencies.
3. The client should be able to reach the call button easily.
4. The client should be taught how to use the call system.

1. *INCORRECT. It is necessary for the safety and well-being of the client to be able to signal for help when needed. The question asks you to select an option that is NOT a true statement about the call system.*
2. ***CORRECT. This question has a false response stem. The call system should be used whenever a client needs help, not only in emergencies. For the safety and well-being of the client, the client should be instructed how to use the system, and should be able to reach it easily and safely.***
3. *INCORRECT. It is necessary for the safety and well-being of the client to be able to reach the call bell easily. The question asks you to select an option that is NOT a true statement about the call system.*
4. *INCORRECT. It is necessary for the safety and well-being of the client to teach the client to use the call system. This question asks you to select an option that is not a true statement about the call system.*

19. A client has just returned to her room after abdominal surgery. She has a nasogastric tube in place and a drain attached to a Hemovac. The Foley catheter is draining clear yellow urine. The nurse understands the reason for maintaining the side rails in the raised position is to:

1. Prevent the urine collection bag and tubing from getting tangled up in the side rails when the client is turned in bed.
2. Prevent the client from falling out of bed after receiving an anesthetic.
3. Provide a place to attach the nasogastric tubing to prevent it from being dislodged.
4. Attach the call light so it is within easy reach.

1. INCORRECT. This option might be a possibility. However, the urine collection bag and tubing can be attached to the side rails even if the side rails are lowered, so this is not a reason for having the side rails up on the bed.

2 CORRECT. ***Post-operative clients who have received anesthesia are usually very sleepy and not aware of their surroundings. The client may fall out of bed if the side rails are not raised. This is the best option because it provides for the safety of the client.***

TEST-TAKING TIP: Note that the other options are concerned with attaching something to the side rails. These similar options can be eliminated.

3. INCORRECT. It is an incorrect nursing action to attach the nasogastric tube to the side rail, because it may become dislodged when the side rail is lowered or raised.

4. INCORRECT. The call light can be attached to the side rail even if the side rails are lowered, so this is not a reason for maintaining the side rails in a raised position.

20. A client is ambulating down the tile hallway in her stocking-covered feet. How should the nurse ensure the client's safety?

1. Remind the client to avoid any wet spots on the floor.
2. Tell the client that she should always wear slippers or shoes when ambulating.
3. Get the client's slippers and have her put them on.
4. No action is necessary, since the client has her feet covered.

1. INCORRECT. Although telling the client to avoid wet spots may help to prevent a fall, it is not the priority nursing action. Stocking feet are very slippery on a tile floor, and this situation needs to be addressed first.

TEST-TAKING TIP: The introductory statement doesn't mention any "wet spots" on the floor — and if there were any wet spots, the appropriate nursing action would be to wipe them up!

2. INCORRECT. The client should be instructed in proper footwear to avoid falling. This action alone, however, will not prevent this client from slipping on the tile floor. This client is at risk for a fall.

3. CORRECT. Making sure that slippers or shoes are worn by the client is the priority action, since it addresses immediately the problem of slipping on the tile floor.

4. INCORRECT. The client should have footwear that protects the client from slipping and falling.

21. A client is very irritable at breakfast. When asked if there is a problem, the client states that he was unable to sleep because of noise made by the staff on the night shift. The best initial response by the nurse is:

1. "It must be very distressing to be unable to sleep at night. Would you like to take a nap this morning?"
2. "I'll report that to the supervisor."
3. "Maybe we can move you to a room further from the nurses' station when one of those rooms becomes available."
4. "Why don't you close your door at night? Sometimes the nurses make noise and don't realize it."

1. CORRECT. Addressing the client's feelings is the first action by the nurse. This response lets the client know that his feelings are important and need to be addressed. This response also addresses the client's physiological need for sleep. Finally, this is also a safety issue: Sleep-deprived clients are at risk for injury related to decreased judgment, slower response time, and slower reflexes.

2. INCORRECT. Although reporting the situation to the supervisor may be appropriate, this response by the nurse is not therapeutic because it does not address the client's feelings or the problem of sleep deprivation, and passes the buck to the supervisor.

3. INCORRECT. Moving the client when a room becomes available does not address the client's present problem of sleep deprivation. Sleep-deprived clients are at risk for injury related to decreased judgment, slower response time, and slower reflexes.

4. INCORRECT. This response is not therapeutic, because it is defensive and attempts to provide justification for the noise. The client, for safety and health reasons, has the right to uninterrupted sleep (unless the physician's orders require that the client be awakened during the night).

22. The physician has determined that a client is extremely dehydrated and in need of intravenous fluids. The client is confused, and she has pulled out one intravenous catheter and caused another intravenous site to become infiltrated. The nurse restarts the IV in the client's left arm. An order for restraints is given. The best nursing action is to:

1. Apply a vest restraint and extremity restraints to ensure that the intravenous site will be protected.
2. Apply a restraint to the left arm.
3. Apply a restraint to the right arm.
4. Apply restraints to the right and left arms.

1. INCORRECT. This option completely restrains the client. The information in the introductory statement indicates that only the intravenous site is in need of being protected. This is an example of over-restraining a client and is inappropriate.

2. INCORRECT. Restraining the left arm allows the client to reach the intravenous site with the right hand. The intravenous site is not protected.

3. INCORRECT. Even though the right hand is restrained, the client can move the left hand over to the right side, which will allow the client to disturb the intravenous site.

4. ***CORRECT. Applying restraints to both upper extremities provides protection for the intravenous site. The client does not have the opportunity to disturb the site.***

23. The physician has ordered extremity restraints for safety reasons for a confused elderly client. After placing the client in extremity restraints, the priority nursing action is to:

1. Release each extremity every two hours for range of motion exercises.
2. Discuss the rationale for the restraints with the family members.
3. Reduce the client's distress by dimming the lights and closing the door.
4. Tie the restraints to the side rails using a half bow knot.

1. ***CORRECT. This is the priority action, because the client with restraints is at risk of circulatory problems and possible permanent injury. Releasing the extremity for range of motion exercises addresses this risk, and allows the nurse to assess for possible injury from the restraints.***
2. *INCORRECT. While it would be important to discuss the use of restraints with the family, it is not a priority action. Actions that ensure the safety of the client take priority.*
3. *INCORRECT. The nurse should never isolate a restrained client by turning the lights off and closing the door. The client's distress might be increased. It is also important to visually check on a restrained client frequently.*
4. *INCORRECT. The half bow knot is correct, but tying the restraints to the side rails is incorrect. The restraints are tied to the bed frame.*

24. An elderly client requires extremity restraints for safety reasons. After applying restraints to the client's extremities, the nurse should consider which of the following as a priority action concerned with the client's safety?

1. Documenting the type of restraints applied to the client.
2. Explaining to family members the reason for the restraints.
3. Checking the restraints for circulatory adequacy once during each shift.
4. Observing the restrained extremities for color and pulses at least every hour.

1. *INCORRECT. The application of and reason for the restraints should be documented in order to help protect the nurse from possible assault and battery charges; however, this option is not a priority action concerned with the client's safety.*

> ***TEST-TAKING TIP:*** Which priority-setting guideline would you use in this question?

2. *INCORRECT. Greater understanding and cooperation can be obtained from the family if they are given an explanation for the restraints placed on a client. This is not the most important action, however, because it does not directly address the safety of the client.*
3. *INCORRECT. Extremity restraints should be checked at least every hour. Allowing eight hours between checks can result in permanent damage to the client if circulation has been compromised by restraints that might be too tight or are improperly applied.*
4. ***CORRECT. This option is the priority action concerned with the client's safety. Observing the extremities for pulses and color allows the nurse to assess the potential for injury to the client that can be caused by the restraints.***

> ***TEST-TAKING TIP:*** This assessment action that provides for the client's safety takes priority over documenting or explaining to the family. This question uses the nursing process and Maslow's Hierarchy of Needs.

25. While caring for a client receiving fluids using an IV pump that is plugged into an electrical outlet, which of the following is the least appropriate nursing action?

1. Palpate the client's IV site while resetting the pump for the next bag of IV solution.
2. Assess the IV site.
3. Change the tubing according to hospital protocol.
4. Observe the pump for correct operation.

1. ***CORRECT. The client should never be touched at the same time that a piece of electrical equipment is being handled. If there were any electrical current leakage from the pump, it would transfer from the nurse to the client.***
2. *INCORRECT. Assessing an IV site for signs of phlebitis or infection should be done on a regular basis. The question asked you to identify an INAPPROPRIATE action, however, so this cannot be the correct answer.*
3. *INCORRECT. Whatever protocol the hospital uses should be carefully followed. The question asked you to identify an INAPPROPRIATE action, however, so this cannot be the correct answer.*
4. *INCORRECT. The pump should be observed to determine if it is operating correctly. The question asked you to identify an INAPPROPRIATE action, however, so this cannot be the correct answer.*

26. The nurse notices a fire in the linen room. Which type of extinguisher should the nurse use?

1. Dry powder.
2. Water.
3. Dry chemical.
4. Carbon dioxide.

1. *INCORRECT. Dry powder is used for metal fires. Think analytically: What kind of fire would likely occur in a linen room?*
2. ***CORRECT. Water may be used on fires, which involve paper, wood or cloth. A soda and acid extinguisher may also be used for this type of fire.***

> ***TEST-TAKING TIP:*** This question isn't really so hard! A cloth fire can be extinguished with water. Go with what you know! (To review the proper uses of the other types of fire extinguishers, read the rationales for the other options).

3. *INCORRECT. Dry chemical extinguishers are appropriate for fires, which involve electrical equipment, or fires, which involve combustible metals. Think analytically: What kind of fire would likely occur in a linen room?*
4. *INCORRECT. A carbon dioxide extinguisher is appropriate for fires, which involve flammable liquids and gases. Think analytically: What kind of fire would likely occur in a linen room?*

27. An confused elderly client has wrist restraints for safety reasons. Which nursing action is the safest?

1. Check the pulse, color, and temperature of extremities every shift and report these findings.
2. Make sure the call light is within the client's reach.
3. Notify the client's family of the restraints and explain the rationale for their use.
4. Remove the restraints at night while the client is sleeping.

1. *INCORRECT. Checking every shift will not be adequate to protect the client from permanent injury, since the client is at risk of decreased circulation. The extremities should be assessed at least every two hours.*
2. ***CORRECT. Even though the client is confused, the call light must be available to allow the client to communicate his or her needs. This option is the best choice because it is the only action that provides for the client's immediate safety.***
3. *INCORRECT. The family should be informed; however, there is another option that is more necessary for the client's immediate safety.*
4. *INCORRECT. If the client requires restraints because of confusion, the restraints should not be removed at night.*

28. A client complains that he is unable to rest because of the noise from his roommate's TV. The best action by the nurse is to:

1. Have the client moved to a private room.
2. Provide ear phones for the client who is watching television.
3. Explain that the roommate is hard of hearing, so the television is louder than usual.
4. Ask the roommate to shut off the television so the client can rest.

1. *INCORRECT. Moving the client to a private room would eliminate the noisy television. The client, however, would need input to determine if his insurance will cover the cost of a private room, and if not, whether he is willing to pay the difference. This is not the best action by the nurse at this time.*
2. ***CORRECT. Providing ear phones provides both clients with an immediate (and low-cost) solution to the problem. This action promotes rest for the client in the question and does not interfere with the roommate's right to watch television.***
3. *INCORRECT. Explaining the action of the roommate indicates to the client that his concerns are not important since nothing is being done to decrease the noise. This action also fails to promote rest for the client.*

> ***TEST-TAKING TIP:*** There is no information in the introductory statement that the roommate is hard of hearing! This cannot be the answer.

4. *INCORRECT. Telling the roommate to turn off the television interferes with his right to watch television. There is a better option.*

29. While bathing a preschooler in a tub, which would be the least appropriate nursing action?

1. Check the temperature of the water with a thermometer.
2. Never leave the child unattended.
3. Make sure the temperature in the room is warm.
4. Allow the child to determine if the water temperature is comfortable by placing the child's feet in the water.

1. *INCORRECT. This action is appropriate. Water temperature should be between 100° and 105° F, since the small child's skin is easily burned at higher temperatures. You are looking for an INAPPROPRIATE action.*
2. *INCORRECT. A small child may be able to turn the water faucet on and may turn on the hot water and receive burn injuries. There also is a danger of drowning when a small child is left unattended.*
3. *INCORRECT. The temperature of the room should be warm, to avoid chilling the child. You are looking for an INAPPROPRIATE action.*
4. ***CORRECT. You have identified the inappropriate action! If the water is too hot, the child may sustain burned feet. Instead, the nurse should use a thermometer to ensure that the temperature is in the correct range of between 100° and 105° F.***

30. The nurse is caring for an elderly client in a long-term care facility. When applying a hot water bottle to the client, it would place the client at risk if the nurse:

1. Wrapped the hot water bottle in a cloth before placing it next to the client's skin.
2. Filled the hot water bottle with as much hot water as it will hold.
3. Eliminated as much air as possible from the hot water bottle.
4. Checked the temperature of the water with a thermometer.

1. *INCORRECT— this is safe! The cover provides comfort and prevents burns, because the cloth acts as an insulator. This question is asking you to select an action that is UNSAFE.*
2. ***CORRECT. This action is unsafe! The bag should be filled only two-thirds full, to keep the bag***

easy to mold and lessen the chances of leakage.

3. *INCORRECT — this is safe. Eliminating excess air is important, since air is a poor conductor of heat. The question, however, asks you to identify an UNSAFE action.*
4. *INCORRECT. The temperature of the water should be close to 115° F, to avoid burning the client. Checking the temperature of the water is a safe nursing action. The question, however, asks you to select an action that is UNSAFE.*

31. The nurse is about to instruct parents of young children about poison control in the home. The nurse should:

1. Instruct the parents to induce vomiting with syrup of ipecac.
2. Instruct the parents to immediately bring the child to the emergency room.
3. Provide labels for the parent's telephone with the Poison Control Center's telephone number, and give instructions to call that number after an accidental ingestion.
4. Notify social services to investigate the home situation for safety.

1. *INCORRECT. In some poisons, such as lye or petroleum products, vomiting is contraindicated! Syrup of ipecac should be available for parents' use, but identification of the poison is most important before treatment can be initiated.*
2. *INCORRECT. Immediate measures usually can be instituted by the parents to lessen the severity of the poisoning by preventing or slowing absorption. The phone number for the Poison Control Center can place the parents in contact with an immediate source of information for initial emergency measures. Depending on the location of the hospital, time may be a factor in the outcome of the situation.*
3. ***CORRECT. The phone number for the Poison Control Center can place the parents in contact with an immediate source of information for initial emergency measures that can be implemented to help decrease the severity of the poisoning prior to transportation to the emergency room.***
4. *INCORRECT. Accidental poisoning often occurs because of a lack of knowledge on the part of the parents. A social service consult is not necessary unless a pattern of practices indicates an unsafe environment for the children. There is no information in the introductory statement to justify this intervention at this time. Do not "read into" the question.*

32. An adolescent client is to have a water system heating device ("K-Pad"), applied to a pulled muscle. The client tells the nurse that the device does not feel very warm. The safest nursing action is to:

1. Tell the client that these heating devices never feel hot.
2. Check the temperature setting on the heating unit and feel the pad for warmth.
3. Call the appropriate repair department and have them fix the unit.
4. Turn the temperature up on the unit if it doesn't feel warm enough to the client.

1. *INCORRECT. Although these heating units do feel warm and not hot, the unit may not be at a therapeutic temperature, and should be assessed to see if it is working properly.*
2. ***CORRECT. The nurse should check that the device is set to the temperature recommended by the manufacturer. The nurse should also assess whether the pad feels warm.***

> ***TEST-TAKING TIP:*** This option includes the only assessment action.

3. *INCORRECT. The unit may not be malfunctioning. It should be assessed by the nurse before any other action is taken. If the unit is malfunctioning, it should be replaced with another unit, and the malfunctioning unit should be sent to the repair department.*
4. *INCORRECT. The temperature should not be set above the recommended setting, to avoid causing a burn to the client.*

33. While working the night shift, the nurse notices a mouse running down the hallway of the clinical unit. The best nursing action is to:

1. Place rat poison in the vicinity where the mouse was seen.
2. Set some mouse traps to catch the mouse, and then dispose of it in a plastic bag labeled as contaminated.
3. Notify the supervisor of the problem.
4. Call the environmental health department of the hospital, and report the incident.

1. *INCORRECT. Poison should not be placed in an area that clients, staff and visitors utilize because of the risk of accidental exposure or poisoning.*
2. *INCORRECT. It is not the nurse's responsibility to catch mice. To prevent infection, however, the nurse must report the problem to the department responsible for rodent control.*
3. *INCORRECT. The supervisor is not responsible for rodent control. If the nurse has a problem getting the department that is responsible for environmental health to take care of the mouse, then the supervisor may be needed to intervene on behalf of the nurse.*
4. ***CORRECT. The department that is responsible for environmental health deals with pest and rodent control and should be notified of this problem.***

34. A vest restraint is placed on a confused elderly client who is at high risk for falling. Which nursing action is the least appropriate?

1. Provide an opportunity for the client to use the bedpan, toilet, or other toilet facilities at regular intervals.
2. Assess the respiratory status of the client frequently.
3. Utilizing help from other nurses, approach the client and apply the vest as quickly as possible, in order to avoid any resistance from the client.
4. Change the client's position at least every two hours.

1. *INCORRECT. Placing a vest restraint on a client results in the client's being dependent on the nurse for many basic needs. This client cannot get a bed pan or go to the bathroom without assistance. This is a true statement, but it is not the correct answer because the question asks you to select an option that is INAPPROPRIATE.*
2. *INCORRECT. A vest restraint can interfere with respiratory effort if the restraint is too tight; therefore, frequent assessment is necessary. This question asks for an INAPPROPRIATE action, however, so this is not the correct answer.*
3. ***CORRECT. The question asks you to identify the inappropriate action. Applying a restraint can be threatening to an agitated or confused client. The client should be approached slowly and calmly, utilizing only as much help as is deemed necessary to ensure the safety of the client and the nurse.***
4. *INCORRECT.. In order to avoid complications that may develop as a result of immobility, the client should have a position change at least every two hours. However, this question asks you to identify an INAPPROPRIATE action, so this is not the correct option.*

35. The nurse discovers a fire in the hospital. Which of the following nursing actions would place the client at risk?

1. Sound the nearest fire alarm.
2. Move clients who are in the immediate area of the fire.
3. Turn off any oxygen or electrical equipment.
4. Open the doors and windows to let the smoke out.

1. *INCORRECT. This is a safe action in case of fire. This question has a false response stem and requires an answer that is unsafe.*
2. *INCORRECT. This is a safe action in case of fire. The stem of this question asks for an option that is NOT safe.*
3. *INCORRECT. This is a safe action in case of fire. This question has a false response stem and asks for an option that is NOT safe.*
4. ***CORRECT. You have identified the unsafe action. Opening doors and windows makes the fire worse by providing more oxygen, which fuels the fire. Doors and windows should be shut.***

36. A client is in the bathroom after taking a shower. The nurse hears a loud thud. The nurse opens the bathroom door to find the client on the floor and a hair dryer in the sink with the basin full of water. The first nursing action is to:

1. Assess the client to determine if she is breathing.
2. Assess the client for a heart rate.
3. Unplug the hair dryer, while taking care not to touch the client or any water or wet surface.
4. Perform a neurological assessment.

1. *INCORRECT. While this is important and should be done, it is not the first action, since the safety of the nurse may also be at stake in this situation.*
2. *INCORRECT. Assessing the heart rate is not the first nursing action during an emergency. The safety of the nurse may also be at stake during this situation.*
3. ***CORRECT. The hair dryer in a basin of water appears to be the cause of this client's problem. The dryer still poses a serious electrical hazard and should be carefully unplugged, so that the nurse does not also become injured.***

> ***TEST-TAKING TIP:*** This is the different option — in this case, the only one that is NOT an assessment action and directly addresses the issue of the electrical hazard.

4. *INCORRECT. While this is an appropriate measure, the safety of the nurse may be at stake in this situation. This is not the first action to initiate.*

37. A young client is paralyzed from the waist down. He has a TV, radio, video tape player, stereo, and video game unit, which are all used throughout the day. The nurse notices that there are not enough electrical outlets, and that extension cords with multiple outlets are in use to accommodate this equipment. The best nursing action is to:

1. Have the client's family take some of the equipment home.
2. Unplug as much of the client's equipment as necessary, after informing the client that an overloaded circuit can cause an electrical fire and that extension cords are not allowed.
3. Tell the client that only single-outlet cords can be used, and that you will check often to see if he wants to use anything not currently connected.
4. Call the maintenance department and have more wall outlets installed in the client's room.

1. *INCORRECT. The client should not be deprived of activities that he finds entertaining. This option does not solve the problem at hand, either, since an electrical fire could occur while waiting for the family to take the equipment home.*
2. *INCORRECT. This action would provide for the client's safety, but it does not provide any alternatives for consideration of the client.*
3. ***CORRECT. This option allows the client the continued use of his electrical devices, and provides for the client's immediate safety by decreasing the possibility of an electrical fire.***
4. *INCORRECT. Revamping the physical structure of a building is an administrative decision. Adding electrical outlets is expensive, and may not comply with fire or electrical codes. Also, this option does not solve the problem at hand, since an electrical fire could occur while waiting for the electrical work to be done.*

38. While caring for a client, the nurse notices that the call light cord is frayed. The nurse should:

1. Tell the client not to use the call light until it is fixed.
2. Remove the call light, and report the problem to the supervising nurse immediately.
3. Tape up the cord until the maintenance people can fix it, so the client will have a call light.

4. Tell the client to call out if he needs help, and to use the call light only in an emergency.

1. INCORRECT. This will not protect the client from potential electrical burns or shocks. A frayed cord is an electrical hazard.

2. CORRECT. Removal of a frayed cord is the only way to protect the client from potential electrical burns or shocks. The supervising nurse will make arrangements for another call light or system for the client.

3. This is not a proper repair, and it will not protect the client from potential electrical burns or shocks.

4. This will not protect the client from potential electrical burns or shocks.

39. An elderly client is scheduled for surgery tomorrow. The nurse enters the client's room and finds that flames are coming out of the waste basket. The nurse would demonstrate an understanding of safety priorities by first:

1. Placing the folded blanket from the client's bed over the entire opening of the waste basket.
2. Finding the nearest fire extinguisher to put the fire out.
3. Telling the client that he is not supposed to be smoking.
4. Pulling the nearest fire alarm.

1. CORRECT. Placing the blanket over the waste basket will eliminate the source of oxygen, which is an element needed for a fire to burn. This is the fastest method in this situation for putting out a small fire.

2. INCORRECT. While an extinguisher will put out this small fire, it is not the best first action in this situation. While you are getting the extinguisher, the fire will increase.

3. INCORRECT. This is not an appropriate first action during this emergency situation! Providing for the immediate safety of the client is most important.

TEST-TAKING TIP: The introductory statement does not tell you that the client has been smoking, and it is incorrect to assume this. Do not "read into" the question!

4. INCORRECT. An attempt should be made to quickly extinguish a small fire at the time it is found, since it can become out of control within ten minutes. The fire alarm should be pulled immediately AFTER appropriate initial measures to extinguish the fire have been implemented.

40. A client spills hot coffee on himself during breakfast. The first action by the nurse is to:

1. Remove the clothing from the burn area and apply cold water to the area.
2. Call the physician.
3. Make out an incident report.
4. Cover the area with sterile towels.

1. CORRECT. Removing the "hot" clothing and applying cold water helps to stop the burning process.

2. INCORRECT. The physician should be notified, but AFTER emergency first aid measures have been initiated.

3. INCORRECT. An incident report should be completed for any client who receives an injury while in a health care facility, but not until AFTER steps have been taken to help the client.

4. INCORRECT. The area should be kept as clean as possible to prevent infection, but this is not the first action in the care of a burn.

41. An elderly client has an IV with an infusion pump. While examining the infusion pump, the nurse experiences a slight tingling sensation in the hand as the plug is checked. What is the safest nursing action?

1. Shut the pump off immediately.
2. Inform the repair department to immediately shut off the pump.
3. Recheck the equipment in one hour.
4. Use a different electrical outlet site.

1. INCORRECT. The question is trying to determine if you know what to do to prevent an electrical injury to the client and yourself. The pump should be turned off, but since the nurse has already felt tingling when she touched the plug, she should not shut the pump off herself! Look for a safer option.

2. CORRECT. The repair department should be notified to immediately shut off the pump to protect the client and nurse from risk of electrical injury.

3. INCORRECT. The pump must be shut off to protect the client from the risk of electrical injury. Leaving the equipment operating and rechecking it in an hour increases risk for the client.

4. INCORRECT. This is an incorrect action that increases the risk of electrical injury for the client. Switching the electrical outlet will not ensure the client's safety. The pump must be shut off to protect the client from the risk of electrical injury.

42. While caring for an infant, the nurse notices that one of the infant's stuffed animals in the crib has eyes that can easily be pulled off. The appropriate nursing action is to:

1. Take the toy out of the crib immediately.
2. Remove the eyes from the stuffed animal and return it to the crib.
3. When the mother comes to visit, show her the eyes and explain that the infant could pull them off and choke on them.
4. Send the toy home with the mother.

1. CORRECT. The stuffed animal has the potential for causing the infant to choke. This is a safety issue, and immediate measures should be taken to prevent an accident from occurring. The nurse can discuss the issue with the mother at her next visit.

2. INCORRECT. Since the introductory statement indicates that the stuffed toy belongs to the infant and not the hospital, the nurse should not remove the eyes unless she discusses it with the mother first.

3. *INCORRECT.. Waiting for the mother to visit before providing for the infant's safety is not appropriate. The situation should be discussed with the mother, but this is not the best initial action. The immediate safety of the infant needs to be addressed.*

> ***TEST-TAKING TIP:*** Options 3 and 4 are similar in that they include waiting for the mother's next visit. Similar distractors can be eliminated.

4. *INCORRECT. The toy can be sent home with the mother, especially if it has sentimental value and can be kept intact until the child is old enough that it is no longer a safety issue. However, the immediate safety of the infant needs to be addressed.*

> ***TEST-TAKING TIP:*** Options 3 and 4 are similar in that they include waiting for the mother's next visit. Similar distractors can be eliminated.

43. A client is to have an electrical heating device applied to his lower back area. The plug on the heating device has three prongs, and the electrical wall outlet available only has two-pronged openings. The client's radio is plugged into a three-pronged outlet. The best action by the nurse at this time is to:

1. Unplug the client's radio, which is plugged into a three-pronged outlet, and use that outlet for the heating device.
2. Obtain an extension cord with a three-pronged outlet on it.
3. Use a 2-pronged adapter to plug into the wall outlet; then plug the heating device into the adapter.
4. Call central supply to see if you can get a heating device with a two-pronged plug on it.

1. ***CORRECT. The third prong on the heating device when plugged into a grounded outlet is the ground, which prevents the client from receiving an electrical injury if the heating device malfunctions and causes a short in the circuit. The grounded electrical outlet provides a pathway for any stray electrical current.***
2. *INCORRECT. Extension cords should be avoided because of the potential for fire. In this situation, the client would not be protected from an electrical injury since there is no ground on the wall outlet or the extension cord. The ground prong on the heating device is thus not in contact with any pathway for stray electricity, which places the client at risk for electrical injury if the heating device shorts out.*

> ***TEST-TAKING TIP:*** Using an extension cord is similar to using an adapter. Options 2 and 3 are similar distractors and can be eliminated.

3. *INCORRECT. Plug adapters or "cheater plugs" should never be used, since they eliminate the pathway for stray electricity, placing the client at risk for an electrical injury if the heating device shorts out.*

> ***TEST-TAKING TIP:*** Using an extension cord is similar to using an adapter. Options 2 and 3 are similar distractors and can be eliminated.

4. *This action is unsafe. Only grounded equipment should be used for any client. A two-pronged plug does not provide a ground to protect the client from an electrical injury.*

44. A client is confused and confined to bed. He has attempted to crawl over the side rails. The safe nursing action is to:

1. Apply restraints to the client immediately.
2. Stay with the client and notify the supervising nurse.
3. Remind the client to stay in bed.
4. Tell the client to stay in bed, or else the nursing staff will have to restrain him.

1. *INCORRECT. Applying restraints unnecessarily can be considered false imprisonment. This client is at risk falling. Can you identify a less restrictive nursing approach to ensure his safety?*
2. ***CORRECT. This client is at risk for falling. Staying with the client protects him from harm. The supervising nurse can then notify the physician and request orders.***
3. *INCORRECT. This action will not provide for the client's safety because the client is confused.*
4. *INCORRECT. Restraints should never be used as a punishment. This response would also be ineffective, because the client is confused. Restraints are to be used only when necessary, to protect the client from harm.*

45. In a hospital pediatric unit, which action by the nurse is best for preventing accidental poisoning to a toddler?

1. Place cleaning supplies on a counter out of reach of the toddler.
2. Do not allow any plant life on the pediatric unit.
3. Place cleaning supplies in a locked cabinet.
4. Place all toddlers in specific rooms where they are supervised frequently.

1. *INCORRECT. A toddler is able to climb and can obtain many things that are "out of reach." Placing cleaning supplies on a high counter does not ensure the safety of the toddler.*
2. *INCORRECT. Some plants are poisonous and should be recognized by the pediatric staff. Many are not poisonous and should not be banned or sent home from a client's room unless there is a safety issue.*
3. ***CORRECT. Cleaning supplies should be locked up to provide for the safety of toddlers. They are very inquisitive and are able to open many doors without difficulty. If the door is locked, the toddler can't open the door.***
4. *INCORRECT. Toddlers need constant — not just frequent — supervision in order to promote a safe environment.*

46. The nurse, walking by a client's room, notices that the top sheet on the client's bed is on fire and the client is in the bed. What is the first action by the nurse?

1. Get a fire extinguisher and spray the entire bed, including the client, who is at risk for burns.

2. Grab a towel and beat the flames out by hitting the burning sheet.
3. Take the blanket at the foot of the bed, place the blanket over the burning sheets to smother the flames, and smooth the blanket to remove any pockets of oxygen.
4. Use the nearest fire hose to extinguish the flames.

1. *INCORRECT. The best action is to put the fire out as fast as possible. Obtaining the fire extinguisher takes time and allows the fire to worsen during that time. Some fire extinguisher chemicals should not come in contact with skin, so spraying the client may cause further injury.*
2. *INCORRECT. Waving an object causes a fire to burn better by creating a fanning of the flames.*
3. ***CORRECT. The blanket will smother the flames by eliminating the source of oxygen. This is the fastest action for putting out this fire.***
4. *INCORRECT. A fire hose has high pressure behind the water and is very difficult for one person to hold under control. In addition, the force of the water could push the client out of the bed and onto the floor, causing further injury.*

47. The nurse notices a crack in an electrical outlet. The IV pump that is plugged into the outlet appears to be working without any problems. Which is the safest nursing action?

1. Use another outlet; then call the maintenance department to have the outlet changed.
2. Since the pump is working, no action is necessary.
3. Test the outlet by moving the plug a bit in the outlet, and observing if this affects the pump.
4. Since the outlet works, continue to use it until maintenance can replace it.

1. ***CORRECT. A cracked electrical outlet should never be used and should be replaced, since it has the potential to start an electrical fire or to cause an electrical shock to any person who attempts to insert a plug.***
2. *INCORRECT. This is unsafe. Although the electrical outlet is presently working, it could quit working or cause a short and start an electrical fire.*

> ***TEST-TAKING TIP:*** This option is similar to option 4, since no safety action would be taken at this time. Similar options can be eliminated.

3. *INCORRECT. This is unsafe. Moving the plug in the outlet may cause the outlet to become further damaged and cause an electrical shock or electrical fire.*
4. *INCORRECT. This is unsafe. A broken electrical outlet should never be used because of the potential for an electrical fire or short.*

> ***TEST-TAKING TIP:*** This option is similar to option 2, since no safety action would be taken at this time.. Similar distractors can be eliminated.

48. The nurse is caring for a client who is scheduled for surgery. When the transporter arrives to take the client to the operating room, the client is seated in a chair. To achieve the client's safe transfer onto the stretcher, the best nursing action is to:

1. Assist the client to get back into bed, and then move her across to the stretcher with the help of a drawsheet.
2. Have the client use the chair to step up onto the stretcher.
3. Assist the client to climb up onto the stretcher.
4. Together with the transporter, lift the client from the chair onto the stretcher, keeping a wide stance and a straight back.

1. ***CORRECT. The client should first get back onto the bed. Then, with the bed raised to the height of the stretcher, the client should slide across to the stretcher. This is the safest option for the client and staff in preventing a fall or back injury.***
2. *INCORRECT. Different items of equipment have specific purposes, and they should be used accordingly. A client could fall when climbing onto or standing on a chair, or the chair could slide out from under the client during the transfer to the stretcher. The client is at risk for a fall.*
3. *INCORRECT. The client could miss the edge of the stretcher and fall, which could result in an injury.*
4. *INCORRECT. Clients should be lifted only when necessary, to avoid a potential fall for the client and back injuries to the staff.*

49. While mixing a solution of bleach and water to be used as a disinfectant spray, the nurse discovers that there is more solution than will fit in the spray bottle. Which of the following actions by the nurse would place the client at risk?

1. Pour the excess solution into an empty container, label the container as to contents, and place it in the cleaning supply closet.
2. Discard the excess solution.
3. Use the excess solution for the immediate cleaning job, then discard what is left.
4. Pour the excess into another cleaning solution container that has only a small amount of an ammonia solution left in the bottom.

1. *INCORRECT. This is an appropriate action. All containers should be labeled with the contents and stored in the appropriate area for the contents. Cleaning supplies and chemicals should not be kept near supplies that are for oral consumption or other uses where a client could be injured by someone picking up the wrong bottle.*
2. *INCORRECT. This is an appropriate action. If there are no available containers that can be safely used, then discarding the solution is the best action in order to avoid poisoning or injury by another person using the unidentified solution for the wrong purpose.*
3. *INCORRECT. This is an appropriate action. If the solution was prepared because of the need to clean a particular area, then the person who prepared the solution can use the excess, then discard what is left after the immediate cleaning task is completed. Any*

solution that is not identified has the potential for being mistakenly misused by another person.

4. ***CORRECT. Mixing chlorine or bleach with ammonia produces toxic fumes that can cause damage to the respiratory tract when inhaled.***

50. During an electrical storm the lights go out for a few seconds. Some of the lights come back on, but the ventilator is not working. What is the first nursing action?

1. Remove the client from the ventilator and ventilate with a bag and mask.
2. Quickly check the electrical outlets to determine if the ventilator is plugged into an emergency power outlet.
3. Call a code.
4. Ventilate the client with oxygen using a positive pressure bag attached to the endotracheal tube, until full power is restored.

1. *INCORRECT. A client on a ventilator has an endotracheal tube in place. A mask cannot be used because a seal cannot be made.*
2. ***CORRECT. All emergency equipment such as ventilators should be plugged into emergency outlets in case of power failure. If the ventilator was not plugged into the appropriate outlet, then the nurse should move the plug to an emergency power outlet.***
3. *INCORRECT. It is not necessary to call a code because of equipment malfunction. A code is to be called only if the equipment cannot be readily restored and the client's condition begins to deteriorate.*
4. *INCORRECT. This option may be necessary if the nurse cannot get the ventilator turned back on. The nurse's first effort, however, should be to restore the functioning of the ventilator.*

Section 3: Preventing the Spread of Infection

1. An HIV positive client is admitted to the hospital with a lung infection. Which of the following isolation categories should be implemented in order to prevent transmission of the HIV virus?

1. Strict isolation.
2. Respiratory isolation.
3. Universal precautions.
4. Enteric precautions.

1. *INCORRECT. Strict isolation prevents transmission of highly contagious infections that are spread by air and contact. It may or may not be appropriate for this client, depending upon the type of lung infection. The question, however, asks about prevention of transmission of the HIV virus, not about the lung infection. How is HIV spread?*

TEST-TAKING TIP: The issue in the question is not always the same as the admitting diagnosis.

2. *INCORRECT. Respiratory isolation prevents transmission of infectious diseases over short distances via air droplets. It may or may not be appropriate for this client, depending upon the type of lung infection. The question, however, asks about prevention of transmission of the HIV virus, not about the lung infection. HIV is not spread by air droplets; therefore, respiratory isolation is not necessary to prevent the spread of HIV.*
3. ***CORRECT. Universal precautions prevent the spread of infections that are transmitted by direct or indirect contact with infectious blood or other body fluids. Since this is the mode of transmission of HIV, this is the appropriate isolation precaution.***

TEST TAKING TIP: The issue in the question is not always the same as the admitting diagnosis. Always check to see what the question is specifically asking about.

4. *INCORRECT. Enteric precautions prevent the spread of infections that are transmitted by direct or indirect contact with feces. Prevention of HIV transmission involves more than protection from feces, so enteric precautions are not adequate protection.*

2. While changing the linen on a client's bed, how should the nurse handle the linen?

1. Hold it close to the body to avoid dropping it.
2. Place soiled linen on the chair until done making the bed.
3. Hold the linen away from the body and uniform.
4. Shake clean linen to unfold it and provide ease in making the bed.

1. *INCORRECT. Holding clean linen next to the body can transfer organisms from the uniform to the clean linen. Holding dirty linen next to the body can transfer organisms from the soiled linen to the uniform. Either action results in contamination and transfer of organisms.*
2. *INCORRECT. Soiled linen is contaminated and will further contaminate the surfaces of the chair. All soiled linen should be placed directly into the laundry hamper in order to prevent contamination of other surfaces.*
3. ***CORRECT. The linen should be held away from the uniform. Since the nurse must go from client to client, any organisms present on the uniform can be transferred from one client to another.***
4. INCORRECT. Opening linens by shaking them causes movement of air. Air currents can carry dust and organisms about the room, resulting in potential infection.

3. A client is recovering from surgery. While changing the linens on the client's bed, the nurse notes that drainage from an infected wound has soiled the bed sheet. What is the best method for changing this linen?

1. Carefully place the soiled sheet in the cloth linen bag and label it as contaminated.
2. Spray the soiled area with a bleach solution prior to placing it in the linen bag.
3. Carefully place the soiled sheet in a moisture-resistant plastic linen bag designated for soiled articles.
4. Discard the sheet into a plastic trash bag.

1. *INCORRECT. A cloth linen bag does not protect the laundry employees from exposure to the soiled sheet and organisms that may be present on the sheet.*
2. *INCORRECT. Spraying the soiled area of the sheet does not destroy any organisms that may be present on other parts of the sheet but cannot be seen. Spraying the sheet is not practical, since the sheet will be effectively disinfected during laundering. Also, using a cloth linen bag does not protect the laundry employees from exposure to the soiled sheet.*
3. ***CORRECT. Placing the sheet in a moisture-resistant plastic bag protects the laundry employees and others that may come in contact with the bag from exposure to organisms that may be present in the soiled linen.***
4. *INCORRECT. Discarding linen is neither appropriate nor cost-effective. Proper handling by placing the linen in a moisture-resistant bag will protect the nurse and other employees, and the sheet will be effectively disinfected during laundering.*

4. The best nursing action to prevent the spread of infection among hospitalized clients is:

1. Using sterile technique when performing any procedure
2. Hand washing before coming in contact with each client.
3. Wearing gloves to perform any procedure.
4. Wearing a mask and gown while performing any procedure.

1. *INCORRECT. Sterile technique is not required for every procedure. Using sterile technique while administering medications or similar interventions is neither necessary nor practical. Aseptic technique is appropriate for most non-invasive procedures.*
2. ***CORRECT. Hand washing has been found to be the most effective action in preventing spread of infection among clients. This activity inhibits the transfer of organisms from one client to another.***

> ***TEST-TAKING TIP:*** This is the only option that repeats the word "client" from the stem of the question. If you didn't know the answer, this would be a clue.

3. *INCORRECT. Gloves should be worn if there is any chance of the nurse coming in contact with body fluids. However, gloves are not necessary for procedures such as administration of oral medications, where exposure to body fluids is not likely to occur.*
4. *INCORRECT. It is not necessary to wear a gown and mask for all procedures. In addition, although wearing a gown and mask protects the nurse, it does not effectively protect the client. This is not the best option.*

5. A client is admitted to the hospital with a diagnosis of active pulmonary tuberculosis. An immediate nursing goal is to control the spread of infection. To control the spread of active tuberculosis, the nurse would:

1. Wear a gown and mask when caring for the client.
2. Recommend that the client wear a mask when she has visitors.
3. Teach the client how to cover her nose and mouth when she coughs or sneezes.
4. Use blood and needle precautions.

1. *INCORRECT. The mask would be appropriate, but there is no need for a gown.*

> ***TEST-TAKING TIP:*** An option which is partially wrong cannot be the correct answer.

2. *INCORRECT. The correct procedure would be for visitors, as well as all health care providers, to wear a mask when in the room — not the client.*
3. ***CORRECT. Teaching this, along with proper handwashing, will help prevent the spread of the infection, which is by droplet nuclei.***
4. *INCORRECT. Tuberculosis is not transmitted via the blood.*

6. When changing dressings for an HIV positive client, the nurse should remember to wash her hands and to:

1. Wear a mask.
2. Wear gloves.
3. Maintain strict isolation.
4. Wear a gown and gloves.

1. *INCORRECT. Masks are not necessary. Goggles should be used if splatter is likely.*
2. ***CORRECT. Gloves are necessary and, besides handwashing, are the best protection from HIV clients.***
3. *INCORRECT. Universal precautions are required to care for HIV positive clients, not strict isolation.*
4. *INCORRECT. This is necessary only if the nurse's clothing may become contaminated.*

7. While starting an intravenous infusion, the nurse's gloved hands get spotted with blood. The client has not been diagnosed with any organisms that are transmitted by way of the blood stream. The first action the nurse should take upon completion of the task is to:

1. Remove the gloves carefully and follow with handwashing.
2. Wash the gloved hands, and then throw the gloves away.
3. Prepare an incident report so that this occurrence will be documented, in case a health care problem develops at a later date.
4. Ask the client to have a blood test to determine if a bloodborne pathogen is present in the client's blood.

1. CORRECT. Universal precautions require the use of gloves and hand washing in the care of all clients. This response addresses the issue in the question.

> ***TEST-TAKING TIP:*** Since hand washing is required in the care of all clients, you know this action is appropriate. When in doubt, "Go with what you know."

2. INCORRECT. Washing the gloves while still on the nurse's hands does not result in clean hands for the nurse. Handwashing is still required for infection control.

3. INCORRECT. Unless there is a break in the nurse's skin, there is no need for an incident report or further investigation. Also, this would not be the nurse's FIRST action. The issue in this question is infection control and blood on the nurse's gloved hands.

4. INCORRECT. This is not a nursing action and therefore cannot be the answer! If there is a concern about transmission of a disease, the nurse should follow the hospital protocol. What is the nurse's FIRST action after getting blood on the hands?

8. While the nurse is caring for a client, the intravenous tubing becomes disconnected from the intravenous catheter, resulting in the client's blood spilling onto the side of the bed and floor. The nurse knows that which solution is recommended for disinfection of blood spills?

1. Betadine solution.
2. Alcohol.
3. Soap and water.
4. Sodium hypochlorite or chlorine bleach solution.

1. INCORRECT. Betadine solution is used for disinfecting skin and is effective after being allowed to dry on the skin surface. It is not appropriate to apply to objects because it stains surfaces with which it comes in contact.

2. INCORRECT. Alcohol is a skin disinfectant. It has not been found to destroy the HIV virus; therefore, it is not effective for blood spills.

3. INCORRECT. Soap and water emulsifies dirt for easy removal of the dirt, but it is not a disinfectant.

> ***TEST-TAKING TIP:*** Does this option address the issue in the question?

4. CORRECT. Chlorine acts as a disinfectant and is recommended for cleansing objects. It is recommended for blood spills because it is effective in killing the HIV virus, which can be found in body fluids such as blood.

9. The nurse would select which infection control precautions as appropriate in caring for an AIDS client?

1. Strict isolation.
2. Respiratory isolation.
3. Contact isolation.
4. Universal blood and body fluid precautions.

1. INCORRECT. Strict isolation is instituted for clients with highly contagious infections spread by air and contact, such as chicken pox and diphtheria. How is the AIDS virus transmitted?

2. INCORRECT. Respiratory isolation prevents transmission of infectious diseases over short distances through air droplets. It is appropriate for pulmonary tuberculosis, measles, mumps, pneumonia, and meningitis. How is the AIDS virus transmitted?

3. INCORRECT. Contact isolation prevents transmission of highly transmissible infections spread by close or direct contact that do not warrant strict precautions. It is appropriate for impetigo, herpes simplex infections, and acute respiratory infections in infants and young children. How is the AIDS virus transmitted?

4. CORRECT. HIV has not been found to be transmitted via the respiratory route, although the virus has been isolated in sputum. It is not a disease of airborne transmission, like tuberculosis. Evidence has indicated that HIV is transmitted only through intimate sexual contact, parenteral exposure to infected blood or blood products, and perinatal transmission from mother to neonate. Universal precautions prevent contact with pathogens transmitted by direct or indirect contact with infective blood or body fluids. Universal precautions include both enteric and secretion precautions.

10. The nurse caring for an AIDS client accidentally pierces her hand with a needle used to give the client his pain medication. The priority nursing action is to:

1. Report the incident to the charge nurse.
2. Cover the wound with a sterile gauze dressing and report the incident to employee health.
3. Complete an incident report.
4. "Bleed" the site and rinse under water, apply an antibiotic ointment, and cover the area with a dry dressing.

1. INCORRECT — this would be the second action taken by the nurse, not the first. What should the nurse do first?

2. INCORRECT. This wound requires more than a sterile dry dressing.

3. INCORRECT — an incident report is indicated, but it is not the first action by the nurse. What should the nurse do first?

4. CORRECT. The initial action is to bleed the area to rid the wound of any pathogens. Then an

antibiotic ointment should be applied and the area protected with a dry dressing.

11. Which exposure would place the nurse at greatest risk for contracting AIDS?

1. Vaginal secretions and semen.
2. Blood.
3. Cerebrospinal fluid.
4. Sputum.

1. *INCORRECT. The virus has been isolated in several body fluids, including sputum, saliva, cerebrospinal fluid, urine, and semen, but its concentration is highest in blood.*
2. ***CORRECT. Blood contains the AIDS virus. Universal precautions must always be used when dealing with blood from any source.***
3. *INCORRECT. The virus has been isolated in several body fluids, including sputum, saliva, cerebrospinal fluid, urine, and semen, but its concentration is highest in blood.*
4. *INCORRECT. The virus has been isolated in several body fluids, including sputum, saliva, cerebrospinal fluid, urine, and semen, but its concentration is highest in blood.*

12. A postoperative client has an infected surgical incision. The area is red and swollen with a small amount of thick, yellow drainage. The correct term for the nurse to use in describing this drainage is:

1. Purulent.
2. Sanguineous.
3. Serous.
4. Serosanguineous.

1. ***CORRECT. Purulent drainage is commonly known as pus, the thick yellow secretion from an infected wound that is composed of bacteria, necrotic tissue, and white blood cells.***

> **TEST-TAKING TIP:** If you did not know the answer, one clue is that options two and four are similar to each other, and also options 3 and 4. This option is different and includes neither blood nor serum.

2. *INCORRECT. "Sanguineous" refers to blood and would designate bleeding from a surgical incision.*
3. *INCORRECT . Serous drainage, typically seen on the original surgical dressing, is clear to light yellow in color with a thin consistency. This drainage is serum, the clear liquid portion of blood that does not contain fibrinogen or blood cells.*
4. *INCORRECT. Serosanguineous drainage contains both serum and blood. It is pink to cherry red in color and does not indicate an infectious process.*

13. In planning to teach a client who has the human immunodeficiency virus (HIV), the nurse should remember to alert the client that the virus can be transmitted:

1. As soon as the client develops symptoms.
2. To anyone having contact with the client's blood.
3. Via the respiratory route, like tuberculosis.
4. Only during the active phase of the virus, but not while it is inactive.

1. *INCORRECT. HIV can be transmitted BEFORE the client develops symptoms of an opportunistic infection or is diagnosed with AIDS. Because the client is asymptomatic and is not aware that he/she has the virus, the virus is usually transmitted during this time.*
2. ***CORRECT. The concentration of the virus is highest in blood, and has been isolated in several body fluids, including sputum, saliva, cerebrospinal fluid, urine, and semen. Clients with HIV are cautioned to practice safe sex and to avoid donating blood or sharing needles with others.***
3. *INCORRECT. HIV has not been found to be transmitted via the respiratory route, although the virus has been isolated in sputum. It is not a disease of airborne transmission, like tuberculosis. Evidence has indicated that HIV is transmitted only through intimate sexual contact, parenteral exposure to infected blood or blood products, and perinatal transmission from mother to neonate.*
4. *INCORRECT. HIV can be transmitted at any time. There is no such thing as an active or inactive phase of transmission of this disease.*

14. Universal precautions requires that a nurse wear which protective equipment when performing a nasogastric tube irrigation on a client with acquired immunodeficiency syndrome (AIDS)?

1. Sterile gloves.
2. Goggles and nonsterile gloves.
3. Nonsterile gown, sterile gloves.
4. Nonsterile gloves.

1. *INCORRECT. Universal precautions does not require the use of sterile gloves when performing a nasogastric tube irrigation, although the nurse must protect herself from contact with blood and certain body fluids.*
2. *INCORRECT. It would not be necessary for the nurse to wear goggles. These are indicated when the nurse can anticipate a splash, such as during a surgical procedure or when suctioning a tracheostomy.*
3. *INCORRECT. It is not necessary for the nurse to wear a gown when performing a nasogastric tube irrigation. The gown is worn when the nurse anticipates being splashed by body fluids or blood. A splash is not likely to occur with this procedure.*
4. ***CORRECT. Universal precautions requires the use of clean gloves and other protective barriers to reduce the risk of occupational exposure to blood and certain body fluids. Nonsterile gloves are indicated for this procedure.***

Section 4: Client Hygiene and Comfort Needs

1. The nurse is caring for a client who is paralyzed on his right side following a stroke. In preparing to give a bed bath to this client, which of the following nursing actions is the most appropriate?

1. Adjust the bed to the lowest position, in case the client falls.
2. Raise the bed to the high horizontal position.
3. Put the bed in low semi-Fowler's position.
4. Unplug the bed.

1. INCORRECT. This action does not permit the nurse to use proper body mechanics.

2. CORRECT. The high horizontal position is the most efficient and safest way for the nurse to bathe the client, since it permits the nurse to use proper body mechanics.

3. INCORRECT, because it does not permit the nurse to use good body mechanics.

4. INCORRECT. Unplugging the bed serves no purpose.

2. A client is in the intensive care unit and is in a coma as a result of a head injury. The most important nursing action in performing mouth care on this client is to:

1. Turn the client to her side before starting mouth care.
2. Use a soft toothbrush.
3. Use a mouth bite to keep her mouth open.
4. Wear gloves.

1. CORRECT. Turning the client on her side is the most important intervention, since it will help prevent aspiration of the fluids used for cleaning the mouth.

> ***TEST-TAKING TIP:*** Note that the test- taking strategy of eliminating similar distractors would identify this option as the correct answer, because the other three options all refer to equipment to be used.

2. INCORRECT. A soft toothbrush is preferred, but this is not the most important action in this procedure. Can you identify an option which provides for the client's safety in this priority-setting question?

3. INCORRECT. This intervention is helpful while cleaning the mouth, but this is not the most important action in this procedure. This question asks you to select priorities. Can you identify an option which provides for the client's safety?

4. INCORRECT. The nurse should wear gloves, but this is not the most important action in this procedure. Can you identify an option which provides for the client's safety in this priority-setting question?

3. When giving a partial bath, which nursing action is the least appropriate?

1. Arrange equipment and linen for easy access.
2. Open the window to let fresh air in.
3. Pull the curtain for privacy.
4. Rinse off all of the soap.

1. INCORRECT. This action results in less disorganization of the bath for the client. However, this question has a false response stem. The correct answer will be something that the nurse should NOT do.

2. CORRECT. Although fresh air is important, it is not appropriate to open the window during a bath, since this can cause chilling of the client. This INAPPROPRIATE action is the correct option because the question has a false response stem.

3. INCORRECT. Privacy is an important issue in care of the client. However, this question has a false response stem. The correct answer will be some thing that the nurse should NOT do.

4. INCORRECT. Rinsing off all of the soap is important in order to avoid irritation and dry skin, which is more prone to skin breakdown. However, this question has a false response stem. The correct answer will be something that the nurse should NOT do.

4. A client with osteoarthritis complains of discomfort when performing exercises prescribed by the physical therapist. Which response by the nurse is most appropriate?

1. "The exercises will prevent pain."
2. "The exercises will prevent worsening of the disease."
3. "The exercises will help to maintain as near normal joint function as possible, as well as range of motion."
4. "The exercises will make you feel better."

1. INCORRECT. This statement is not true, and the exercises themselves may cause some mild discomfort.

> ***TEST-TAKING TIP:*** Note that this option is similar to option 2. These similar distractors can be eliminated.

2. INCORRECT. The exercises will not prevent worsening of the disease. There is no cure for osteoarthritis.

> ***TEST-TAKING TIP:*** This option is similar to option 1 and can be eliminated.

3. CORRECT. The exercises will help maintain joint function and range of motion if done on a regular basis. This response is therapeutic because it provides correct information about the rationale for the exercises.

4. INCORRECT. The exercises may help the client to feel better, but this sounds like a cliché and is not the most appropriate response.

5. An elderly client is to receive a bath. In preparing the bath, which action would place the client at risk?

1. Check the temperature of the tub room.
2. Gather and take all of the necessary equipment to the tub room prior to the bath.
3. Test the temperature of the bath water by having the client place his hand in the water.
4. Place a mat or towel in the bottom of the tub.

1 INCORRECT. The tub room should not be too cold or too hot, since the client may become chilled or too warm. This safe action is not the correct answer because the question is asking you to choose an UNSAFE action.

TEST-TAKING TIP: Remember the critical elements! What type of stem does this question have?

2. INCORRECT. All of the supplies should be available before taking the client to the tub room. This safe action is not the correct answer because the question is asking you to choose an UNSAFE action. This question has a false response stem.

3. CORRECT. This is an unsafe action. Sensitivity to hot and cold decreases as part of the aging process. There is a potential for the client to become chilled or to incur a burn when he tests the bath temperature. Also, the skin of elderly clients is often thin and fragile, which puts them at a high risk for burns.

4. INCORRECT. A mat or towel will help prevent a slip or fall as the client gets into or out of the tub. This safe action is not the correct answer because the question is asking you to choose an UNSAFE action. Always identify the type of stem!

6. The nurse caring for a client who is unconscious would place the unconscious client in which position?

1. Semi-Fowler's.
2. Trendelenburg.
3. Prone.
4. Supine.

1. INCORRECT. A semi-Fowler's position is a sitting position with the head of the bed elevated 45-60 degrees. An unconscious client cannot swallow and may therefore choke on saliva or secretions in this position. The client may also slump to one side or the other. This position would be unsafe.

2. INCORRECT. A Trendelenburg position requires that the lower extremities be elevated 20 degrees above the rest of the body. This position is used for clients who are in shock. This option does not address the issue in the question.

3. CORRECT. The prone position consists of placing the client on the abdomen. An unconscious client cannot swallow and is at risk for choking. This position facilitates drainage of saliva and secretions. The lateral or side-lying position may also be used to provide a change in position for the unconscious client.

TEST-TAKING TIP: The other options all involve placing the client on his back. This is the option that is different. If you didn't know the answer to this question, this strategy would be a good clue.

4. INCORRECT. The supine position involves placing the client on his back. Since the unconscious client cannot swallow, choking on saliva or secretions can occur.

Section 5: Physical Assessment of the Client and Basic Skills

1. A female client returns to the postoperative unit following abdominal surgery. She has a nasogastric tube to low continuous suction and complains of a sore throat. She asks the nurse when the nasogastric tube will be taken out. Which response by the nurse is most appropriate at this time?

1. "The doctor will discontinue the tube when your bowel sounds return."
2. "The tube probably will be removed tomorrow, but you'll remain NPO for three to five more days."
3. "The tube will be removed when peristalsis returns through the entire GI tract, usually in three to five days."
4. "You'll have to ask that question of your doctor. He's the one who has to give the order to discontinue the tube."

1. INCORRECT. This is only part of the conditions that must be present. Think about the return of total peristalsis and how that might be evidenced.

2. INCORRECT. The client will need the nasogastric tube for a longer period of time, because gastric and intestinal juices are still being produced, even with the NPO status. Without the tube, the accumulation of these secretions would lead to nausea/vomiting and increased discomfort for the client.

3. CORRECT. The return of peristalsis will be evidenced not only by the return of bowel sounds, but also by the passing of flatus through the rectum. It is then deemed safe to pull the nasogastric tube and begin the client on a progressive diet from sips of clear liquids to a regular diet.

4. INCORRECT. This statement gives no information to the client. Based on your knowledge of postoperative management of clients with a nasogastric tube, there is some information that you can share with her. This statement also uses the communication block of referring to an inappropriate person (the doctor).

2. The physician orders a stool specimen to be collected for ova and parasites. What is the proper procedure for collection of this specimen by the nurse?

1. Send the entire stool immediately to the lab.
2. Use a sterile container.
3. Take feces from several areas of the bowel movement.
4. Refrigerate the specimen until it can be delivered to the lab.

1. ***CORRECT. A stool specimen for ova and parasites should be collected in its entirety, placed in a dry container free of urine, labeled correctly, and sent immediately to the laboratory.***
2. *INCORRECT. A sterile container is not necessary. The feces should be collected in a dry container free of urine.*
3. *INCORRECT. Taking samples from various areas of the stool is done when a stool for occult blood is ordered.*
4. *INCORRECT. Refrigeration will kill the parasites and definitely alter the test results.*

3. A client is admitted to the hospital, and a urine specimen is ordered. When obtaining a urine specimen from the client, which action should be avoided?

1. Place the urine cup in the client's bathroom.
2. Take the full specimen cup to the lab pick up area and then place it in a clean plastic bag.
3. Attach the client's name to the specimen cup.
4. Explain to the client the procedure for obtaining a urine specimen.

1. *INCORRECT. This is an appropriate action. The specimen cup should be placed in the client's bathroom so that it is readily available when the client has the urge to void. You are looking for an action that is INAPPROPRIATE.*
2. ***CORRECT. It is inappropriate for the nurse to carry the specimen cup out of the client's room without first placing it in a clean bag to prevent possible spread of organisms. The ideal method of transporting the specimen cup is for the nurse to place it in a clean bag for transportation to the lab pick up area.***

> ***TEST-TAKING TIP:*** This question has a false response stem.

3. *INCORRECT. This is an appropriate action. The specimen cup should be labeled with the client's identification in order to prevent erroneous reporting or mix-up of specimens in the lab. You are looking for an action that is INAPPROPRIATE.*
4. *INCORRECT. This is an appropriate action. Teaching the client how to obtain the specimen is part of the nurse's responsibility in order to provide the best specimen for the test. The question has a false response stem, you are looking for an action that is INAPPROPRIATE.*

4. A child weighing 1800 gm is admitted. The nurse knows that the infant's weight in pounds is:

1. 3.9 lbs.
2. 8.1 lbs.
3. 18 lbs.
4. 36 lbs.

1. ***CORRECT. One kilogram is equal to 2.2 pounds. The correct weight in pounds is calculated by multiplying the weight in kilograms by 2.2. There are 1000 grams in a kilogram. 1.8 kg x 2.2 = 3.96 lbs.***

> ***TEST-TAKING TIP:*** Know your equivalent measures!

2. *INCORRECT. Remember that one kilogram is equal to 2.2 pounds. Therefore, the correct weight is calculated by multiplying the weight in kilograms by 2.2. There are 1000 grams in a kilogram. 1.8 kg x 2.2 = 3.96 pounds.*
3. *INCORRECT. One kilogram is equal to 2.2 pounds. The correct weight in pounds is calculated by multiplying the weight in kilograms by 2.2. There are 1000 grams in a kilogram. 1.8 kg x 2.2 = 3.96 lbs.*

> ***TEST-TAKING TIP:*** Know your equivalent measures!

4. *INCORRECT. One kilogram is equal to 2.2 pounds. The correct weight in pounds is calculated by multiplying the weight in kilograms by 2.2. There are 1000 grams in a kilogram. 1.8 kg x 2.2 = 3.96 lbs.*

5. Which approach by the nurse is best when taking the blood pressure of a client with hypertension?

1. Measure the blood pressure under the same conditions each time.
2. Take the blood pressure with the client sitting on the side of the bed.
3. Place the blood pressure cuff on the right arm above the elbow.
4. Measure the blood pressure with the client in supine position.

1. ***CORRECT. The nurse should record the client's position in the chart so that the next reading may be done with the client in the same position.***

> ***TEST-TAKING TIP:*** The other three options are similar to each other in that they each describe a specific position or method. This option is a broader or more global response.

2. *INCORRECT. The client may be sitting, lying or standing when blood pressure is measured. The nurse should record the client's position in the chart so that the reading may be done with the client in the same position each time.*
3. *INCORRECT. The blood pressure cuff may be placed above the elbow on either the right or left arm.*
4. *INCORRECT. The client may be sitting, lying or stand-*

ing when blood pressure is measured. The nurse should record the client's position in the chart so that the reading may be done with the client in the same position each time.

6. The nurse has just collected a liquid stool specimen for ova and parasites. The test results may not be accurate if the nurse:

1. Places the specimen into a clean container.
2. Puts the collected specimen in the refrigerator.
3. Instructs the client to defecate into a bedpan.
4. Sends only the bloody and mucoid portions of the stool.

1. *INCORRECT — This question has a false response stem. This option describes proper procedure, and this action would not negate the test results. Ova and parasites are detected by microscopic examination. A sterile container is needed for specimens that are to be cultured. You are looking for an action that will make the test results INACCURATE.*
2. ***CORRECT — You have identified the incorrect action. A liquid stool specimen for ova and parasites must be sent immediately to the lab and examined within 30 minutes, to preserve the "life" of any ova. If it cannot be examined within 30 minutes, then some of the specimen should be placed in a preservative, not refrigerated.***
3. *INCORRECT. This would not affect the test results. The client could be instructed to use a bedpan or bedside commode to collect the stool specimen. The specimen, however, must remain free from urine contamination.*
4. *INCORRECT. This would be the correct portion of the specimen to collect if the entire stool cannot be sent to the laboratory. You are looking for an action that will make the test results INACCURATE.*

7. The physician has ordered a sputum specimen to be collected for culture and sensitivity. The nurse is aware that the preferable time to collect this specimen is:

1. In the morning.
2. In the evening, after forcing fluids all day.
3. After antibiotics have been started.
4. After the client has taken an expectorant.

1. ***CORRECT. Generally, the deepest specimens are obtained in the early morning. The client is instructed to rinse his mouth prior to expectorating into the sterile container. It's preferable to collect the specimen before breakfast.***
2. *INCORRECT. Although forcing fluids (especially clear liquids) will help to thin the secretions, the evening hours are not the best time.*
3. *INCORRECT. Recall that any specimen ordered for culture and sensitivity should be obtained before antibiotic therapy is started in order to prevent interference with test results.*
4. *INCORRECT. This is not the best time. Expectorants can contaminate the specimen.*

8. To assess for correct placement of a nasogastric tube, the nurse should:

1. Instill 30 ml of saline to assess client tolerance.
2. Instill 10 ml of air into the tube and listen for gurgling sounds with a stethoscope over the gastric area.
3. Aspirate stomach contents with a syringe.
4. Place the end of the tube in water to assess for bubbling.

1. *INCORRECT. A hazardous procedure! This could be dangerous if the tube was in the lungs and not the stomach.*
2. *INCORRECT. This method does not provide for a sufficient amount of air to reach the stomach and make any gurgling sounds. At least 30 ml of air is needed. There is a safer and more reliable method among the options given.*
3. ***CORRECT. Placement should be checked by aspirating gastric contents with a syringe and testing the pH of the aspirate.***
4. *INCORRECT. This could be dangerous to the client if the tube was incorrectly positioned in the lungs. The client could aspirate the water in the glass.*

9. When obtaining a urine specimen from an indwelling catheter for culture and sensitivity, the nurse should:

1. Empty the drainage bag from the urometer port.
2. Wear sterile gloves.
3. Cleanse the entry site on the catheter prior to inserting the needle.
4. Drain the bag and wait for a fresh urine sample to send from the drainage bag.

1. *INCORRECT. The urometer port can only be used to obtain a non-sterile specimen. You cannot obtain a urine culture and sensitivity from this port.*
2. *INCORRECT. Sterile gloves are unnecessary when obtaining a specimen for culture and sensitivity since the nurse does not disrupt the closed system except with a sterile needle.*
3. ***CORRECT. Disinfecting the needle insertion site removes or destroys any microorganisms on the surface of the catheter, thereby avoiding contamination of the needle and entrance of microorganisms into the catheter.***
4. *INCORRECT. Urine obtained from the drainage bag is unsterile because the bag contains microorganisms. Urine from the drainage bag cannot be used for culture and sensitivity.*

10. When collecting a urine specimen for a routine urinalysis, which of the following nursing actions is the most important?

1. Label the container with the client's room number.
2. Check the identification of the client.
3. Avoid using gloves when handling a urine specimen.
4. Instruct the client to put the specimen on the counter at the nurses' station for pick up.

1. *INCORRECT. This is appropriate, but it is not the most important measure and it is not sufficient for identifying the specimen.*
2. ***CORRECT. In order to avoid errors, the most important thing to do is to identify the client. Then, after the client is identified, the next action is to make sure the specimen label has the client's name and room number.***
3. *INCORRECT. Gloves should be worn when handling any specimen.*
4. *INCORRECT. The nurse should take the specimen container to the dirty utility room.*

11. In obtaining a blood pressure measurement, the most appropriate nursing action is to:

1. Obtain the proper equipment, place the client in a comfortable position, and record the appropriate information in the client's chart.
2. Measure the client's arm, if you are uncertain of the size of cuff to use.
3. Have the client recline or sit comfortably in a chair with the forearm at the level of the heart.
4. Document the measurement, which extremity was used, and the position that the client was in during the measurement.

1. ***CORRECT. This is a general or comprehensive statement about the correct procedure, and it includes the basic ideas that are found in the other options.***
2. *INCORRECT. This option is a possibility. The correct size cuff is necessary in order to obtain a reliable measurement. However, this is not the best option.*
3. *INCORRECT. The client should be relaxed and comfortable for a reliable reading. However, this is not the best option.*
4. *Documentation of these parameters is essential. However, this is not the best option.*

12. The physician requests a stool specimen for culture, for an alert and ambulatory client. The nurse would give which directions to the client for proper stool collection?

1. Restrict food and liquids the night before the collection.
2. Maintain a sterile procedure.
3. Require the collection of specimens on three consecutive days.
4. Retrieve from the toilet with sterile gloves and then place in the container.

1. *INCORRECT. There are no food or fluid restrictions involved in the collection of a stool specimen.*
2. *INCORRECT. This is not possible. However, the client should use a procedure that will ensure that the specimen is not contaminated when transferred to the container.*
3. ***CORRECT. This is normal procedure for a stool culture in order to detect pathogens of the gastrointestinal tract.***
4. *INCORRECT. The stool specimen should not be immersed in water, and certainly not in the toilet. It should be placed directly into the specimen container.*

13. Assisting the doctor in examining a two-year-old who has otitis media, the nurse should have the child:

1. Lie down on the examining table while his throat and ears are examined, and then allow him to sit up for the rest of the exam.
2. Lie down on the examining table, while the physician starts with examining the head and proceeds downward with the exam.
3. Sit in his mother's lap while the heart and lungs are auscultated, and then examine the rest of his body, doing the throat and ears last.
4. Allow him to sit in his mother's lap while his ears are examined with an otoscope, and then take his BP and vital signs.

1. *INCORRECT. This approach is likely to have the child crying and upset.*
2. *INCORRECT. In young children it is not recommended to start at the head and work down. This method is recommended for school age and above.*
3. ***CORRECT. This is the correct sequence, leaving the most invasive procedures until last.***
4. *INCORRECT. This may result in inaccurate vital signs, or great difficulty in even obtaining them. Following the exam of the ears, the child is likely to be upset and crying.*

14. A postoperative client has an electronic blood pressure machine automatically measuring her blood pressure every 15 minutes. The nurse notes that the blood pressure machine is reading the client's blood pressure at more frequent intervals, and that the readings are not similar. The nurse checks the machine settings and observes additional readings, but the problem continues. At this time, the best nursing action is to:

1. Record only those blood pressures that are needed for the 15-minute intervals.
2. Disconnect the machine and measure the blood pressure with a sphygmomanometer and stethoscope.
3. Turn on the machine every 15 minutes to obtain the client's blood pressure.
4. Measure the blood pressure manually and compare readings obtained by the machine with readings obtained manually.

1. *INCORRECT. Although blood pressure readings are being obtained, the fact that the machine is taking the blood pressure more frequently and the measurements obtained are not similar suggests that the machine is malfunctioning and is in need of repair. A malfunctioning machine may present an electrical hazard.*

TEST-TAKING TIP: Remember — Safety first! Also, note that options 1 and 3 are similar and can be eliminated.

2. ***CORRECT. If there is a question concerning the reliability of the monitoring equipment, a manual check should be made, so that a client does not receive medical treatment because of an erroneous measurement. Also, a malfunctioning machine may present an electrical hazard and should be disconnected.***
3. *INCORRECT. Since the measurements and the operation of the machine appear to be questionable, the machine should be taken out of service and repaired. A malfunctioning machine may present an electrical hazard.*

> ***TEST-TAKING TIP:*** Remember — Safety first! Also, note that options 1 and 3 are similar and can be eliminated.

4. *INCORRECT. Although this option appears to provide a means of checking the machine, the fact that it is not operating correctly suggests that it should be disconnected and not used until it has been checked by a biomedical technician. A malfunctioning machine may present an electrical hazard.*

15. Six hours into the collection of a 24-hour urine specimen, one voided specimen is accidentally discarded by the client. The nurse should:

1. Continue the collection, noting the loss on the lab slip.
2. Notify the nurse in charge.
3. Discard the previously collected urine and start the collection again.
4. Notify the lab so that the collection can be reduced to six hours.

1. *INCORRECT. This action would give false results because the values would be still based on less than a 24-hour collection of ALL voided urine.*
2. *INCORRECT. There is an action that the nurse can take independently prior to notifying the nurse in charge.*
3. ***CORRECT. If a specimen is lost or contaminated in any way during the 24-hour collection, the process must begin again. ALL urine voided in 24 hours must be collected or the test results will not be valid. Remember that lab values are being monitored based on the average elimination of those elements in a 24-hour time period.***
4. *INCORRECT. 24-hour collections are designed to be just that: no less and no more. Lost specimens mean delays and time lost in the analysis of the urine.*

16. The physician orders a urine test. The nurse understands that specific gravity of urine is used to determine the amount of:

1. Proteins in the urine.
2. Uric acid crystals in the urine.
3. Solutes in the urine.
4. Epithelial cells in the urine.

1. *INCORRECT. Although proteins may be present in the urine, they are not measured in this test.*
2. *INCORRECT. Although uric acid crystals may be present in the urine, they are not measured in this test.*
3. ***CORRECT. Specific gravity varies with fluid intake and the quantity of solutes dissolved in the urine. Normal value is 1.005 to 1.025.***
4. *INCORRECT. Although epithelial cells may be present in the urine, they are not measured in this test.*

Section 6: Growth and Development

1. The nurse is preparing a seven-year-old female for hospitalization. The child had a previous hospital experience. To best prepare this child, the nurse would:

1. Suggest a role play and provide materials.
2. Remind the child of the experience of her past hospitalization.
3. Read her a story about another child having a similar operation.
4. Tell her she is only going in to have her throat checked.

1. ***CORRECT. Concrete experiences are the most meaningful learning for a school-aged child. This is the rationale for pediatric orientation programs. If there is inadequate time for her to participate in such a program, a shortened version where she could practice with a mask and other equipment in a non-threatening environment would be helpful.***

> ***TEST-TAKING TIP:*** This is the only option that involves DOING something with the child, instead of just talking with her.

2. *INCORRECT. Past experiences may not have been positive, and may even have been traumatic. Don't read into the question!*
3. *INCORRECT. This isn't the best response. This is somewhat abstract, and abstract thinking is not highly developed in the seven-year-old child. Think about how you learned what an operation was really like for a client.*
4. *INCORRECT. Never lie to a child. This is inappropriate under any circumstances.*

2. A nephrectomy (removal of the kidney) is scheduled tomorrow on a three-year-old client. How would the nurse best prepare this child for this procedure?

1. On the evening before the procedure, demonstrate by pointing on the child's body where the incision will be made.
2. Give the preoperative sedation as ordered with a small needle so that a Band-Aid will not be needed.
3. Ask the child's parents to leave the room while the preoperative medication is administered.

4. Explain the procedure to the child in simple sentences just before giving the preoperative sedation.

1 *INCORRECT. This action will increase anxiety. Also, the evening before surgery is too long before the procedure to explain to a three-year-old child. Did you read all the options before choosing your answer?*

2. *INCORRECT. The child does need a Band-Aid because at the age of three the child has fears of mutilation.*

> ***TEST-TAKING TIP:*** Note that this option concerns the preoperative medication, not the more general issue of preparing the child for surgery.

3. *INCORRECT. The child needs the parents for support during the pain of the injection and for immediate comfort following it. Parents should only leave the room if that is their preference.*

> ***TEST-TAKING TIP:*** Note that this option and option 2 both concern the preoperative injection and can be eliminated.

4. ***CORRECT. The child should have an explanation at an age appropriate level just before the nurse is going to follow through. This approach promotes trust and avoids unnecessary anxiety.***

> ***TEST-TAKING TIP:*** Note that options 2 and 3 are both specifically concerned with the preoperative injection and can be eliminated.

3. During a well-child visit, the mother of a five-year-old expresses concern that her son refuses to wear his helmet while riding his bicycle. What is the appropriate nursing response?

1. "Tell him the bike doesn't leave the garage without the helmet."
2. "It isn't that important, since he won't be riding in the road."
3. "Gradually encourage the wearing of the helmet with small rewards."
4. "I'll explain to him the potential for injury without a helmet."

1. ***CORRECT. Even though this may sound very tough, it is direct, and it is an appropriate method of obtaining compliance. The parent must believe that the helmet is necessary and apply the rule consistently. This question requires an understanding of growth and development issues for a young school-age child.***

> ***TEST-TAKING TIP:*** This is the only option that provides for the child's safety.

2. *INCORRECT. Any fall anywhere can potentially cause a head injury. Also, there is no information about where the child will ride.*

> ***TEST-TAKING TIP:*** Option 2 and Option 3 would both result in the child not wearing the helmet when riding. Similar options can be eliminated.

3. *INCORRECT. This response implies inconsistency. Children respond more favorably to consistency. A reward system should not be necessary, since this is expected rather that an optional behavior. This child is at risk for head injury.*

> ***TEST-TAKING TIP:*** Option 2 and Option 3 would both result in the child not wearing the helmet when riding. Similar options can be eliminated.

4. *INCORRECT. The nurse's explanation is not likely to be effective and will not provide for the safety of the child. This child is at risk for head injury. This question requires an understanding of behavior and developmental issues for a young school-age child, who needs strict limit setting.*

4. On the tenth day of hospitalization, an 11-month-old child is quiet and sad when his mother leaves. The nurse knows this behavior indicates:

1. An understanding of his mother's need to leave.
2. Despair at his mother's absence.
3. Protest that his source of emotional support is gone.
4. Developing autonomy.

1. *INCORRECT. Did you note the age of this child?*
2. ***CORRECT. This is an indication that separation anxiety has progressed beyond the stage where protest is demonstrated. This may have consequences after hospitalization.***
3. *INCORRECT. Look at the behaviors that are stated in the question.*
4. *INCORRECT. This child is too young to be working on the development of autonomy. He is still in the stage of trust development with his primary caregiver.*

5. A 30-month-old male is being admitted with asthma. To decrease the stress of hospitalization for the toddler, the nurse should:

1. Explain procedures and routines.
2. Encourage contact with children of the same age.
3. Provide for privacy.
4. Encourage rooming-in.

1. *INCORRECT. You can explain procedures, but this is not the best answer. This becomes a more appropriate stress-reducing technique as the child matures into school age and adolescence.*

> ***TEST-TAKING TIP:*** Identify the critical elements! The issue is stress of hospitalization. What is the age of the client?

2. *INCORRECT. The peer group is not the major support for the toddler. This would be a more successful plan with the school age or adolescent client.*

> ***TEST-TAKING TIP:*** Identify the critical elements! The issue is stress of hospitalization. What is the age of the client?

3. *INCORRECT. Adolescence is the age in which stress may be reduced by providing privacy in order for them to cope more effectively.*

> **TEST-TAKING TIP:** What is the age of the client?

4. ***CORRECT. Rooming-in is the most effective means of providing emotional support for the toddler. The family's presence provides a sense of security that will increase the child's ability to cope in an unfamiliar environment. This is well supported by nursing research.***

6. A disruptive 10-year-old child is having difficulty interacting with other children on the unit. Which nursing action would be best initially?

1. Have a unit conference with other staff members and discuss strategies to solve the problem.
2. Talk to the child about the behavior that is causing the problem and identify possible solutions.
3. Tell the other children to stop teasing the client and to observe for changes in the client's behavior.
4. Tell the client's mother that she needs to talk to her son about his disruptive behavior.

1. *INCORRECT. The client in this question is the disruptive 10-year-old child, and the issue is disruptive behavior. This option is only indirectly related to the client.*
2. ***CORRECT. The disruptive 10-year-old child is the client in this question, and the issue is the child's behavior. This option deals directly and therapeutically with the issue of the client's behavior.***

> **TEST-TAKING TIP:** This is the only option that involves the nurse talking directly with the client. In all the other options, the nurse will talk to someone else instead.

3. *The client in this question is the disruptive 10-year-old child, not the other children on the unit. The answer should be related to the client. Also, "telling" the other children what to do about the problem is characteristic of an authority figure and is not therapeutic in the nurse-client relationship. The nurse's response must be therapeutic for the client.*
4. *INCORRECT. This option focuses on inappropriate person, the client's mother. Also, "telling" the client's mother what she "needs" to do is characteristic of an authority figure and is not therapeutic in the nurse-client relationship.*

7. In caring for a preschooler who is being admitted the evening before surgery, the nurse knows that which activity is least appropriate for reducing the stress of hospitalization?

1. Explaining the surgical procedure.
2. Playing "surgery" with cap and masks.
3. Showing her the call light and bathroom.
4. Having her mother undress her.

1. ***CORRECT. The evening before surgery is too early to explain the procedure to a preschooler.***

> **TEST-TAKING TIP:** This question has a false response stem.

2. *INCORRECT. The question has a false response stem, and this action is an appropriate stress-reducing activity for a preschool child. Play is practice/learning for young children, and this will help prepare the child for the experience of surgery.*
3. *INCORRECT. The question has a false response stem, and this action is an appropriate stress-reducing activity for this preschool child. The purpose of this nursing action is to increase the client's feelings of security and control, and to provide a safe environment for the client.*
4. *INCORRECT. This action will help the child feel safe and more comfortable in this "foreign" environment. Also, the mother will feel more capable of nurturing her child. This action is an appropriate stress-reducing activity for a preschooler — and the question has a false response stem.*

8. A four-year-old is visiting his brother who is critically ill and may be dying. In talking with this young visitor, the nurse is aware that he would be least likely to believe that death is:

1. Like going to sleep.
2. The result of magic.
3. Permanent and lasting.
4. The result of a wish.

1. *INCORRECT. Children may frequently make this comparison, since they have little experience with death. This may make it frightening for a preschooler.*

> **TEST-TAKING TIP:** This question has a false response stem. Select again.

2. *INCORRECT. A child this age may see death as the result of magic, since it is not well understood.*

> **TEST-TAKING TIP:** Options 2 and 4 are very similar — so neither can be the correct answer. Which belief is least likely in a four-year-old child?

3. ***CORRECT. This question has a false response stem. Four year olds have difficulty understanding the concept of time and are therefore not likely to believe that death is permanent.***
4. *INCORRECT. Preschoolers do believe that their thoughts and wishes can make things happen, since they are egocentric. This is one reason why the death of a family member can be very difficult for a child this age.*

> **TEST-TAKING TIP:** Options 2 and 4 are very similar -- so neither can be the correct answer.

9. Anticipatory guidance is given to the parents of a 10-year-old girl. The nurse knows the parents understand this information if they say they will reinforce:

1. Sex education and self breast exam.
2. The need for increased caloric intake.
3. The child's increasing need for sleep.
4. The need for fewer dental visits.

1. ***CORRECT. "Anticipatory guidance" means family/client teaching about the next developmental stage. Since puberty is usually attained between 10 and 12 for females, the most important information is about her developing sexual body.***
2. *INCORRECT. The most important nutritional information at this age is the need for increased sources of iron.*
3. *INCORRECT. Sleep requirements diminish from birth to adulthood. This is mainly due to the maturing body's ability to get into REM sleep more quickly.*
4. *INCORRECT. Although permanent teeth are in by this age, this is all the more reason to have regular check-ups and good oral hygiene, which includes brushing and flossing. These habits will help the child keep these teeth for a lifetime.*

10. The nurse knows that which of the following behaviors would indicate regression in a hospitalized five-year-old?

1. Bedwetting several times a day.
2. Crying when mother leaves.
3. Eating only food from home.
4. Wanting his teddy bear for bedtime.

1. ***CORRECT. You would expect a five-year-old to be toilet trained. Incontinence is a commonly seen sign of regression in young children.***
2. *INCORRECT. This is a sign of separation anxiety, which is seen in children between the ages of six months and five years. This is within normal for this child's age and is not a sign of regression for this child.*

> ***TEST-TAKING TIP:*** The stem of the question is specifically asking about regression.

3. *INCORRECT. This is normal behavior, not a sign of regression. Children frequently do not eat foods that are different. Sick children particularly do not make changes in their dietary habits.*
4. *INCORRECT. This is normal behavior, not a sign of regression. Many young children are attached to a familiar object from home, which is referred to as a transitional object.*

11. A nine-year-old girl is admitted with asthma. In planning her care, the nurse should anticipate that the child will prefer to:

1. Play with another girl her age.
2. Be with older girls.
3. Associate with small groups of boys and girls.
4. Have male companions.

1. ***CORRECT. The school age child is in the latent psychosexual stage according to Freud, and would feel most comfortable with a peer of the same age and sex.***
2. *INCORRECT. This isn't the school age child's group of choice.*

> ***TEST-TAKING TIP:*** To answer this growth and development question, think about the activities that children of this age enjoy. This may help you know who they would be most comfortable with socially.

3. *INCORRECT. Younger children will socialize in this way, not really caring if the companions are male or female.*

> ***TEST-TAKING TIP:*** To answer the question, think about the activities that children of this age enjoy. This may help you know who they would be most comfortable with socially.

4. *INCORRECT. This would be way ahead of this child's psychosexual developmental stage. Adolescents, not school age children, prefer gender opposites.*

12. In caring for elderly clients, the nurse understands that the aging process generally results in:

1. A decline in physiological and sensory systems of the body.
2. A decreased skin resilience.
3. A diminished hearing acuity.
4. An absence of sexual interest and activity.

1. ***CORRECT. This is a general statement about the effects of aging.***

> ***TEST-TAKING TIP:*** The test-taking strategy of looking for a global response option would identify this option as the correct answer. Note that this option includes the correct ideas in options 2 and 3.

2. *INCORRECT. Loss of skin resilience is a normal finding in the elderly; however, this is not the best option. Read the other options, and try to select the best one using a test-taking strategy.*
3. *INCORRECT. Many elderly clients experience some hearing loss; however, this is not the best option. Read the other options, and try to select the best one using a test- taking strategy.*
4. *INCORRECT. Sexual interest and activity does not cease in the elderly.*

13. A four-year-old is admitted to the hospital with croup. When the mother comes to visit the next day, she finds the nurse changing the bedding after the client has wet the bed. The mother says, "He never wets the bed at home. I am so embarrassed." Which nursing response is most helpful to the mother?

1. "I know this can really be embarrassing, but I have kids myself, so I understand and it doesn't bother me."
2. "It is not uncommon for children to regress during a hospitalization. His toileting skills will return when he is feeling better."
3. "It's probably due to the medication we are giving him for his infection."
4. "I plan to discuss your child's incontinence with the physician, as this may require further investigation."

1. INCORRECT. Even though you may have heard nurses say this, it is not therapeutic communication, since it offers no information about the source or treatment of the incontinence.

> **TEST-TAKING TIP:** This response cannot be correct because it uses the communication block of referring to inappropriate persons (the nurse and the nurse's children).

2. CORRECT. A recently gained skill such as toilet training is often temporarily lost due to the stress of hospitalization. It is appropriate to reassure the mother that this is an expected behavior in young children and that continence will be regained when his health is regained.

> **TEST-TAKING TIP:** The mother is the client in this communication question. This response addresses the client's concern uses the therapeutic communication tool of giving information.

3. INCORRECT. The medications most likely to be administered for croup would be antibiotics and acetaminophen; neither have side effects of incontinence.

> **TEST-TAKING TIP:** How old is the child?

4. INCORRECT. Are you reading into the question? Symptoms such as hematuria, abdominal pain, or pain during urination would be necessary to warrant follow-up from this one episode of bedwetting in a four-year-old child.

14. In developing a plan to improve the self-image of an eight-year-old client with asthma, the nurse should consider that:

1. The client is not able to understand the causes or limitations of chronic illness.
2. The client's peers, parents, and teachers should be instructed in strategies for encouraging her.
3. Teaching the client self-care skills will increase her sense of control.
4. The client should be told about all potential long-term complications.

1. INCORRECT. This child is in third grade at school, where science is part of the curriculum. Cause and effect is understood if the terms used are appropriate.

> **TEST-TAKING TIP:** This option does not address the issue in the question, which is self-esteem.

2. INCORRECT. Her peers are also eight years old, and they are not necessarily supportive or encouraging. These are all external sources of approval, not a measure of self-esteem.

3. CORRECT. Teaching her about her medications and how to handle her asthma attacks will increase her sense of control over her illness, thereby improving her self-esteem.

> **TEST-TAKING TIP:** Note that the word "self" occurs in the question and in this option. This is a clue that this option may be the correct answer.

4. INCORRECT. School age children cannot comprehend long-term complications. This would not improve her self-esteem, either, so this option does not address the issue in the question.

15. The mother of a two-year-old who is hospitalized asks how she should handle her son's temper tantrums. The nurse should advise the mother to:

1. Restrain the child physically.
2. Ignore the behavior.
3. Let the child know his temper tantrums are not acceptable.
4. Play a game with him, or rock him quietly.

1. INCORRECT. This may actually cause the behavior to intensify. Select an option that will diminish the behavior.

2. CORRECT. This is the recommended approach, since it does not reinforce the behavior. Ignoring a negative behavior is a basic concept in behavior modification.

> **TEST-TAKING TIP:** The other options all include an action in response to the tantrums. This option is the one that is different.

3. INCORRECT. This behavior is due to lack of self-control, which is gradually being gained at this age.

4. INCORRECT. This would reinforce the negative behavior, so it is incorrect.

16. A hospitalized eight-year-old is losing a game of checkers. He stands up and says, "I quit." The nurse understands that this behavior probably is:

1. A personality change due to hospitalization.
2. Immaturity for his age.
3. A sign that this game is too hard for him.
4. Normal for his social development.

1. INCORRECT. This behavior is probably not a change.

> **TEST-TAKING TIP:** Consider the age of the client in this question, and look for another reason for this behavior. Are you "reading into" the question?

2. INCORRECT. This behavior is not unusual at this age.

TEST-TAKING TIP: Consider the age of the client in this question, and look for another reason for this behavior.

3. *INCORRECT. This is an age-appropriate activity. Remember, play is the way children learn..*

TEST-TAKING TIP: Don't "read into" the question! The introductory statement tells you that the client is losing the game; it does not tell you that the client does not understand how to play. Consider the age of the client and look for another reason for this behavior.

4. ***CORRECT. Children will frequently "quit" at this age if they cannot succeed, until they learn that the social interaction is more important than winning.***

TEST-TAKING TIP: This is the "different" option — the only one that does not indicate that there is a problem. If you were unsure of the answer, this is a clue.

17. The nurse is evaluating the effectiveness of the teaching performed for the mother of a six-month-old who is teething. The nurse would consider the teaching to be successful if the mother:

1. Provides the infant with a hard rubber toy to bite.
2. Places aspirin against the erupting tooth.
3. Rubs a topical anesthetic on the sensitive area.
4. Places sherry and water mixture on gums at bedtime.

1. ***CORRECT. This is safe and will speed the tooth's erupting by providing a firm surface to help the tooth break through the skin.***

TEST-TAKING TIP: The issue in the question is teething, and the correct action must, above all, be safe. Also, note that this option is the "different" option because the others involve the use of an anesthetic or analgesic.

2. *INCORRECT. This is unsafe, since the infant may aspirate the aspirin.*

TEST-TAKING TIP: The issue in the question is teething. Remember, "Safety first!" Look for an option that addresses the issue is a safe manner.

3. *INCORRECT. Topical anesthetics are not to be taken internally or used in the mouth. Only oral anesthetics can be used safely.*
4. *INCORRECT. Although many parents will remember someone in the family using alcohol to reduce teething pain, this is never recommended for children.*

TEST-TAKING TIP: The issue in the question is teething. Remember, "Safety first!"

18. At nine months of age, an infant has been in the hospital four times for a total of 42 days. The nurse notices that the infant does not seem upset when her parents leave. The nurse would evaluate this behavior as:

1. An infant with an easy temperament.
2. A mature infant who is very secure.
3. A strong attachment to the nurse.
4. Experiencing detachment.

1. *INCORRECT. Even children with an easy temperament would not normally feel comfortable with parents leaving them. Fear of abandonment is strong at this age.*

TEST-TAKING TIP: The question is about the infant's behavior "when her parents leave." The issue in this growth and development question is separation anxiety.

2. *INCORRECT. There is no reason to believe this is a true statement. This child has had four interruptions in a sensitive period of development: the period where trust in the primary care giver needs to be developed.*
3. *INCORRECT. The infant must first develop a sense of trust with one individual (the primary care giver) before meaningful relationships can occur with others. Due to many separations, this child has not had the opportunity to develop that trust.*

TEST-TAKING TIP: There is no information to indicate that the child has developed an attachment to the nurse, so you know this option has to be incorrect.

4. ***CORRECT. Although the characteristic superficial interaction with the environment might appear to be an acceptance by the child of being left by parents, this infant is exhibiting the third stage of separation anxiety, which is detachment.***

TEST-TAKING TIP: The question is about the infant's behavior "when her parents leave." The issue in this growth and development question is separation anxiety. Note also that this is the only option that identifies a problem.

19. The father of a four-year-old son tells the nurse that his child believes there are monsters in his closet at bedtime. The nurse's best suggestion for dealing with this problem is:

1. Letting the child sleep with his parents.
2. Keeping a night light on in the child's bedroom.
3. Tell the child that these fears are not real.
4. Staying with the child until he falls asleep.

1. *INCORRECT. This suggestion is inappropriate. The child is apt to develop a habit that will interfere with the parents' need for privacy and the child's ability to settle himself for sleep.*
2. ***CORRECT. After the parent reassures the child, the light helps the child "see" for himself that there is nothing hiding in the shadows.***

TEST-TAKING TIP: Using your understanding of growth and development, you recognize that the child of age four has difficulty distinguishing between real and make-believe.

3. *INCORRECT. Although the "monsters and bogeymen" are not real, the child's fears are! This is not the best suggestion for the child of age four, who has difficulty distinguishing between real and make-believe.*
4. *INCORRECT. This encourages procrastination going to sleep. This easily becomes a habit that is difficult to break.*

TEST-TAKING TIP: In normal growth and development, the child of age four has difficulty distinguishing between real and make-believe. This option does not address this issue.

20. A three-year-old is brought to the clinic for evaluation because he is thin and his mother is concerned about his appetite. The best response the nurse can give his mom is:

1. "His appetite should be increasing, so he needs to be fed."
2. "You should discourage food rituals."
3. "His growth is slow, and so his appetite is, too."
4. "If this continues, he will need testing."

1. *INCORRECT. Three year olds do not like being fed. They want to do it themselves. Use your knowledge of growth and development.*
2. *INCORRECT. Food fads and rituals are a normal part of the developing toddler. Ignoring these behaviors is recommended, rather than drawing attention to them.*
3. ***CORRECT. The term for this is "physiologic anorexia." The child's appetite decreases in response to the plateau of growth at this age.***
4. *INCORRECT. Think about the norms for this age child.*

21. In caring for a confused elderly client, which statement by the nurse indicates the best understanding of the principles of reality orientation?

1. "Good morning, Mr. Jones. Did you sleep well? It's time to get dressed."
2. "Good morning. This is your second day in Shady Pines and I am your nurse for the day."
3. "Do you remember who I am? We met yesterday when you were admitted."
4. "Good morning, how are you today? I am your nurse for the day. My name is Mrs. Smith."

1. *INCORRECT. It does not actually orient the client to anything other than his name. Also, the nurse should wait for the client to answer her initial question before telling him it is time to get dressed. Short statements, made one at a time, should be used with persons who have memory and other cognitive deficits.*
2. ***CORRECT. This statement orients the client to time of day, place, and the nurse's identity. It also is a clear statement that does not contain any irrelevant information that could be confusing to the client.***

TEST-TAKING TIP: Focus on the issue in the question!

3. *INCORRECT. The client with memory deficits will probably not recognize the nurse or remember meeting her the previous day. The question does not orient the client to time or place, and even fails to identify the nurse.*
4. *This greeting does not orient the client to place. There is a better option.*

22. The nurse caring for clients in a long-term care facility understands that remotivation therapy is used to:

1. Stimulate and encourage social participation.
2. Reorient clients with cognitive problems.
3. Encourage clients to share memories of past experiences and events.
4. Resolve emotional problems.

1. ***CORRECT. The goals of remotivation therapy are to stimulate and encourage social participation using structured group approaches.***

TEST-TAKING TIP: "Stimulate" and the word motivate or "remotivate" in the stem have somewhat similar meanings. This is a clue that this option might be the answer.

2. *INCORRECT. This option describes reality orientation programs.*
3. *INCORRECT. This option describes reminiscence therapy.*
4. *INCORRECT. Psychotherapy, either individual or group, is used to assist clients to resolve emotional and psychological difficulties. This is not the rationale for remotivation therapy.*

23. An elderly client is able to walk with a cane and enjoys ambulating in the hall. Since he has memory problems, he has great difficulty remembering which room is his. What nursing action would best alleviate this problem?

1. Assign him a room close to the nursing station so staff members will be available to help him.
2. Assign him to a room with a roommate who can watch out for him.
3. Do not allow him to leave his room unaccompanied.
4. Put his picture and his name written in large letters on the door to his room.

1. *INCORRECT. This action is not feasible in most settings, and even if it were, would only serve to make him more dependent on the nursing staff. Read all the options before selecting the best!*
2. *INCORRECT. The nursing staff is responsible for assuring the client's safety, not the roommate. This action would also foster increasing dependency and loss of a sense of control.*
3. *INCORRECT. It is unnecessarily restrictive and would foster increasing dependency. The client "is able to*

walk with a cane and enjoys ambulating." The client should be assisted to maintain his level of independence.

4. ***CORRECT. This is an orienting device that would allow the client to locate his room independently. This will assist the client to maintain his level of independence. This option is therapeutic for the client.***

> ***TEST-TAKING TIP:*** This is the only option that assists the client to deal with his "memory problem" as identified in the introductory statement.

24. While working in a pediatric unit, the nurse encounters all ages of children. The nurse knows that a child's social interactions with peers are very important. During which periods of a child's life is this need greatest?

1. Preschool and school age.
2. Toddler and preschool.
3. School age and adolescence.
4. Late adolescence and early adulthood.

1. *INCORRECT. Think about the type of interactions a child has at each age.*

> ***TEST-TAKING TIP:*** The key word in the introductory statement is "peers."

2. *INCORRECT. The toddler's world is still the family.*

> ***TEST-TAKING TIP:*** The key word in the introductory statement is "peers."

3. ***CORRECT. School age children begin to extend beyond the nuclear family, while adolescents need peers to help them develop their identity and independence.***
4. *INCORRECT. Note that young adulthood is beyond childhood. This is a clue that this option is not the best choice in this question situated in a pediatric ward!*

25. The nurse knows that it is characteristic of the development of a 30-month-old child to:

1. Tell tall tales.
2. Have a command vocabulary of about 10 words.
3. Weigh double his birth weight.
4. Have achieved complete primary dentition.

1. *INCORRECT. This is true of children of about four years old.*
2. *INCORRECT. Language is much more developed at this age; the child's vocabulary consists of approximately 300 words.*
3. *INCORRECT. This important developmental milestone should be attained by six months.*
4. ***CORRECT. The 20 primary teeth should be erupted by approximately 30 months.***

> ***TEST-TAKING TIP:*** There are no clues in this question! You need to know your growth and development milestones.

26. In developing a plan for perioperative teaching for an adolescent, the nurse should be guided by the knowledge that:

1. He may act as if he knows much more than he actually does.
2. He will only be interested in reassurance that things will go well.
3. The major part of the teaching should be delayed until after the surgery.
4. His parents should be the major focus of the teaching.

1. ***CORRECT. Adolescents may have a difficult time asking questions or being open to explanations. This is part of their struggle for independence.***

> ***TEST-TAKING TIP:*** The indefinite word "may" is a clue that this MAY be the correct answer. And here's another tip: Since this describes a tendency in adolescent behavior, "go with what you know."

2. *INCORRECT. Adolescents are capable of abstract thought and realize that there are risks.*

> ***TEST-TAKING TIP:*** The restrictive word "only" is a clue that this option is incorrect.

3. *INCORRECT. The timing and content of perioperative teaching for an adolescent should be similar to that of an adult, since they have the ability to understand the concept of time as well as abstract reasoning. The adolescent will want to know and understand what will happen; this is part of their struggle for independence.*
4. *INCORRECT. In adolescence, health professionals should switch the direction of teaching to the client. This does not mean that parents are excluded, but that they are no longer the focus, as they were in earlier periods.*

27. The nurse would best describe the most important aspect of planning the discipline of a hospitalized toddler as:

1. Consistency in enforcing the rules.
2. Delaying punishment for wrong doing until parents are present.
3. Eliminating discipline while the child is ill.
4. Giving several warnings before actually disciplining.

1. ***CORRECT. Although this may be a "hard sell" to parents who have guilty feelings about the hospitalization, parents need to be reminded that discipline communicates love to children.***
2. *INCORRECT. This is inappropriate and would be ineffective with a toddler. Rules should be consistently maintained, even in the parents' absence.*
3. *INCORRECT. This is inappropriate, even though some parents feel that this is appropriate.*

> **TEST-TAKING TIP:** This option seems to contradict the issue in the question, which is discipline! If in doubt, rule it out.

4. *INCORRECT. This is inappropriate part of a disciplinary plan for a toddler because it encourages testing on the child's part to determine the limits. It could actually be dangerous, depending on the behavior.*

28. In caring for the elderly, the nurse is guided by Erikson's observation that the elderly need to resolve conflicts between:

1. Ego integrity and despair.
2. Intimacy and isolation.
3. Generativity and stagnation.
4. Identity and isolation.

1. ***CORRECT. Integrity requires the acceptance of one's life, the ability to give up fantasies and goals that could not be achieved, making peace with oneself, and taking responsibility for how one's life has turned out. Failure to reach this level of self-acceptance may result in despair, contempt for others, and fear of death.***

> **TEST-TAKING TIP:** There are no clues here! There is no substitute for knowing developmental stages. The nurse needs this knowledge to be therapeutic.

2. *INCORRECT. Intimacy versus isolation is the psychosocial crisis associated with adulthood. What is the characteristic challenge of old age?*
3. *INCORRECT. Generativity versus stagnation is the psychosocial crisis associated with middle age. What is the characteristic challenge of old age?*
4. *INCORRECT. Identity versus isolation is the psychosocial crisis associated with adolescence. How would you describe the characteristic challenge of old age?*

29. The nurse has been caring for an elderly client who was admitted for hip replacement and is disoriented to time and place. The nurse requests to be assigned to stay with the client when she returns to the unit after her surgery. The rationale for this request is:

1. The elderly client requires close postoperative supervision because of her unpredictable preoperative behavior.
2. The elderly client will most likely be agitated when she regains consciousness after surgery.
3. The many stresses associated with surgery could lead to further cognitive impairment in this elderly client.
4. Elderly clients are particularly vulnerable to the development of postoperative complications.

1. *INCORRECT. The client had disorientation to time and place preoperatively, but she was not described as "unpredictable." Do not read into the question!*
2. *INCORRECT. This client is at risk for many problems, including agitation, postoperatively. Note, however, that the client exhibited disorientation to time and place preoperatively, but she was not described as agitated.*
3. ***CORRECT. The many stresses, both physiological and psychological, associated with surgery, place this client at risk for further cognitive impairment postoperatively. Her postoperative behavior requires ongoing nursing assessment and intervention. This can be best provided by a nurse in constant attendance. The continuity of care with the nurse who attended the client before surgery may also help the client in maintaining orientation.***
4. *INCORRECT. This is a true statement, but it does not specifically address the issues and risk factors in this question.*

30. The nurse working with elderly clients knows that organic mental disorders:

1. Are the most prevalent type of psychiatric problem in this age group.
2. Are almost always chronic.
3. Need careful evaluation as they may be caused by a medical problem that could be treated effectively.
4. Can be controlled with supportive and behavioral approaches, but eventually will lead to further deterioration and death.

1. *INCORRECT. About 4% of persons over the age of 65 suffer from a dementia, with this percentage increasing with age to about 20% of those over the age of 80. Depression is a psychiatric problem that is much more common in elderly persons, with an estimated 15% to 20% of older adults affected at any point in time.*
2. *INCORRECT. Many of the organic mental disorders are acute and reversible.*
3. ***CORRECT. Cognitive changes, such as memory problems, disorientation, and confusion, require careful evaluation to determine whether a physiological or medical condition is responsible. The client's cognitive state will return to normal when the underlying cause is identified and effectively treated.***
4. *INCORRECT. Chronic and irreversible organic mental disorders, such as Alzheimer's disease and AIDS dementia complex, are called dementias. However, there are some dementias that can be reversed when treated, such as the dementia caused by hypothyroidism. Delirium, a third type of organic mental disorder, has a rapid onset and is reversible.*

31. The nurse working with elderly clients should remember that dementia in the elderly:

1. Is easy to distinguish from depression.
2. May coexist with depression.
3. Is not affected by medications.
4. Cannot be concealed by the client.

1. *INCORRECT. Many times the symptoms of depression in an elderly client are mistaken for those of*

dementia. Symptoms found in both conditions include apathy, memory loss, and disorientation. A thorough assessment is needed to identify the appropriate disorder and treatment.

2. CORRECT. Persons with dementia, especially in the early stages of the disorder, may suffer a depression when the individual becomes aware of his or her memory loss and other cognitive problems. Treatment of the depression will improve the client's cognitive functioning, but will not return it to a pre-dementia level.

> **TEST-TAKING TIP:** The indefinite word "may" in this option is a clue that it MAY be correct.

3. INCORRECT. Certain medications, such as sedatives and hypnotics, affect alertness and other cognitive functioning, and can make the symptoms of a dementia worse.

4. INCORRECT. Denial is a common defense mechanism used by a client with dementia to deal with the anxiety of the memory loss and other signs and symptoms of dementia.

32. At what age would the nurse expect that the anterior fontanel would be closed?

1. Three weeks.
2. Three months.
3. Eighteen months.
4. Four years.

1. INCORRECT. This is too young and would not allow the brain to grow normally.

> **TEST-TAKING TIP:** There are no clues here! You need to know your developmental milestones.

2. INCORRECT. Perhaps you were thinking about the posterior fontanel.

> **TEST-TAKING TIP:** Identify the key words.

3. CORRECT. A child with premature or delayed closure needs follow-up.

4. INCORRECT. The anterior fontanel should be closed well before this age.

> **TEST-TAKING TIP:** You need to know your developmental milestones.

33. When working with three-year-olds, which speech patterns does the nurse expect to observe?

1. Speech that is not understood by strangers.
2. Sentences average four to five words.
3. Only direct commands are understood.
4. Practices speech by talking constantly.

1. INCORRECT. This is the level of language for two-year-olds.

2. INCORRECT. Three-year-olds would tend to use three words in a sentence.

3. INCORRECT. This is below the level of three-year-olds, who should be beginning to understand concepts, such as time.

4. CORRECT. Ask anyone with a three-year-old! They practice speech by talking non-stop and asking many questions. Go with what you know!

34. The mother of a four-year-old says that she is worried about her son's fine motor development. The nurse expects the child to be able to:

1. Tie shoelaces.
2. Copy a square and circle.
3. Draw a stick man with seven to nine parts.
4. Print name without errors.

1. INCORRECT. This is a skill expected of five-year-olds.

2. CORRECT. This is a tough question. Copying a simple shape is achieved at age four. Know your developmental milestones!

3. INCORRECT. This would be the expectation for a five-year-old.

4. INCORRECT. Preschoolers often may reverse letters or capitalize incorrectly.

> **TEST-TAKING TIP:** This option does not actually address the issue in the question, which is fine motor development, not reading and writing skills.

35. The nurse observes that, in the first few days of hospitalization, an 18-month-old client sits quietly sucking her thumb in the corner of her crib. When the nurse approaches the crib, the client shyly turns her head away from the nurse. The nurse understands that the toddler's behavior:

1. Indicates a pathological reaction to being hospitalized.
2. Indicates that the relationship between parents and child should be assessed.
3. Demonstrates an anxiety reaction to the stress of hospitalization.
4. Is an example of negative behavior and a beginning attempt at autonomy.

1. INCORRECT. At 18 months, the client is able to identify the nurse as a stranger. Her behavior is appropriate. There is no evidence of pathology.

> **TEST-TAKING TIP:** Identify the key words.

2. INCORRECT. No data about the relationship between the client and her parents is provided. The conclusion that the relationship between parents and child needs to be evaluated is an assumption.

> **TEST-TAKING TIP:** Do not "read into" the question!

3. CORRECT. Hospitalization is stressful, regardless of the age of the hospitalized client. The nurse needs to be aware of this stress and how

it may be evidenced at different developmental levels. For an 18-month-old, separation from her parents adds to that stress. The client is demonstrating an anxiety reaction to the stress of hospitalization.

> ***TEST-TAKING TIP:*** The key word "shyly" is a clue!

4. *INCORRECT. Erikson's development theory identifies the developmental conflict for children age one to three as autonomy versus shame and doubt. An 18-month-old may be beginning to develop autonomy. However, since the client is hospitalized, her behavior has most likely regressed to the developmental conflict of trust versus mistrust.*

> ***TEST-TAKING TIP:*** The key word "shyly" is a clue that this behavior is not a demonstration of autonomy.

36. A client is in the hospital, and he is dying. He is very weak, tired, and short of breath. The nursing plan of care for the client and his family should emphasize:

1. Limiting visiting hours to help conserve his energy.
2. Having the client do as much as he can for himself to increase his self-esteem and independence.
3. Encouraging the family to spend as much time as possible with him and do whatever they feel comfortable with in caring for him.
4. Planning to perform as much of his care as possible at one time, so he can rest for long intervals.

1. *INCORRECT. The question tells you that the client is dying. Limiting visiting hours serves no purpose and denies the client, family and friends valuable time together.*
2. *INCORRECT. The client is weak and short of breath. Self-care activities will increase oxygen needs and cause more physiological distress for the client.*
3. ***CORRECT. This plan provides support systems for the client and allows the family to spend as much time as possible with the client before his death, which is important when working through the grieving process.***
4. *INCORRECT. This will further exhaust the client and increase oxygen consumption. A better approach is to provide frequent rest periods.*

Section 7: Meeting Basic Needs of Fluids, Nutrition, Elimination and Oxygenation

1. An elderly male is admitted to the hospital with complaints of abdominal pain and distention. He has a history of no bowel movement for the past 10 days. After a diagnostic evaluation, it is determined that the client has a fecal impaction. Which treatment can the nurse anticipate will be ordered initially?

1. Soap suds enemas until clear.
2. Bisacodyl (Dulcolax) suppository.
3. Oil retention enema.
4. Tap water enema.

1. *INCORRECT. The issue in this question is fecal impaction. This treatment would not be ordered initially, due to the impaction of the stool. The soap suds solution would not be able to bypass the stool to facilitate elimination.*
2. *INCORRECT. The issues in this question is fecal impaction. The suppository would stimulate peristalsis, but initially would be ineffective in moving the impacted stool.*
3. ***CORRECT. The initial administration of an oil retention enema will help to lubricate the impaction so that it can pass more readily through the intestine. After the mineral oil enema is given, the client is asked to retain it for 30-60 minutes. This enema then is followed with saline or soap suds enemas until the bowel is clear. At times, a digital extraction of the stool is necessary. Unless adequate lubrication is used, bowel perforation can occur with manual extraction.***

> ***TEST-TAKING TIP:*** This is the only option that addresses the issue in the question, which is fecal impaction.

4. *INCORRECT. Tap water enemas are rarely used because of their hypotonic nature, which could upset the client's fluid and electrolyte status.*

2. Following a stroke that affected the left side of the brain, an elderly client had the tube feeding removed and is ready to begin oral feedings. Which of the following combinations of nursing measures would be best?

1. Feed from right side of mouth; upright position; mouth care before feeding.
2. Verbal encouragement; check gag reflex; feed thinned foods and liquids.
3. Check gag reflex; feed on left side of mouth; upright position.
4. Sensory stimulation; verbal encouragement; favorite foods.

1. *INCORRECT. The key words "left side of the brain" identify that the client's right side would be affected. This option suggests feeding on his affected side.*
2. *INCORRECT. Thinned foods and liquids are poorly handled by the client with any dysphagia. Thickened liquids and soft foods are best.*
3. ***CORRECT. The key words "left side of the brain"***

includes the important points of checking to make sure the client will be able to sense the food and approaching from the unaffected side. Feeding in the upright position best avoids choking.

4. *INCORRECT. Sensory stimulation may actually be counterproductive, and the other measures, although generally helpful, do not specifically address the issue of oral feeding after left-sided brain injury. The correct answer must address the issue in the question.*

3. A client is recovering from surgery. The nurse is preparing to irrigate his urinary catheter. To prevent injury to the mucosa of the bladder when irrigating the catheter, the nurse should:

1. Gently compress the ball of the syringe to instill the irrigating solution.
2. Quickly instill the irrigating solution, using some pressure to loosen any clots or mucous.
3. After instilling the solution, apply gentle pressure to remove the irrigating solution from the bladder.
4. Place a sterile cap on the end of the drainage tubing to protect it from contamination.

1. ***CORRECT. Gentle instillation creates a flow that helps to dilute and free sediment or debris within the lumen of the catheter, while avoiding any force or suction, which could injure the mucosa of the bladder. Note that this is the only option that specifically addresses the issue of preventing injury to the mucosa.***
2. *INCORRECT. Using force can injure tissue or cause the solution to leak from the connection. Any suction should be avoided because the mucosa of the bladder is easily injured. Removing the syringe from the catheter will break any suction created by vacuum.*

> ***TEST-TAKING TIP:*** Note that both this option and option 3 include the use of pressure — and both are wrong.

3. *INCORRECT. Using force can injure the mucosa of the bladder.*

> ***TEST-TAKING TIP:*** Option 2 also involves the use of pressure, and both of these options are wrong.

4. *INCORRECT. A sterile cap can help prevent a potential infection but does not protect the mucosa of the bladder from injury during irrigation. This option does not address the issue in the question.*

4. Postural drainage with percussion is ordered for a client with pneumonia. What would the nurse include in the plan for this procedure?

1. Perform this procedure before meals.
2. Cup and clap lightly, to avoid causing redness to the client's skin.
3. Administer bronchodilators after percussion and before postural drainage.
4. Provide analgesia prior to each treatment.

1. ***CORRECT. To facilitate the client's ability to tolerate the procedure, an empty stomach is recommended.***

> ***TEST-TAKING TIP:*** If in doubt, use common sense and "go with what you know." This option is good common sense.

2. *INCORRECT. Percussion, when performed correctly, causes a slight redness, even though the client's gown or a towel is placed between the percussor's hands and the client's skin.*
3. *INCORRECT. Bronchodilators would be given approximately 20-30 minutes before the treatment to facilitate the drainage of secretions.*
4. *INCORRECT. This would be counterproductive. This procedure is not considered painful, and the ability of the client to cough effectively following the treatment may be diminished with analgesia.*

5. At a boy scout camp the nurse encounters a child who exhibits a high-pitched inspiratory sound, and cyanosis. Describe the procedure that the nurse should perform.

1. Stand behind the child and apply an upward thrust below the xiphoid.
2. Monitor the child, and if respirations cease, use the Heimlich maneuver.
3. Bend the child forward and deliver back blows to dislodge the object.
4. Begin cardiopulmonary resuscitation.

1. ***CORRECT. You have correctly evaluated the data as a child with an inadequate gas exchange, and then selected the correct procedure for the Heimlich maneuver on a child.***
2. *INCORRECT, do not delay treatment! The cyanosis and high-pitched inspiratory sound indicate an inadequate gas exchange. This child needs assistance now!*
3. *INCORRECT. This is the treatment for an infant with an airway obstruction. Identify the treatment for a school age child.*
4. *INCORRECT. There is no indication in the assessment that a cardiac arrest has occurred, and the child has distinct signs of an airway obstruction and inadequate gas exchange. Most children are primary respiratory arrests. This is not the correct emergency intervention for the situation described in the introductory statement, and it does not address the issue in the question.*

6. The nurse takes precautions to prevent constipation and fecal impaction in an immobilized client. The nurse is aware that, if a client develops a fecal impaction, what serious complication could result?

1. Intestinal obstruction.
2. Bowel perforation.
3. Peritonitis.
4. Rectal bleeding.

1. ***CORRECT. A fecal impaction is the presence of either hardened or putty-like feces in the rectum and sigmoid colon. If the condition is not relieved, intestinal obstruction can occur.***
2. *INCORRECT. Although this complication could occur during digital removal of the fecal impaction, it is not a complication of the impaction itself. This option does*

not specifically address the issue in the question.

3. *INCORRECT. Peritonitis is an inflammation of the peritoneum caused by the introduction of bacteria into the abdominal cavity. A fecal impaction is contained within the bowel and therefore cannot cause peritonitis.*
4. *INCORRECT. Rectal bleeding is seen in clients with hemorrhoids or certain types of bowel pathology, but a fecal impaction does not cause rectal bleeding.*

7. A person in a restaurant puts his hand to his throat. A nurse who sees this happen begins to administer the Heimlich maneuver. After the client falls to the floor, the nurse should take the following initial action:

1. Check for the pulse.
2. Sweep the mouth.
3. Attempt to ventilate.
4. Administer five abdominal thrusts.

1. *INCORRECT. If there is no air moving it is not appropriate to progress to the pulse check.*
2. ***CORRECT. The mouth sweep is performed in case the object is high enough in the oral cavity to allow for removal.***
3. *INCORRECT. This is not the correct sequence as taught by the American Heart Association or the Red Cross. What must the nurse do first?*
4. *INCORRECT. Not yet. Several steps are missing.*

8. The physician has ordered an indwelling urinary catheter for a male client. Where should the nurse tape the catheter to prevent pressure on the urethra at the penoscrotal junction?

1. Medial thigh.
2. Upper abdomen.
3. Mid-abdominal region.
4. Lateral thigh.

1. *INCORRECT. Taping in this area would not eliminate the penoscrotal angle and could lead to a fistula.*
2. *INCORRECT. This section of the abdomen would not be possible to reach without putting undo pressure on the catheter and the retention balloon.*
3. *INCORRECT. The mid-abdominal region would not be comfortable for the client nor would it allow for the downward flow of urine via gravity into the drainage bag.*
4. ***CORRECT. The lateral thigh or lower abdomen are the recommended sites to eliminate the penoscrotal angle and prevent the formation of a urethrocutaneous fistula.***

9. During a home visit, the wife of your client collapses. There is no pulse or respirations. Which of the following accurately describes the CPR the nurse would provide?

1. 5 to 1 ratio of compressions to ventilations, at a rate of 100 beats/min.
2. 15 to 2 ratio of compressions to ventilations, at a rate of 80 beats/min.
3. 15 to 2 ratio of compressions to ventilations, at a rate of 100 beats/min.
4. 5 to 1 ratio of compressions to ventilations, at a rate of 80 beats/min.

1. *INCORRECT. Go back and reread the question.*
2. *INCORRECT. You have selected the correct ratio, but the rate is not fast enough.*
3. ***CORRECT. One-person CPR is performed with 15 compressions and 2 ventilations. It is necessary to give the compressions at a rate of 100 per minute, since you are pausing after every 15 compressions to give the ventilations. This actually results in approximately 60 compressions per minute to the client.***
4. *INCORRECT. This is not one-person CPR.*

10. A client has just been catheterized and has an indwelling Foley catheter in her bladder. If all of the following actions were taken, improper technique was used when the nurse:

1. Cleansed the client's urinary meatus with soap and water prior to inserting the catheter.
2. Placed the client in the lithotomy position.
3. Inserted the catheter one to two inches further into the urinary meatus when urine was observed in the catheter tubing.
4. Used sterile normal saline to inflate the retention balloon on the catheter.

1. ***CORRECT. This question has a false response stem, and this action is incorrect! Even if this was done prior to beginning the procedure, the cleansing of the urinary meatus must be done with an antiseptic solution to decrease the chance of bacteria being introduced into the urinary meatus.***

> ***TEST-TAKING TIP:*** Always determine the type of stem before selecting your answer!

2. *INCORRECT. This is proper technique. The lithotomy position provides for the best visualization of the urinary meatus. Most clients are placed in the dorsal recumbent position with knees bent and legs apart, but the lithotomy position is appropriate and would not be judged improper technique. This question has a false response stem, and you are looking for an action that is incorrect.*
3. *INCORRECT. This is proper technique. It allows for advancement of the catheter and the retention balloon, which is distal to the openings on the end of the catheter. Advancing the catheter further after urine is sighted in the tubing prevents the retention balloon from remaining in the urinary meatus, which can cause pain for the client if inflated in this area. This question has a false response stem, and you are looking for an action that is incorrect.*
4. *INCORRECT. This is proper technique. Sterile normal saline can be used to inflate the retention balloon. The key word in this option is STERILE. This question has a false response stem, and you are looking for an action that is incorrect.*

11. When inserting a nasogastric tube in a comatose client for internal tube feedings, it is least appropriate for the nurse to:

1. Measure the amount of the tube to be inserted.

2. Lubricate the distal portion of the tube.
3. Tilt the client's head back when inserting the tube.
4. Check placement of the tube.

1. *INCORRECT. This action is appropriate. Measurement from the tip of the client's nose to the ear lobe to the xiphoid process is the measurement considered to be approximately equal to the distance necessary for stomach placement. This question is asking for something that is NOT appropriate to do.*
2. *INCORRECT. Remember, this question has a false response stem and is looking for something NOT to do when inserting a nasogastric tube. Lubricating the tube allows it to pass through the nostril easier. This is an appropriate nursing action.*
3. ***The question has a false response stem, and this action is inappropriate. Tilting the client's head back makes it difficult to swallow, and increases the likelihood of introducing the tube into the trachea. This action is unsafe.***
4. *Wrong choice. Remember, this question has a false response stem. This is a correct action, because placement needs to be verified to ensure that the tube is not in the trachea or lungs. This question asked for something that was NOT appropriate to do.*

12. A client is in the hospital and has weakness on her left side because of a stroke. She becomes upset when eating because liquids drool out of her mouth on her weak side. What is the best nursing intervention?

1. Provide only pureed and solid foods to prevent drooling, so the client will not become upset.
2. Have a member of the family assist with the client's feedings.
3. Teach the client how to drink fluids on the unaffected side to prevent drooling.
4. Have the client use a syringe to squirt liquids into the back of her mouth.

1. *INCORRECT. Eliminating liquids from the client's diet is inappropriate, since fluids are a basic physiological need.*
2. *INCORRECT. This option does not solve the problem of the drooling fluids and does not promote independence in this client. This option does not correctly address the issue in the question.*
3. ***CORRECT. This action promotes independence and addresses the problem of drooling. The client still has control over swallowing and tongue motion on the unaffected side, which will address her concerns. This question reflects the implementation phase of the nursing process.***
4. *INCORRECT. Although this may help eliminate some drooling, it does not promote normalcy during eating, which can result in a decrease in self-esteem.*

13. Which nursing action is contraindicated for a client with an indwelling Foley catheter?

1. Instill sterile distilled water in the catheter.
2. Use minimal pressure to clear the catheter of clots or mucous plugs.
3. Use sterile equipment for irrigation.
4. Use the flow of gravity for return of the irrigant.

1. ***CORRECT. Sterile solution is necessary. However, distilled water is hypotonic and may be absorbed by body tissues. Sterile normal saline is the solution of choice, since it is the most similar to normal body tissue fluid.***

> **TEST-TAKING TIP:** This option is different from the other three and is an incorrect action. Note that this planning question has a negative response stem.

2. *INCORRECT. This action is appropriate. Minimal pressure is used to clear clots, in order to avoid trauma to the bladder tissue. This option is not the correct selection because this question has a false response stem.*
3. *INCORRECT. This action is appropriate. The bladder is a sterile cavity, and any procedure that introduces foreign substances into it should utilize surgical asepsis. This question has a false response stem.*
4. *INCORRECT. This action is appropriate. The option correctly states that the irrigant should be allowed to return by the flow of gravity. The nurse knows that negative pressure or suction is not used because it can cause injury to bladder tissue. However, this question has a false response stem, so this is a wrong choice.*

14. A client has a nasogastric tube in place following abdominal surgery. Which nursing action would the nurse avoid when planning the care for a client with a nasogastric tube?

1. Attach the nasogastric tube to high suction.
2. Provide frequent oral hygiene.
3. Measure the amount of drainage from the nasogastric tube.
4. Attach the nasogastric tube to the client's gown in order to prevent pulling at the insertion site.

1. ***CORRECT. This action is inappropriate for inclusion in the nursing plan of care because this is not an independent nursing action. The amount of suction is determined by the physician and should be a part of the medical plan that is implemented by the nurse. This planning question has a false response stem.***
2. *INCORRECT. This action is appropriate. Frequent oral hygiene provides comfort for the client, since the mucous membranes of a client with a nasogastric tube in place can become dry and uncomfortable. The question asks for an INAPPROPRIATE action.*
3. *INCORRECT. This action is appropriate. Drainage from a nasogastric tube should be measured, since it represents a fluid loss for the client. This needs to be considered by the physician when determining fluid replacement therapy. The question asks for an INAPPROPRIATE action.*
4. *INCORRECT. This action is appropriate. A nasogastric tube that is not secured can cause irritation to the nares as a result of the tube being pulled and caught on the bed or other equipment. The tube also can be accidentally dislodged if not properly secured. The question asks for an INAPPROPRIATE action.*

15. The nurse is assisting a frail elderly client to eat. The client begins to choke and indicates to the nurse that she cannot talk. The first nursing action is to:

1. Perform the Heimlich maneuver to obtain a patent airway.
2. Begin mouth to mouth resuscitation.
3. Place an oxygen mask on the client.
4. Go to the nurses' station to get some help.

1. ***CORRECT. The client is beginning to choke, which is a life-threatening situation. Performing the Heimlich maneuver on this client may alleviate the obstruction and provide the client with a patent airway.***
2. *INCORRECT. Because the client does not have a patent airway and is conscious, mouth to mouth resuscitation is an inappropriate first nursing action.*
3. *INCORRECT. Oxygenation correctly identifies a physiological need in this question. However, administering oxygen to a client who does not have a patent airway is inappropriate. There is no access for air exchange, so the oxygen is of no value to this client.*
4. *INCORRECT. Leaving a client who is in distress is very inappropriate! If immediate nursing measures are ineffective, help can be summoned without leaving the client. The nurse can summon help by calling out, using the call system, or using the emergency call system.*

16. CPR has been initiated on a client in the emergency room. Which finding by the nurse would indicate effective cardiac compressions?

1. An EKG pattern with each compression.
2. Compression depth of 1 1/2 to 2 inches.
3. A palpable femoral pulse during each compression.
4. Pupils changing from pinpoint to dilated.

1. *INCORRECT. The EKG only indicates an electrical impulse; it does not guarantee that there is contraction of the myocardium, because there will be an electrical pattern generated by any movement of the chest wall by the compressor. This option does not address the specific question asked in the stem.*
2. *INCORRECT. This is the proper CPR technique, but this is not an evaluation of effective compression. This option does not address the specific question asked in the stem.*
3. ***CORRECT. To evaluate cardiac compression, the nurse should place several fingers on the femoral pulse during artificial compressions. If a pulse is generated with the compression, it is considered effective in circulating blood.***
4. *INCORRECT. This is backwards! If the pupils change from pinpoint to dilated, this would indicate that the brain is not receiving adequate oxygen due to inadequate ventilations or compressions.*

17. A client who is incontinent of stool has been placed on a bowel training program. The nurse understands that the goal of bowel training is to:

1. Prevent soiling of the bed.
2. Prevent cancer of the colon.
3. Prevent loose stools.
4. Provide the client with control over his bowels.

1. *INCORRECT. Bowel training will help the client to avoid soiling of the bed, but preventing soiling of the bed is not the goal of bowel training.*
2. *INCORRECT. Bowel training does not prevent cancer.*
3. *INCORRECT. Loose stools cannot be prevented by bowel training.*
4. ***CORRECT. The bowel training program provides the client with the ability to control bowel elimination.***

> ***TEST-TAKING TIP:*** Note that options 1, 2 and 3 all concern preventing something — and this is the option that is different. Also, the word "bowels" in this option is the same as "bowel" in the stem, which is a clue that this might be the answer.

18. A client is scheduled for bowel surgery . The doctor orders a cleansing enema for the morning of surgery. The best nursing approach is to:

1. Wear gloves to insert the tubing.
2. Use universal precautions and provide comfort measures to help the client relax during the procedure.
3. Lubricate the tubing well prior to insertion.
4. Position the client on his side and drape the client for warmth and privacy.

1. *INCORRECT. Gloves should be worn to prevent contamination. This is a correct nursing action. However, there is a better statement of the best nursing approach.*

> ***TEST-TAKING TIP:*** Always read all of the options before choosing the best one!

2. ***CORRECT. This is a comprehensive statement of the best nursing approach. Using universal precautions and providing comfort measures will prevent contamination and provide for the well-being of the client.***

> ***TEST-TAKING TIP:*** This is the global response option.

3. *INCORRECT. Lubricating the tube provides for the safety and comfort of the client by facilitating insertion.*
4. *INCORRECT. Positioning and privacy are important aspects of administering an enema. However, there is a better statement of the most appropriate nursing intervention.*

19. The client is admitted with anorexia nervosa. A nasogastric tube is to be inserted. In preparing the client for this procedure, what would be the initial nursing action?

1. Assist the client to a sitting position.
2. Explain the procedure to the client.
3. If the client has dentures, make sure that they are in place in the client's mouth.
4. Have a stethoscope available to listen for proper placement.

1. *INCORRECT. This is an appropriate position, but it is not the initial nursing approach.*

> ***TEST-TAKING TIP:*** Note that the word "first" is a key word in the stem of the question.

2. ***CORRECT. Informing the client reduces fear and is helpful in gaining the cooperation of the client, which is necessary for implementation of this procedure.***
3. *INCORRECT. This would be unsafe. The procedure may induce gagging, and dentures may become dislodged and cause the client to choke. Dentures should be removed before inserting a nasogastric tube.*
4. *INCORRECT. The issue in the question is insertion of a nasogastric tube, and the stem asks for the first nursing action in preparing the client. Although a stethoscope is necessary to allow the nurse to hear air that might be instilled into the stomach, this measure does not prepare the client for the procedure.*

20. A 10 year old is overweight. He has no dietary restrictions. The nurse is helping him make out his menu. Which diet should the nurse encourage?

1. A glass of whole milk, hot dog on a roll with pickles, and a candy bar.
2. A glass of skim milk, baked fish sandwich on whole wheat roll with lettuce, and a medium apple.
3. A glass of diet lemonade, hamburger and roll, medium orange and mashed potatoes.
4. A salad plate of low fat cottage cheese, potato salad, and macaroni salad with a croissant and water.

1. *INCORRECT. This diet is not well balanced and lacks vitamins and minerals. There is also an excess of carbohydrates and fats in the candy and hot dog.*
2. ***CORRECT. The menu includes selections from several food groups, has complex carbohydrates, and is low in fat, which should be encouraged during weight reduction.***

> ***TEST-TAKING TIP:*** Always identify the client and the key words. The client is 10 years old and overweight.

3. *INCORRECT. This diet doesn't include an adequate source of calcium for this 10 year old and has fairly high carbohydrates.*
4. *INCORRECT. This may look OK at first, but there is too much fat in the ingredients of the salads and croissant. This choice also lacks fruit and has no green vegetable.*

21. A client develops a fecal impaction. Before digital removal of the mass, what type of enema is usually given by the nurse to loosen the feces?

1. Fleets.
2. Oil retention.
3. Soap suds.
4. Tap water.

1. *INCORRECT. A Fleets enema, which is a hypertonic solution, is given to cleanse the bowel. It is usually given after digital removal of the impaction.*

> ***TEST-TAKING TIP:*** The key word in the question is "before."

2. ***CORRECT. Before digital removal of the fecal mass, an oil retention enema is often given to soften the stool. This makes the digital removal less painful for the client.***
3. *INCORRECT. A soap suds enema acts as an irritant to increase peristalsis and thus facilitate the removal of stool. The soap suds enema is usually given after the fecal impaction has been digitally removed in order to completely cleanse the bowel.*

> ***TEST-TAKING TIP:*** The key word in the question is "before."

4. *INCORRECT. Tap water enemas were previously used to cleanse the bowel, but now are contraindicated because of the possibility of fluid and electrolyte imbalances. Tap water, which is hypotonic, can be drawn into the cells, causing a fluid overload (hypervolemic state).*

22. During the resuscitation of a client, the physician orders the client to be defibrillated by receiving a controlled electrical shock. The nurse knows that it would place the client at risk to:

1. Move away from the bed while the client is defibrillated.
2. Observe the other nurses to be sure they are not in contact with the client or the bed during defibrillation.
3. Hold the IV pole out of the way while the client is defibrillated.
4. Make sure the client's chest is dry, except where the electrode paste or pads are applied for placement of the defibrillator paddles.

1. *INCORRECT. This is a safe action, and, therefore, not the answer to this question. Touching the bed or the client may result in the nurse receiving an electrical shock, since the electricity the client receives can be conducted to anything with which the client is in contact.*
2. *INCORRECT. This is a safe action, and, therefore, not the answer to this question. You should observe for other nurses who may be so involved in performing a particular task, such as starting an intravenous line, that the physician's order may not be heard. Observing their actions and alerting them may protect them from an electrical injury.*
3. ***CORRECT. This action is unsafe, so this is the correct answer in this question with a false response stem. The IV pole may conduct electricity by way of the IV fluid that the client is receiving. Touching the pole could result in an electrical shock to the nurse.***
4. *INCORRECT. This is a safe action, and, therefore, not the answer to this question. Moisture is an excellent conductor of electricity. During defibrillation, the electricity will follow the path of least resistance, including any moisture on the chest, which could result in burns to the chest area where the moisture is present.*

23. A trauma client, admitted through the Emergency Room, has a urinary catheter inserted to monitor kidney function and assess for early signs of shock. The nurse would report which urinary output measurements as suggestive of cardiac failure or hypovolemia?

1. 20 ml/hour.
2. 35 ml/hour.
3. 40 ml/hour.
4. 50 ml/hour.

1. ***CORRECT. Normal urine flow is 50 ml/hour. A urinary output of 30 ml/hour or less is suggestive of cardiac failure or inadequate volume replacement.***
2. *INCORRECT. The client should be monitored closely to watch for further changes, but this output would be within safe parameters.*
3. *INCORRECT. This urinary output amount is within safe limits. The client will need continued monitoring to evaluate further changes in urinary output.*
4. *INCORRECT. Normal urine flow is 50 ml/hour. This output would suggest normal kidney function.*

> ***TEST-TAKING TIP:*** You are looking for an output measurement which is outside of normal limits. Did you misread the question?

24. The nurse is assessing an immobilized client for symptoms of a fecal impaction. The most definitive symptom is:

1. The absence of bowel sounds.
2. Diarrhea stools with abdominal cramping.
3. A rigid board-like abdomen.
4. Constipation with liquid fecal seepage.

1. *INCORRECT. Absence of bowel sounds is seen in a paralytic ileus when peristalsis has stopped. That is not the problem with a fecal impaction.*
2. *INCORRECT. Diarrhea stools with abdominal cramping are often caused by gastroenteritis. Although both signs and symptoms may be present in the case of a fecal impaction, they are not the "most definitive" assessments that can be made.*

> ***TEST-TAKING TIP:*** Did you identify the key words in the stem? Did you read all the options before choosing the best one?

3. *INCORRECT. A rigid, board-like abdomen is seen in peritonitis, an inflammation of the peritoneum. As the affected area of the abdomen becomes extremely tender, the muscles become rigid, giving the board-like appearance to the abdomen.*
4. ***CORRECT. These are the classic symptoms of a fecal impaction. Other symptoms of a fecal impaction include painful defecation, a feeling of fullness in the rectum, abdominal distention, and sometimes cramps and watery stools. Very often, liquid fecal material may bypass the hardened mass.***

25. The physician has ordered a urine specimen to be sent to the lab for analysis of specific gravity. How should the nurse collect the specimen?

1. Clean-catch midstream urine.
2. Catheterized urine specimen.
3. Random urine sample.
4. 24-hour urine collection.

1. *INCORRECT. A clean-catch midstream urine would be collected if the physician is looking for a causative organism for a urinary tract infection. Specific gravity measurements do not detect bacteria.*
2. *INCORRECT. A catheterized specimen is ordered the least frequently because of the chance of introducing bacteria into the urinary system.*
3. ***CORRECT. Only a random sample is needed to test for specific gravity of urine, which measures the concentration of the urine and can give a clue as to the body's hydration status. At least 10 ml should be obtained. A fresh morning specimen is preferred, but the urine can be collected at any time.***
4. *INCORRECT. 24-hour urine collections are not necessary when testing for specific gravity.*

26. The nurse is instructing the client regarding good food sources for potassium. Which menu choice by the client indicates to the nurse that the client has understood the instruction?

1. Baked chicken, boiled potato, pudding.
2. Boiled chicken, rice, cranberry juice.
3. Broiled meat, baked potato, citrus fruit salad.
4. Beef stew, bread and butter, jello.

1. *INCORRECT. Chicken and potato are both good sources of potassium, but since the potato is boiled it has lost significant amounts of potassium. Milk products contain some potassium but are not considered a good source.*

> ***TEST-TAKING TIP:*** Always read all the options before selecting the best one. Is this menu selection the best source of potassium?

2. *INCORRECT. Chicken is a good source of potassium, but since it is boiled it has lost significant amounts of potassium. Rice and cranberry juice contain only small amounts of potassium.*
3. ***CORRECT. Broiled meat, baked potato and citrus fruit salad are all good sources of potassium and the cooking methods have not depleted this nutrient.***
4. *INCORRECT. Beef is a good source of potassium, but bread, butter and jello are not.*

27. A client in an extended care facility is in the dining room, having dinner with the other clients. The client has stopped eating, is grasping his throat with his hands, and cannot talk. The first and most effective action by the nurse is to:

1. Call a code and obtain assistance, before taking further action.

2. Perform the Heimlich maneuver.
3. Place the client on the floor and begin mouth-to-mouth resuscitation.
4. Slap the client on the back several times.

1. INCORRECT. It is not necessary to call a code at this time. Also, choking requires immediate intervention. Waiting for help places the client at further risk.
2. CORRECT. The Heimlich maneuver is the most effective method to clear an obstructed airway of a choking person.
3. INCORRECT. This action is inappropriate and might cause further danger to the client. Mouth-to-mouth resuscitation is indicated after the airway has been cleared, for a client who has ceased breathing. Mouth-to-mouth resuscitation performed on a choking client could lodge the food even further into the airway.
4. INCORRECT. The client is choking. Slapping a person on the back is not the best intervention for choking.

28. The nurse is assisting an elderly client to eat. The client suddenly coughs a few times, then appears to be attempting to cough, making a whistling sound as he inhales. When using the Heimlich maneuver on a conscious client, which of the following nursing actions is most effective?

1. Ask the client what he is choking on.
2. Place your arms around the client and position your fist in the abdomen, between the bottom of the breast bone and the navel.
3. Slap the client on the back until the object is expelled or until the client becomes unconscious.
4. Stand in front of the person.

1. INCORRECT. This is not appropriate because the client requires immediate assistance to dislodge the object that is obstructing the airway. It does not matter what the client is choking on, and the client will be unable to speak if he is choking.
2. CORRECT. This is the proper placement of the fist in the Heimlich maneuver: above the navel and below the end of the sternum or breast bone. This is the necessary emergency action by the nurse.
3. INCORRECT. It is not helpful to slap someone who is choking. The client requires immediate assistance to dislodge the object that is obstructing the airway.

> ***TEST-TAKING TIP:*** The stem asks for an action used in performing the Heimlich maneuver.

4. INCORRECT. This choice is the same as doing nothing at all! The client requires immediate assistance to dislodge the object that is obstructing the airway, and the stem asks for an action used in performing the Heimlich maneuver — which is done with the nurse standing behind the client.

> ***TEST-TAKING TIP:*** When selecting a nursing action to answer a question, ask yourself what is the rationale for your answer?

29. The nurse is caring for a client who is on a moderate sodium diet. Which of the following lunch selections by the client would signify an understanding of the diet?

1. Grilled cheese sandwich and tomato soup.
2. Bologna sandwich and dill pickles.
3. Chinese vegetables with soy sauce.
4. Chicken salad sandwich with tossed salad.

1. INCORRECT.. Most processed and canned foods are high in sodium. The cheese in the sandwich and the soup are both high in sodium.
2. INCORRECT. Most cold cuts are high in sodium, and the dill pickles are very high.
3. INCORRECT. The Chinese vegetables are safe, but the soy sauce is very high in sodium.

> ***TEST-TAKING TIP:*** If one part of an option is incorrect, look for a better choice.

4. CORRECT. Chicken salad and tossed salad are both low in sodium.

30. During cardiopulmonary resuscitation (CPR), the nurse should assess the adult's pulse by feeling the:

1. Carotid pulse in the neck.
2. Brachial pulse in the arm.
3. Femoral pulse in the groin.
4. Radial pulse in the wrist.

1. CORRECT. The carotid area is the pulse of choice because of its closeness to the heart and the ease with which it can be assessed after establishing an airway and giving the rescue breaths.

> ***TEST-TAKING TIP:*** The issue in this question is pulse during CPR, and the client is an adult.

2. INCORRECT. This not correct in an adult — but it is the correct pulse site to assess in the infant when performing CPR.

> ***TEST-TAKING TIP:*** Always identify the client in the question.

3. INCORRECT. The femoral site is not preferred because of its distance from the heart and difficulty in palpating quickly during the pulse check, which occurs after four cycles of 15 compressions and two breaths, and every few minutes thereafter.
4. INCORRECT. The radial pulse is one of the most distant from the heart and is not as reliable as another site that is closer to the heart.

> ***TEST-TAKING TIP:*** The issue in this question is pulse during CPR.

31. In the initiation of cardiopulmonary resuscitation (CPR), which assessment must be made by the nurse PRIOR to beginning chest compressions?

1. Absence of respirations.
2. Dilated pupils.
3. Absence of pulse.
4. Unresponsiveness.

1. *INCORRECT. The nurse would assess for absence of respirations prior to beginning mouth-to-mouth resuscitation.*

> ***TEST-TAKING TIP:*** The issue in this question is CPR, and the key words in the stem are "must" and "prior." What is the essential nursing action prior to beginning chest compressions in CPR?

2. *INCORRECT. Dilated pupils (failure of the pupils to react to light) will eventually occur as the brain is deprived of its oxygen supply, but this is a late sign and is not assessed in the early initiation of CPR. What is the essential nursing action prior to beginning chest compressions in CPR?*
3. ***CORRECT. Prior to beginning chest compressions, it is essential that the nurse assess for the absence of a pulse. She assesses for five to 10 seconds. If she feels no pulse, then chest compressions are begun. Doing chest compressions on a client who has a pulse can lead to cardiac arrhythmias and death.***
4. *INCORRECT. Establishing unresponsiveness is the first step in CPR. It is done prior to establishing an airway or beginning ventilations. Only after two breaths are given does the nurse do a further assessment. Remember the ABC's of CPR!*

32. When an infant is choking and turning blue, but still is conscious, the best initial action by the nurse is to:

1. Turn the child on his back and attempt mouth-to-mouth ventilation.
2. Support the child in a prone position with the head down and give four back blows.
3. Perform the Heimlich maneuver.
4. Call an ambulance.

1. *INCORRECT. Mouth-to-mouth ventilation is done for a choking infant after he becomes unconscious, in an attempt to deliver some air around the obstruction. This infant is still conscious. What should the nurse do first?*
2. ***CORRECT. In the conscious infant that is choking, four back blows are the first action to attempt to dislodge the object. If this fails, then four chest thrusts are delivered. The infant's mouth is visually examined for the object. If the object is seen, it is removed. If it is not seen, then the sequence of four back blows, four chest thrusts and visual examination of the mouth is repeated until the object is dislodged or the infant becomes unconscious.***
3. *INCORRECT. The Heimlich maneuver involves administering abdominal thrusts, which can injure the liver or spleen of an infant; therefore chest thrusts are only used, if necessary, after back blows have been delivered.*
4. *INCORRECT. Emergency measures should be initiated first. If the infant does not respond immediately to emergency measures, then an ambulance or rescue unit should be contacted.*

33. During cardiopulmonary resuscitation (CPR), the preferred method that the nurse should use for opening the airway is to:

1. Turn the head and open the mouth.
2. Perform a finger sweep of the mouth.
3. Use the jaw thrust and head tilt method.
4. Tilt the head and lift the chin.

1. *INCORRECT. This is not the preferred method for opening the airway, because the tongue may still be blocking the airway.*
2. *INCORRECT. This method will not change the position of the tongue, which is the most common cause of airway obstruction.*
3. *INCORRECT. Although the head tilt is part of the correct method, the jaw thrust is not as successful at bringing the tongue forward as another technique. The jaw thrust method is recommended when there is suspicion of neck injury, because it does not alter the alignment of the cervical spine.*
4. ***CORRECT. The head tilt/chin lift method is preferred when establishing an open airway in the initiation of CPR. This maneuver repositions the trachea and tongue so that the airway is open.***

34. The nurse is to insert a Levin nasogastric tube. The nurse understands that an inappropriate use of the NG tube is:

1. Maintaining NPO status.
2. Decompression.
3. Lavage.
4. Gavage.

1. ***CORRECT. Maintaining NPO status is an inappropriate use of the NG tube. However, it is true that the nurse would not offer any food or liquids to the client while he/she is NPO.***
2. *INCORRECT. Using the NG tube to relieve abdominal distention by removing secretions and gaseous substances from the GI tract is an appropriate and common use of the NG tube. This question has a false response stem.*
3. *INCORRECT. Irrigation of the stomach in cases of active bleeding, poisoning, or gastric dilation is an appropriate and common use of the NG tube. This question has a false response stem.*
4. *INCORRECT. Instillation of liquid nutritional supplements of feedings for clients unable to swallow fluid is an appropriate and common use of the NG tube. This question has a false response stem.*

Section 8: Administration of Medications

1. A 12-year-old child is being discharged from the hospital with a diagnosis of asthma. She is to be maintained on metered dose inhalers at home. The nurse is preparing a care plan on the use of cromolyn (Intal). Which of the following nursing instructions to the parents should the nurse avoid including in the client's care plan?

1. Intal will decrease the inflammation in your child's bronchioles.
2. Do not rely on Intal for relief of an acute attack.
3. Have your child rinse her mouth after using the puffer.
4. Your child should breathe more easily after a dose of Intal.

1. *INCORRECT. Intal is a mast cell inhibitor and decreases inflammation in the bronchioles. This information is correct and should be included in the care plan. You are looking for the option that would NOT be included.*
2. *INCORRECT. This is true and should be included in the care plan. Intal has a slow onset and will not relieve an acute asthma attack. A fast-acting bronchodilator should be given. You are looking for the option that would NOT be included.*
3. *INCORRECT. Intal may cause throat and mouth irritation. Rinsing or gargling after the medication will help relieve the irritation. Remember, this question has a false response stem and is asking for an answer that is NOT true.*
4. ***CORRECT. This question has a false response stem, and you correctly picked the answer that is NOT true. Intal is a prophylactic medication and the client will not "feel better" after any single dose. This can lead to noncompliance. Clients need to be aware that the Intal is necessary even though its effect is not immediately felt.***

2. The nurse is to apply topical ointment to the client's skin for a dermatological condition. Which action should the nurse avoid?

1. Massaging the ointment into the skin.
2. Removing excess ointment.
3. Applying ointment with ungloved fingertips.
4. Documenting a description of the skin prior to application of the ointment.

1. *INCORRECT. This action is appropriate. Massaging the ointment into the client's skin provides for penetration of the ointment into the skin. This is not the answer because the question has a false response stem; you are looking for an action to AVOID.*
2. *INCORRECT. Excess ointment should be removed, since it may stain clothing or come into contact with other areas of the body, or with other objects or people. This is not the answer because the question has a false response stem; you are looking for an action to AVOID.*
3. ***CORRECT. Applying ointment with ungloved fingertips allows for absorption of the medication through skin pores on the fingertips, which may cause some undesirable effects to the person applying the ointment.***
4. *INCORRECT. The skin should be described to determine if the ointment is having a positive effect. However, this is not the answer because the question has a false response stem; you are looking for an action to AVOID.*

3. During the administration of a medication, a 19-year-old client asks the nurse if this is a "new pill" and tells the nurse that he has never had that particular pill before. The safest nursing action is to:

1. Check the client's identification bracelet again.
2. Review the physician's orders to see if this is a new medication.
3. Assure the client that the medication package has his name on it.
4. Ask the client to take the medication, since the identification bracelet and medication administration record indicate the client is to receive the medication.

1. *INCORRECT. Rechecking the client's identification bracelet does not resolve the question of a "new pill" for the client.*
2. ***CORRECT. Checking the physician's orders will confirm if this is a new medication ordered for the client. This action addresses the client's concern and provides for the client's safety, by addressing the possibility of a medication error.***

> ***TEST-TAKING TIP:*** The words "new medication" in this option are similar to the words "new pill" in the stem of the question. This is a clue that this might be the correct answer.

3. *INCORRECT. The client's name on the medication label does not address the client's concern about a "new pill." Mistakes can be made with medications. The situation needs to be clarified further in order to provide for the client's safety and to reassure him that he is supposed to receive this pill.*
4. *INCORRECT. The person responsible for transcribing the physician's orders onto the medication administration record could have made an error. The situation needs further clarification.*

4. A child with a rectal temperature of 39° C has an order for acetaminophen (Tylenol) 280 mg by mouth. The label on the bottle reads 160 mg/5 cc. How many cc's should the nurse give to the child?

1. 8.8 cc.
2. 1.8 cc.
3. 7.0 cc.
4. 12.7 cc.

1. ***CORRECT. Use the formula: desired amount (280 mg) divided by amount on hand (160 mg) multiplied by the volume (5 cc).***

2. *INCORRECT. This number is too low. Use the formula: desired amount divided by amount on hand, multiplied by volume.*
3. *INCORRECT. This amount is too low. Use the formula: desired amount divided by amount on hand, multiplied by volume.*
4. *INCORRECT. This amount is too high. Use the formula: desired amount divided by the amount on hand, multiplied by volume.*

5. A concerned mother calls the physician's office. Her child has a respiratory infection and a temperature of 39° C orally. She needs to give her son 240 mg of acetaminophen (Tylenol). The label on her bottle at home reads 160 mg/5 cc. The nurse's accurate response is:

1. Give 1/2 teaspoon.
2. Give 1 1/2 teaspoons.
3. Give 1 1/2 cc.
4. Give 15 cc.

1. *INCORRECT. Too little. 240 mg/160 mg x 5 cc = 7.5 cc. There are 5 cc in a teaspoon. 7.5 cc/5 cc x 1 tsp = 1 1/2 tsp.*
2. ***CORRECT. 240 mg/160 mg x 5 cc = 7.5 cc. There are 5 cc in a teaspoon. 7.5 cc/5 cc x 1 tsp = 1 1/2 tsp.***
3. *INCORRECT. 240 mg/160 mg x 5 cc = 7.5 cc. There are 5 cc in a teaspoon. 7.5 cc/5 cc x 1 tsp = 1 1/2 tsp.*
4. *CORRECT. 240 mg/160 mg x 5 cc = 7.5 cc. There are 5 cc in a teaspoon. 7.5 cc/5 cc x 1 tsp = 1 1/2 tsp.*

6. During administration of medications to a client, the priority nursing action is to:

1. Help the client swallow medications without aspirating by keeping the head in a neutral position.
2. Identify the client by checking the client's identification bracelet and asking for his name.
3. Keep all prepared medications in sight.
4. Check the client for desired or undesired drug effects within an hour after administration of the medication.

1. *INCORRECT. Maintaining the head in a neutral or slightly flexed position is an appropriate nursing action that facilitates the movement of tablets or capsules down the esophagus and into the stomach. This question, however, requires use of the nursing process. This option is an implementation action, not the priority assessment action.*
2. ***CORRECT. Identification of the client helps to ensure that the medication will be given to the right client. This is one of the "five rights" to be checked before administering medications: the right client, the right drug, the right dose, the right route, and the right time.***
3. *INCORRECT. Keeping prepared medications in sight is important in assuring that the right medication will be administered in the right dose. The nurse can ensure that the medications will not be disturbed and will not be taken by others. However, this nursing action is part of the implementation phase of the nursing process. Can you identify the priority assessment action?*
4. *INCORRECT. Evaluating the client's response to a medication is important for identifying undesired signs of toxicity or side effects. For example, after administering a narcotic pain medication, the nurse might observe signs of respiratory depression. The nurse may also evaluate whether the medications are helpful, which can be seen in relief of pain. Evaluation, however, is the last phase of the nursing process. Can you identify the priority assessment action?*

7. A 10-month-old client is scheduled for OR. The preoperative medication is ordered IM, and the volume will amount to 1.5 cc. The nurse should give the injection in the:

1. Deltoid muscle.
2. Gluteus maximus.
3. Rectus femoris.
4. Vastus lateralis.

1. *INCORRECT. This muscle in the arm is too small and undeveloped in the infant. It is sometimes used to give small doses of emergency medications that are to be absorbed quickly and in small volume.*
2. *INCORRECT. Until a child walks, the gluteus maximus (buttocks) is too undeveloped, and this child is only 10 months old.*
3. *INCORRECT. This doesn't even exist! If you've never heard of an answer, it's probably not correct. In other words, "go with what you know" when answering test questions.*
4. ***CORRECT. This is the preferred site for this injection in the infant. This is the lateral aspect of the thigh.***

8. The nurse discovers that the wrong medication was given to a confused client who answered to the name stated when the nurse entered the room. The physician is notified and states that the medication that the client received will not harm him and nothing needs to be done. The priority nursing action after notifying the physician is to:

1. Apologize to the client involved.
2. Make out an incident report documenting the occurrence.
3. Try to avoid being responsible for administering medications again, since this could have been a terrible situation.
4. Realize that everyone makes mistakes, and continue to administer the rest of the medications to the other clients.

1. *INCORRECT. Since the client is confused, he will not know what the apology is about. This action may make the nurse feel better but will not be of any value to the client.*

> ***TEST-TAKING TIP:*** Be sure to identify the client and to read all the options before selecting the best one!

2. ***CORRECT. An incident report should be initiated whenever an error is made involving a client. If an adverse effect results and the caregiver needs to remember the events at a later date, the documentation will be available***

to refresh the memory. The incident reports are also used for statistical purposes in determining the types of incidents that occur. They help administrators to recognize when a particular problem occurs and to help prevent reoccurrences.

3. *INCORRECT. Refusing to administer any more medications again is not realistic or practical. Although the outcome could have been terrible, accepting responsibility for the error and learning from the situation is important. What is the nurse's next action?*
4. *INCORRECT. Although no one is perfect, the fact that the error was made should be acknowledged through documentation. The error may have been made because of understaffing or a variety of other factors that need to be addressed by administration. The error may have been carelessness on the part of the caregiver, which may be a pattern of behavior that needs to be changed for safe client care.*

> ***TEST-TAKING TIP:*** Just accepting what happened and administering the rest of the medications does not address the issue in the question.

9. The nurse is preparing medications for administration in a pediatric unit. Of the following nursing actions, which would be inappropriate?

1. Prepare medications for one client at a time.
2. Calculate correct drug dosage.
3. Open unit dose tablets and place medications in medication cup.
4. Avoid touching tablets or capsules with the hands.

1. *INCORRECT. This action is appropriate. Preparing medications for one client at a time helps prevent preparation errors such as inadvertently placing one client's medication into another client's medication cup. You are looking for the option that is INAPPROPRIATE.*
2. *INCORRECT. This action is appropriate. Calculation of drug dosage should be done prior to administration, when the information from the drug label is readily available. You are looking for the option that is INAPPROPRIATE.*
3. ***CORRECT. You have identified the inappropriate action. Unit dose medications should remain in their wrappers to maintain cleanliness, to better identify the medication and to avoid waste if the medication is not given.***
4. *INCORRECT. This action is correct. Using aseptic technique maintains cleanliness of the medications and prevents possible absorption through contact with the nurse's skin. You are looking for the option that is INAPPROPRIATE.*

10. The nurse is preparing to administer medication to a client who is scheduled to receive his insulin at 8:00 a.m. The best nursing approach is to:

1. Read the label three times.
2. Check the client's identification bracelet.
3. Administer the correct medication to the right client.
4. Check the dosage prescribed.

1. *INCORRECT. Checking the label is important in preparing the correct medication, but this option is not the "best nursing approach." Read all the options before selecting the best one!*
2. *INCORRECT. Checking the client's identification is important in ensuring that the medication is administered to the right client, but this option is not the "best nursing approach." Read all the options before selecting the best one!*

> ***TEST-TAKING TIP:*** When two or more of the options are possible answers, look for a more global option that includes the same concepts.

3. ***CORRECT. Administering the right medication to the right client is the "best nursing approach" because it includes the correct concepts in all of the other options.***

> ***TEST-TAKING TIP:*** This option is more comprehensive than the other options. This is the global response option.

4. *INCORRECT. Checking the prescribed dosage is important in correct administration of a drug, but this option is not the "best nursing approach."*

> ***TEST-TAKING TIP:*** When two or more of the options are possible answers, look for a more global option that includes the same concepts.

11. While caring for the client with an IV, it is most important for the nurse to:

1. Report any signs of infection to the charge nurse.
2. Record the condition of the IV site and the rate of infusion, and report any unusual findings.
3. Record intravenous intake.
4. Ask the client if the IV site is painful or tender.

1. *INCORRECT. This is an appropriate nursing action, since the charge nurse may need to contact the physician to provide orders to alleviate the problem. However, this is not the best option.*
2. ***CORRECT. Observing the site and infusion rate is part of providing safe care to the client receiving intravenous therapy. This option is the most comprehensive and includes the ideas in the other options.***
3. *INCORRECT. This action is standard care for the client receiving intravenous therapy and is a possible choice. However, this is not the best option.*
4. *INCORRECT. This action is part of assessing the site for possible infiltration or phlebitis. This is an appropriate action, but there is a better choice.*

12. When administering ear drops with a dropper, which nursing action best prevents contamination of the bottle of medication?

1. Thorough handwashing prior to preparing the medication.
2. Hold the dropper with the tip above the ear canal.
3. Wash the client's ear prior to instilling the medication.
4. Fill the dropper with only the prescribed number of drops.

1. INCORRECT. This is not the best option. Hands should be washed before preparing any medication, but the tip of the dropper should not come in contact with the hands.

2. CORRECT. Holding the dropper above the ear canal prevents the tip of the dropper from touching the ear. Touching the dropper tip to the skin will contaminate the end of the dropper, which will contaminate the solution when the dropper is placed in the bottle.

3. INCORRECT. The ear may be cleansed if dried secretions or drainage will interfere with absorption of the medication. However, this action will not protect the bottle of solution from contamination.

4. INCORRECT. It is difficult to determine how many drops are available in every size of dropper. Instead, the dropper should be filled with sufficient medication to ensure that enough drops are available for use at the time of instillation. Even if it were possible to predetermine the number of drops, though, this would not protect the bottle of solution from contamination.

13. The nurse is to administer an intramuscular injection. The most important action by the nurse to prevent introduction of the medication into the venous system is to:

1. Inject the medication slowly to allow for slow absorption.
2. Insert the needle at a 45-degree angle where there are fewer blood vessels.
3. Use the Z track method of injection.
4. Aspirate the drug after insertion of needle.

1. INCORRECT. Injecting the medication slowly decreases trauma at the site and minimizes discomfort for the client. It does not prevent medication from entering the venous system.

TEST-TAKING TIP: This is an appropriate nursing action, but this action does not address the issue in the question. What is the question specifically asking?

2. INCORRECT. An intramuscular injection is administered at a 90-degree angle. A subcutaneous injection is administered at a 45-degree angle. Neither position will prevent the medication from entering the venous system.

3. INCORRECT. The Z track method is used for irritating medications. It does not prevent medication from entering the venous system.

TEST-TAKING TIP: This may be an appropriate nursing action, but this action does not address the issue in the question. What is the question specifically asking? The question does not indicate that the medication is irritating. Be careful not to "read into" the question!

4. CORRECT. The drug is aspirated to determine if any blood is in the syringe. If blood is seen, the medication will enter the venous system if it is injected. Many intramuscular medications are not safe for intravenous administration.

14. While preparing to give a morning medication, the first nursing action is to:

1. Read the label.
2. Check for the right dose.
3. Wash hands.
4. Check for the right time.

1. INCORRECT. This is an important part of avoiding medication errors. However, it is not the first thing that the nurse should do.

2. INCORRECT. It is important to have the right dose to prevent over or under dosing the client. However, this is not the first step in preparing medications.

3. CORRECT. Handwashing is the first action prior to performing any procedure.

TEST-TAKING TIP: If you are confused by a question or do not know the answer, "Go with what you know."

4. INCORRECT. The time for administration of the medication is very important, but this is not the first thing that the nurse should do.

15. A client is admitted to the hospital for cataract surgery of the left eye. The physician has ordered eye drops to be administered to both eyes at frequent intervals prior to surgery. Which nursing action is most appropriate?

1. Use aseptic technique and avoid dropping the medication onto the cornea.
2. Gently wash away any crust along the eyelid margin with warm water.
3. Have the client look up toward the ceiling prior to instillation of drops.
4. Drop prescribed number of drops into the conjunctival sac.

1. CORRECT. Aseptic technique is always used when you are administering medications. The cornea is very sensitive to anything applied to it and dropping medication onto it should be avoided.

TEST-TAKING TIP: This option includes correct actions described in the other options. This is the global response option.

2. INCORRECT. Cleansing of the eyelid provides a clean area for instillation of the drops. This is an appropriate nursing action but it is not the best choice.

3. INCORRECT. Having the client look up protects the cornea from the drops landing on it. This is an appropriate nursing action but it is not the best choice.

4. INCORRECT. The drops should be instilled into the conjunctival sac to avoid placement on the cornea, which is very sensitive. This is an appropriate nursing action but it is not the best choice.

16. A client has left her used insulin syringe on the bedside table. What is the best action by the nurse to help prevent spread of infection by way of the contaminated needle?

1. Explain to the client that the syringe should be disposed of in the garbage can, to avoid a potential needle stick by someone providing care for the client.
2. Cap the syringe and take it to the needle disposal container.
3. Place the uncapped syringe in the needle disposal container.
4. Have the nurse administer the injection next time, since the client is not responsible enough to follow through with the correct procedure.

1. INCORRECT. The syringe should not be disposed of in the garbage can because the employees that take care of the trash can incur a needle stick while handling the trash. Furthermore, needles should NOT be recapped, since there is a potential risk of sticking oneself during this action. Look for the action that protects everyone from potential needle sticks.
2. INCORRECT. Needles should not be recapped because there is a potential risk of sticking oneself during this action.
3. CORRECT. Special containers are available for syringe and needle disposal. These containers should be utilized.
4. INCORRECT. The client should be reminded or taught about the potential injuries and infections that can result from a needle stick. The client should continue to administer the insulin, with closer supervision by the nurse concerning disposal of the needle and syringe.

> ***TEST-TAKING TIP:*** This option does not address the issue in the question, which is the safety hazard posed by the used syringe on the bedside table.

17. An elderly client is admitted to the hospital. She brings all of her medicines, including a bottle with no label. She says this is her cough medicine, which she put in a small bottle so it would fit in her purse. At this time, the safest nursing action is to:

1. Pour the liquid down the drain, since it has no label.
2. Instruct the client concerning safety issues related to this practice, and suggest that she have the pharmacy put the medication in smaller containers that will fit in her purse.
3. Send the bottle home with a family member.
4. Tell the client that this is a dangerous practice, which could result in the death of one of her small grandchildren.

1. INCORRECT. Although placing medication in an unlabeled container is not a safe practice, the medication belongs to the client and may be expensive. The nurse should not dispose of it without the client's consent. The client should be informed of the hazard and told of safer alternatives.
2. CORRECT. Instructing the client regarding safety issues and discussing alternatives allows the client to participate in health care decisions, which results in a higher rate of compliance.

> ***TEST-TAKING TIP:*** This option uses the therapeutic communication tool of giving correct information.

3. INCORRECT. The bottle can be sent home with a family member. However, this is a safety issue that should be discussed with the client. In addition, sending the bottle home with a family member will not resolve the problem of medication in an unlabeled bottle.
4. INCORRECT. Using fear as an approach is not appropriate, and this response by the nurse is not therapeutic. In addition, labeling the bottle will not prevent small children from ingesting the contents if given access to the medication. All medications must be kept out of the reach of children.

> ***TEST-TAKING TIP:*** The introductory statement does not mention any small grandchildren! Don't read into the question.

18. A 16-year-old male is to receive an intramuscular injection. To gain cooperation with this procedure, the nurse's first intervention is to:

1. Tell him what he will feel.
2. Explain the purpose of the medication.
3. Offer him a choice of injection sites.
4. Describe the steps in the procedure.

1. INCORRECT. Think about what is said when you go into an adolescent's room. Do you start off saying it's going to hurt?
2. CORRECT. After identifying the client, you state the purpose of the medication. An adolescent is capable of understanding and cooperating based on this information.
3. INCORRECT. This choice may be offered, but it is not the first intervention, especially with an adolescent.
4. INCORRECT. This is unnecessary and may increase anxiety. Many clients don't want to know all the details.

19. A client is seen in the health clinic and is diagnosed with conjunctivitis of the right eye. An antibiotic ophthalmic ointment has been ordered. Which instruction would be appropriate for the nurse to give to this client?

1. Use a sterile glove and applicator to apply the antibiotic ointment.
2. When washing your face, wash the infected eye first.
3. Other family members may share your washcloth as long as you rinse it out first.
4. Apply the ointment in a thin line, beginning at the inner corner and proceeding outward.

1. INCORRECT. Ophthalmic ointments are applied directly from the tube, using clean technique. The tube should not be allowed to touch the eye and should be recapped as soon as the ointment has been applied.
2. INCORRECT. Remember the basic principle of asepsis: clean to dirty. The client should be taught to wash the unaffected eye first, then wash the infected eye. This prevents cross-contamination.
3. INCORRECT. This would not be good aseptic practice. Conjunctivitis is highly contagious. The washcloth used by the client should NOT be used by any other family member. In fact, washcloths should not be shared even in the absence of an infection.
4. CORRECT. This is the proper procedure for ap-

plying ophthalmic ointment. Always proceed from the inner to the outer eye corner, to prevent the medication from entering the lacrimal duct and thus the general circulation.

> **TEST-TAKING TIP:** If you knew that this is standard procedure but were unsure of the correct answer, "going with what you know" would work well in this question.

20. A client is admitted to the hospital with a compound fracture. While making the client's bed, the nurse finds a capsule of medication in the sheets. The nurse knows that it would be least appropriate to:

1. Administer the medication to the client.
2. Notify the physician of the missed dose.
3. Determine what medication the capsule contains.
4. Document the incident in the nurse's notes.

1. ***CORRECT — this action might endanger the client! The nurse does not know which dose of the medication was not taken by the client. Giving the client the capsule may result in an overdose if a capsule of the same medication has recently been administered.***

> **TEST-TAKING TIP:** Remember to identify the critical elements. This question has a false response stem.

2. *INCORRECT. The physician should be notified to determine if the medication should be repeated. You are looking for something the nurse should NOT do.*

> **TEST-TAKING TIP:** Did you notice that this question has a false response stem?

3. *INCORRECT. Determining what the capsule contains is necessary to determine if the client is at risk for injury if a dose was missed. Some medications are very critical for a client's well-being. You are looking for something the nurse should NOT do.*

> **TEST-TAKING TIP:** Did you notice that this question has a false response stem?

4. *INCORRECT. All incidents that can affect the client should be charted in the nurse's notes, in order to reflect any changes that may occur as a result of the incident. You are looking for something the nurse should NOT do.*

21. Acetaminophen (Tylenol) is ordered for a nine-year-old child with a temperature of 102° F. The nurse preparing to administer the medication to the client realizes that he looks very thin for his age. What action would the nurse take first?

1. Give him one-half the ordered dose.
2. Give the prescribed dose.
3. Measure his weight and calculate the dosage range.
4. Call the doctor and question the dosage.

1. *INCORRECT. This is illegal. It is not within the nurse's capacity to alter the dosage prescribed, so this CANNOT be the correct answer.*
2. *INCORRECT. Just because it is ordered by a physician and the child has a fever, it is not necessarily correct to administer the drug. The nurse has an obligation to the client to safeguard his safety. What should the nurse do first?*
3. ***CORRECT. Perhaps the client looks thin for his age but is within the normal range. Measuring his weight and calculating the dosage will tell the nurse if the medication is within the safe dosage range.***

> **TEST-TAKING TIP:** Note that this option includes an assessment action. The nurse needs more information at this time, before deciding to implement any nursing action. The nurse must always assess first.

4. *INCORRECT. There is another action the nurse should take first, to verify the observation that was made. Then, if necessary, the nurse should instead report to the charge nurse, who would make the decision to call the doctor.*

Section 9: Perioperative Nursing Responsibilities

1. A client is recuperating from abdominal surgery performed under general anesthesia. The nurse should encourage the client to use the incentive spirometry a minimum of how many times per hour?

1. Two.
2. Five to 10.
3. 10 to 15.
4. 20 to 25.

1. *INCORRECT. Twice an hour would not be an efficient use of incentive spirometry to decrease the risk of atelectasis and pneumonia.*
2. ***CORRECT. Clients should use incentive spirometry five to 10 times every hour. This device is designed to motivate the client to take deep breaths, and should be included in the postoperative plan of care. Postoperative breathing exercises must be balanced with turning, coughing, and the client's need for rest.***
3. *INCORRECT. This number of times may tire the postoperative client and lead to decreased compliance. Postoperative breathing exercises must be balanced with turning, coughing, and the client's need for rest.*
4. *INCORRECT. This is beyond the reasonable expectation for a postoperative client. Postoperative breathing exercises must be balanced with turning, coughing, and the client's need for rest.*

2. An adolescent client had surgery on his foot and has just been returned to his room from the recovery room. The initial assessment indicates that he is stable. An hour later, his roommate turns on the call light and tells the nurse that the client has gotten up and hopped on one foot to the bathroom, using his IV pole for support. What is the priority nursing action?

1. Open the bathroom door to assess if the client is okay.
2. Help the client back to bed and get him a urinal.
3. Explain to the client that it is not safe for him to be hopping around on one foot.
4. Get a wheelchair and help the client back to bed when he is done in the bathroom.

1. INCORRECT. Even though the client should not have hopped to the bathroom, the nurse should respect his privacy and knock on the door to determine if he is okay.
2. INCORRECT. The client will have to hop back to bed with the nurse helping him, which is not a very stable method of ambulation. This is not safe.
3. INCORRECT. This intervention is appropriate, but it is not the priority action. Getting the client safely back to bed is the priority issue for the nurse.
4. CORRECT. Since the client is already in the bathroom, allow him to void, and then return him to his bed safely in a wheelchair. This is an implementation question, and the stem asks you to prioritize the actions. This option meets the physiological and safety needs of the client.

3. A male client was admitted to the hospital for possible abdominal surgery. Following x-ray and diagnostic procedures, the doctor decided that the surgery was necessary. The nurse's preoperative teaching should include which information?

1. Most clients are admitted to the intensive care unit after abdominal surgery.
2. Minor discomfort is expected in the operative site during the first few postoperative days.
3. Moving as little as possible will decrease the discomfort following this procedure.
4. Learning to cough and deep breathe will help prevent postoperative respiratory breathing complications.

1. INCORRECT. Following abdominal surgery clients usually return to the general nursing unit from the post anesthesia recovery room. This option is a distractor.
2. INCORRECT. Following abdominal surgery clients usually experience acute pain in the operative site for several days.

TEST-TAKING TIP: Options 2 and 3 concern "discomfort" following surgery. These similar distractors can be eliminated.

3. INCORRECT. Moving as little as possible is <u>contraindicated</u> following surgery because it contributes to the complications associated with immobility. Clients are encouraged to turn, cough, deep breathe, and ambulate postoperatively to decrease the possibility of complications. Acute postoperative discomfort can be managed by giving medications as ordered.

TEST-TAKING TIP: Options 2 and 3 concern "discomfort" following surgery. These similar distractors can be eliminated.

4. CORRECT. A demonstration and return demonstration of coughing and deep breathing will facilitate the client's ability to participate in her care postoperatively. Coughing and deep breathing helps prevent postoperative respiratory complications.

TEST-TAKING TIP: Options 2 and 3 concern "discomfort" following surgery. These similar distractors can be eliminated.

4. A postoperative client is to ambulate for the first time after surgery. The nurse understands that which of the following would place the client at risk?

1. Have the client get up and sit in the chair next to the bed.
2. Have the client sit on the edge of the bed with his feet down for a few minutes before he starts to ambulate.
3. Have the client stand at the side of the bed for a few minutes before taking his first steps.
4. Encourage the client to try to walk straight ahead while you assist him with his walking.

1. CORRECT. You have identified the UNSAFE action. Note also that if a client is to ambulate, placing him in a chair next to the bed does not meet the requirements for preparing for ambulation.
2. INCORRECT. The question asks you to select an UNSAFE option and this action is safe. Having the client sit at the edge of the bed with his feet dangling allows assessment of the client for weakness and dizziness, which, if present, would place the client at increased risk of falling.
3. INCORRECT. The question is asking for an UNSAFE action and this action is safe. Having the client stand at the edge of the bed allows for assessment of the client's tolerance of this activity. He is still close to the bed, so if he becomes faint or weak he can easily be assisted back to bed.
4. INCORRECT. A client should be assisted during the initial ambulation following surgery so that assessment can be made of the client's tolerance to this activity. You are, however, looking for an UNSAFE action.

5. A client is scheduled for left below-the-knee amputation in the morning. Before surgery, the preoperative teaching plan included deep breathing and coughing. In evaluating the effectiveness of preoperative teaching, the nurse should ask the client:

1. "Do you understand what we have just discussed about deep breathing and coughing?"

2. "Do you think that you will need to have a sedative to help you sleep tonight?"
3. "Will you demonstrate for me the correct method of deep breathing and coughing?"
4. "Do you have any questions concerning your scheduled surgical procedure?"

1. *INCORRECT. This question asks the client about the content of the preoperative teaching in the form of a closed question, which requires only a "yes" or "no" answer. The client could answer "yes" regardless of the true state of his understanding. This is not the best question to ask.*

> ***TEST-TAKING TIP:*** Read all the options before selecting the best one.

2. *INCORRECT. The test question asks you to select a question that the nurse should ask to evaluate preoperative teaching. In this option, the nurse is asking about the need for a sedative, not about the client's understanding of preoperative teaching. Although the question is an appropriate question for the nurse to ask at this time, it is not the correct answer because it does not relate to the issue in the question.*

> ***TEST-TAKING TIP:*** Focus on what the stem of the question is specifically asking.

3. ***CORRECT. This question asks the client about the content of the preoperative teaching. In addition, the question requests a return demonstration of deep breathing and coughing. If the preoperative teaching has been effective, the client will be able to do the return demonstration. If additional teaching is required, the client will be unable to do the return demonstration properly. This is the best question for evaluating the effectiveness of preoperative teaching.***
4. *INCORRECT. This question is an appropriate question for the nurse to ask at this time. It is not the correct answer, however, because the stem of this test question asks you to select a question that the nurse should ask to evaluate preoperative teaching. Here, the nurse is asking about the client's understanding of the surgical procedure. The client's questions concerning the surgical procedure should be referred to the doctor.*

> ***TEST-TAKING TIP:*** Focus on what the stem of the question is specifically asking.

6. A client is seen in the emergency room for abdominal pain and is scheduled for emergency surgery. In preparing to do the client's preoperative teaching, the nurse knows that it is most important to:

1. Explain the hospital billing process for clients receiving surgery.
2. Teach deep breathing and coughing with abdominal splinting.
3. Obtain the surgical consent.
4. Explain where the incision will be and how much drainage to expect on the dressing after surgery.

1. *INCORRECT. Explaining this process to the client is informative, but it is not appropriate prior to emergency surgery. This option does not address the issue in the question, which is preoperative teaching.*
2. ***CORRECT. Any client having abdominal surgery should be taught deep breathing and coughing.***
3. *INCORRECT. Obtaining the surgical consent is not a part of preoperative teaching, which is the issue in this question.*
4. *INCORRECT. There is not enough information to permit the nurse to explain the location of the incision and amount of drainage. There is another option that is more important in preoperative teaching.*

7. While changing a surgical dressing, the nurse notes green, foul-smelling drainage at the incision site. Another postoperative client is sharing the same room with this client. The most appropriate nursing action is to:

1. Place the client with the drainage in a private room.
2. Institute drainage and secretion precautions.
3. Move the other client to another room.
4. Place the client in strict isolation until the organism has been cultured and identified.

1. *INCORRECT. A client with a wound infection does not need a private room. However, the integrity of the other client in the room needs to be taken into consideration. The nurse should institute measures that will meet the basic needs of both clients.*

> ***TEST-TAKING TIP:*** Options 1 and 3 are very similar and can be eliminated.

2. ***CORRECT. Implementing drainage and secretion precautions protects not only the client with the wound infection, but other clients and the nurse as well. This option meets the physiological needs of all of the people mentioned in the introductory statement by maintaining their physiological integrity in preventing the spread of infection.***
3. *INCORRECT. Moving the other client is not appropriate in the care of a client with a wound infection. Other, less drastic nursing measures can be instituted that will meet the basic needs of both clients.*

> ***TEST-TAKING TIP:*** Options 1 and 3 are very similar and can be eliminated.

4. *INCORRECT. Placing the client in strict isolation is not an appropriate nursing action for a client with a wound infection. Strict isolation is used to prevent the transmission of highly communicable diseases. A wound infection is not considered to be highly communicable. Other nursing measures can be instituted to prevent possible spread of the infection.*

8. The nurse is planning discharge teaching for a client following abdominal surgery. Which of the following instructions about changing dressings in the home would the nurse consider most appropriate?

1. The appropriate opening of bandages to maintain their sterility.

2. Proper aseptic technique.
3. Proper gloving technique.
4. Good handwashing technique.

1. *INCORRECT. The client is at risk for the transmission of microorganisms that may cause infection. However, very often the home environment does not lend itself to the practice of aseptic technique, so the nurse must help the client improvise with the resources available.*
2. *INCORRECT. The client is at risk for the transmission of microorganisms that may cause an infection. However, very often the home environment does not lend itself to the practice of aseptic technique, so the nurse must help the client improvise with the resources available.*
3. *INCORRECT. The client is at risk for the transmission of microorganisms that may cause an infection. However, very often the home environment does not lend itself to the practice of aseptic technique, so the nurse must help the client improvise with the resources available.*
4. ***CORRECT. Handwashing is the most important and most basic technique in preventing and controlling the transmission of pathogens, and it should be practiced in every case. The client is at risk for the transmission of microorganisms that may cause an infection. The home environment may not lend itself to the entire practice of aseptic technique, so the nurse must help the client improvise with the resources available.***

> ***TEST-TAKING TIP:*** Handwashing is absolutely essential in infection control! Go with what you know.

9. The nurse is caring for a client who had abdominal surgery two days ago. The nurse should be most concerned about which finding?

1. A urinary drainage bag with 100 ccs of straw colored urine.
2. A wound dressing with thick, light green drainage.
3. A blood pressure reading of 98/66.
4. Shallow respirations, with a rate of 30.

1. *INCORRECT. The amount of urine in the drainage bag does not provide any useful data, since the introductory statement does not include a time frame for measuring the client's output. More information is needed.*
2. ***CORRECT. Thick, light green drainage is indicative of an infection and should be reported to the physician immediately. The stem of the question requires analysis of the data by the nurse. This option also addresses a client safety issue, which requires an immediate response by the nurse.***
3. *INCORRECT. Since baseline data is not provided in the question, the nurse cannot determine whether or not the blood pressure reading is normal for this client. Further assessment is needed.*
4. *INCORRECT. Shallow respirations are not unusual for the client who has undergone abdominal surgery. Although the nurse needs to address this issue by having the client deep breathe and cough, it is not the priority action.*

10. A client fell at home and fractured her hip. She is to have surgery in the morning. In preparing the client for surgery, which option is outside the scope of the nurse's responsibilities?

1. Assessing the health status of the client.
2. Explaining the operative procedure and any risks that may be involved with the procedure.
3. Determining that the history, physical, and specific laboratory tests have been ordered or completed according to hospital protocol.
4. Determining that a signed surgical consent form is completed.

1. *INCORRECT. Assessing health status is an expected standard of care for the preoperative client. The is not the correct option, however, because this question has a false response stem.*
2. ***CORRECT. Explaining the procedure and risks is a physician responsibility. This is not a nursing responsibility. Since this question has a false response stem, this is the correct option to choose.***
3. *INCORRECT. This action is a nursing responsibility that is part of record keeping and helps assure the safety of the client. This is not the correct option, however, because the question has a false response stem.*
4. *INCORRECT. A signed surgical consent is necessary for this case situation. It is a nursing responsibility to assure that the signed consent form is on the client's chart prior to surgery. This true statement is not the answer, however, since this question has a false response stem.*

11. A client is scheduled for a colostomy after being diagnosed with cancer of the large intestine. The nurse should begin client teaching about the ostomy:

1. Postoperatively, after the pain has subsided, when the client will be better able to concentrate.
2. Postoperatively, after meeting with the ostomy nurse.
3. When the client demonstrates an interest in learning about the ostomy.
4. Preoperatively, to involve the client in his care and give him a sense of control over his life.

1. *INCORRECT. Teaching begins before the operation has occurred, not postoperatively.*

> ***TEST-TAKING TIP:*** This option is very similar to Option 2. Two options that use similar ideas are probably both wrong and can be ruled out as possible answers.

2. *INCORRECT. Teaching begins before the operation, not postoperatively. Consultation with the ostomy nurse is also done preoperatively.*

> ***TEST-TAKING TIP:*** This option is very similar to Option 1. Two options that use similar ideas are probably both wrong and can be ruled out as possible answers.

3. *INCORRECT. The client may be in denial, but the*

nurse has the responsibility to educate the client, using patience and empathy.

4. ***CORRECT. Teaching always begins in the preoperative period. Preparation of the client, mentally, emotionally, and physically, is one of the nurse's primary responsibilities.***

12. In planning preoperative care for a client, the nurse is aware that obtaining legal, informed consent to perform surgery is the responsibility of:

1. The nurse.
2. The surgeon.
3. The client's family physician.
4. The client.

1. *INCORRECT. The nurse's responsibility is to ensure that a signed informed consent is in the chart. The nurse may present a form for the client to sign, and the nurse may sign the form as a witness to the signature. However, this does not transfer legal liability for informed consent for medical care to the nurse.*
2. ***CORRECT. To attain the right to operate, it is necessary for the surgeon to obtain a voluntary and informed consent form from the client. Before the client signs the consent form, the surgeon should inform the client in clear and simple terms what a reasonable person would want to be told, including an explanation of what the surgery will entail, as well as the possible risks and complications of the surgical procedure.***
3. *INCORRECT. The client's family physician does not have responsibility for obtaining the informed consent. The family physician's role is purely advisory in this situation.*
4. *INCORRECT. The client cannot give himself informed consent! He needs information from the expert in the clinical area.*

13. Before giving preoperative medication to a client going to surgery, the nurse must make sure that:

1. The client has an empty bladder.
2. Vital signs are documented on the preoperative check list.
3. Dentures are removed.
4. The consent form has been signed.

1. *INCORRECT. The key word in this question is "must." This assessment is desirable <u>but not critical</u> prior to administering the preoperative medication. If a client expresses the need to urinate after the preoperative medication has been given, then the urinal or bedpan would be used. Remember that, for safety reasons, the client cannot get out of bed after the preoperative medication has been given.*
2. *INCORRECT. The key word in this question is "must." This is important prior to the client's transport to the surgical suite, but it's <u>not necessary</u> that the data be <u>documented</u> prior to giving the preoperative medication. What would be important is the fact that the vital signs were TAKEN prior to the administration of the medication.*
3. *INCORRECT. The key word in this question is "must." It is not critical that the dentures be removed at this time. The client may keep the dentures in place until called to the operating room, if he wishes.*
4. ***CORRECT. The nurse must always check to see that a consent form has been signed before giving the preoperative medication. For legal purposes, the client cannot be under the influence of narcotics or sedatives when signing the consent form, or the client's "mental competence" could be challenged.***

14. A postoperative client should be assessed frequently for any manifestation of hemorrhage, which can lead to hypovolemic shock. In hypovolemic shock, which assessment would most likely be made by the nurse?

1. Rising blood pressure.
2. Hyperthermia.
3. Bradycardia.
4. Tachypnea.

1. *INCORRECT. As the client's blood volume decreases, the cardiac output decreases, causing a decrease in arterial and venous blood pressure.*
2. *INCORRECT. One of the clinical manifestations of hypovolemic shock due to hemorrhage is a falling body temperature, not hyperthermia.*
3. *INCORRECT. In the case of hemorrhage, the pulse rises (tachycardia) as the body attempts to compensate for decreased cardiac output and falling blood pressure, which result in tissue hypoxia.*
4. ***CORRECT. In hypovolemic shock, the respirations are rapid and deep, often of the gasping type spoken of as "air hunger." As shock worsens, the respirations become increasingly shallow and rapid. Tachypnea is the body's attempt to provide more oxygen to the cells.***

15. A postoperative client's knee dressing becomes completely saturated with blood one hour after returning to the clinical unit. The nurse's first priority action would be to:

1. Reinforce the knee dressing.
2. Apply a tourniquet around the closest artery.
3. Apply direct pressure to the knee.
4. Apply ice to the knee.

1. *INCORRECT. This would not be effective. This action is more for cosmetic purposes and does not reflect the seriousness of the client's condition. Something must be done to stop or slow the bleeding.*
2. *INCORRECT. This is not appropriate at this time. This action is somewhat drastic and should only be used as a last resort when the hemorrhage cannot be controlled by any other method. What should the nurse do first?*
3. ***CORRECT. Almost all bleeding can be stopped by direct pressure, except when a major artery has been severed. The charge nurse should then be notified, so that appropriate action can be taken by the surgeon. The client usually has to return to surgery for ligation of the bleeder(s).***
4. *INCORRECT. This is inappropriate in this situation — even though ice is a vasoconstrictor and will help decrease edema and hematoma formation. Something must be done to stop or slow the bleeding.*

16. A client who had surgery 24 hours ago is experiencing dyspnea and tachycardia, and has developed a fever. The nurse suspects atelectasis. If this complication is present, the nurse's auscultation of the client's lung sounds would reveal:

1. Diminished breath sounds.
2. Rhonchi.
3. A pleural friction rub.
4. Absent breath sounds.

1. ***CORRECT. Assessment of atelectasis (collapse of lung tissue) would include increased pulse and temperature, and decreased breath sounds or fine crackles on auscultation.***
2. *INCORRECT. Rhonchi are coarse, low-pitched, sonorous rattling sounds caused by secretions in the larger air passages. They are heard in clients with bronchitis, pulmonary edema, and resolving pneumonia.*
3. *INCORRECT. A pleural friction rub, which is a grating or scratchy sound similar to creaking shoe leather, occurs when irritated visceral and parietal pleura rub against each other, as in pleurisy.*
4. *INCORRECT. Lung sounds would be absent in the case of a pneumothorax, which is the presence of air or gas within the pleural cavity.*

17. The nurse is planning to reinforce the doctor's preoperative teaching. The child is seven years old and is scheduled for abdominal surgery. The best nursing approach is to:

1. Explain the procedure to the child by pointing to the child's abdomen.
2. Discuss the procedure only with the child's parents.
3. Tell the child about the procedure using an age-appropriate explanation.
4. Demonstrate the procedure to the child using a drawing or doll.

1. *INCORRECT. Pointing or touching the child during explanations is considered to be a threatening approach.*
2. *INCORRECT. The seven-year-old child is old enough to understand age-appropriate information. The child will be less fearful and more cooperative if taught what to expect.*
3. *INCORRECT. Just "telling" is not the best choice at this age, and retention is not the best with verbal instructions.*
4. ***CORRECT. This approach incorporates a non-threatening approach and visual props, which will increase learning.***

Section 10: Therapeutic Communication

1. A client is sitting by his food tray, pushing the food around on his plate. He says to the nurse, "I hate hospital food. Is this the only thing that I can get to eat?" The nurse's best response is:

1. "What is it about the food that you dislike?"
2. "Well the other clients haven't complained about the food. Is something else bothering you?"
3. "I'll call the kitchen and order something else for you."
4. "Is there something special that you would like to eat?"

1. ***CORRECT. The client has stated that he hates "hospital food," not just this particular meal. This is a possible indicator of other problems. This response promotes communication by addressing the feelings that the client has about the food, and by asking for clarification of the statement made by the client. Clarification is a tool that promotes therapeutic communications.***

> ***TEST-TAKING TIP:*** If you weren't sure of the answer, this option contains a clue—the word "dislike" in this option is similar to the word "hate" in the introductory statement and obviously addresses the client's feelings.

2. *INCORRECT. This response includes several communication blocks. If is defensive, focuses on inappropriate persons (other clients) and tells the client that his feelings about the food are not valid. Asking the client if something else is bothering him may elicit an expression of feelings by the client, but it actually changes the subject. This approach is not therapeutic.*
3. *INCORRECT. This response does not promote further communication by the client. Therapeutic communication is not developed when the nurse attempts to solve a problem without clarifying exactly what the problem is.*
4. *INCORRECT. The response doesn't focus on the client's feelings. He states that he hates "hospital food," not just this particular meal. This is a possible indicator of other problems. The nurse needs to explore the client's feelings before offering to get other food for him. This is not the best "initial" response.*

2. When the nurse is making morning rounds, a client says, "I almost died last night." The most therapeutic nursing response is:

1. "You made it through the night."
2. "Patients do have dreams that they die when they are hospitalized."
3. "Are you feeling okay now?"
4. "That must have been frightening for you. Tell me more about it."

1. *INCORRECT. At best, this response may appear to be reassuring, but in fact it does not place any value on the client's concerns or feelings. At worst, it appears to make light of what might have been a serious situation! Therapeutic responses focus on the client's feelings and promote further communication with the nurse. This is not therapeutic.*
2. *INCORRECT. This response focuses on inappropriate persons ("clients" in general). It is a generalization that offers false assurance and actually*

contradicts the client, since he did not state that he had a dream. The nurse needs to validate and clarify the client's concerns.

3. *INCORRECT. This is not the most therapeutic response. The nurse may appear to be addressing the "here and now," but this simple "yes or no" question does not address the client's concern and thus does not encourage communication. The client might even infer that the nurse thinks his concern about dying is not valid if he is "okay" now! Although the client should be assessed for his present status, his comment to the nurse indicates that he is concerned most about "almost dying." The nurse's response should address that concern.*
4. ***CORRECT. This response directly addresses the concern of the client. The nurse uses the communication tool of empathy in responding to this client's concerns and encourages further communication with the client about them.***

3. A client is told by her doctor that he has found a lump in her breast and that a biopsy would have to be done. The client states to the nurse, "Do you think it is cancer?" The best initial response by the nurse is:

1. "You seem to be worried about what the doctor may find."
2. "Do you have a family history of breast cancer?"
3. "We won't know anything until the biopsy is done."
4. "Most lumps are not cancerous, so you really shouldn't worry."

1. ***CORRECT. Communication theory states that the nurse should first focus on the client's feelings. This therapeutic response uses the communication tools of empathy and restatement to address the "here and now."***
2. *INCORRECT. This response focuses on the client's family history, not the client's feelings. This information may be obtained after the client's feelings are addressed in order to provide data concerning the incidence of breast cancer in families.*

> ***TEST-TAKING TIP:*** Always look for the key words in the question! The stem of the question asks which is the "best INITIAL response." Communication theory states that the nurse should first focus on the client's feelings.

3. *INCORRECT. This response does not answer the client's question or promote further expression of the client's feelings. This communication block puts the client's feelings of fear on hold.*

> ***TEST-TAKING TIP:*** Options that include communication blocks cannot be correct.

4. *INCORRECT. This response offers false assurance and does not encourage the client to express her feelings concerning the fear of cancer. Saying "Don't worry" devalues the client's feelings.*

> ***TEST-TAKING TIP:*** Options that include communication blocks cannot be correct.

4. An elderly client is constantly putting her call light on. When the nurse answers the light, the client does not appear to need anything. Which action by the nurse is least appropriate?

1. Ask the members of the family if they can spend more time with the client.
2. Remove the call light from easy reach of the client.
3. Make frequent visits to the client's room.
4. Spend more time in the client's room while charting.

1. *INCORRECT. This action is appropriate. Family members are often willing to help in caring for a client if they are asked or given some direction. You are looking for an INAPPROPRIATE action.*
2. ***CORRECT. The call light should NEVER be taken from a client! The client could fall trying to reach for the call light or attempting to get out of bed in order to get someone's attention. This action does not provide for the client's safety.***

> ***TEST-TAKING TIP:*** This action is obviously not client-centered! The answer must be helpful for the client.

3. *INCORRECT. This action is most appropriate. Frequently stopping by the client's room provides the client with some reassurance that someone is available to assist if needed. Many times clients feel alone and isolated, and use the call bell to get attention. You are looking for an INAPPROPRIATE action.*
4. *INCORRECT. This action would be quite appropriate. To help alleviate the client's feelings of isolation, the caregiver can perform tasks such as charting while sitting in a chair in the client's room, rather than at the nurses' station. You are looking for an INAPPROPRIATE action.*

5. A client is taught to do colostomy care for herself prior to discharge. She says to the nurse, "I don't think that I will be able to take care of this colostomy myself." Which of the following is the most helpful response by the nurse?

1. "Don't worry about it. Most clients feel like that at first."
2. "What part of the colostomy care are you having trouble with?"
3. "In time, you will become better at this than I am."
4. "A home health nurse will be visiting you, so if you have any problems, she can help you."

1. *INCORRECT. This response may appear to be reassuring to the client, but it actually inhibits further communication be devaluing the client's feelings. The client is saying "I can't," and the nurse is saying, "Don't worry about it." This is not a therapeutic response.*
2. ***CORRECT. Addressing the client's concerns is a goal of therapeutic communication. The communication tool that is used in this response accepts the client's feelings and seeks clarification of the client's concerns.***
3. *INCORRECT. This response contradicts the client and devalues the client's feelings. The client is saying "I can't," and the nurse is saying, "Yes, you can." This response also refers to an inappropriate person—the nurse. This is not a therapeutic response.*

4. *INCORRECT. This is a common practice for a client with a colostomy. However, this response does not obtain further information about the client's feelings. Clarification of the client's concerns is necessary for further interventions that meet the client's needs.*

6. A client is in the hospital because of severe weight loss and refusal to eat. The physician ordered the insertion of a nasogastric tube for feeding. The nurse finds the client with the tube removed. The client tells that nurse that he "doesn't need that thing." The most appropriate response by this nurse is:

1. "You shouldn't have done that! Now I have to put it down again."
2. "Why did you pull that tube out? Do you want to die?"
3. "Tell me what you don't like about the tube."
4. "Your doctor is going to be very upset with you for doing this."

1. *INCORRECT. This response indicates that the nurse is inconvenienced by the client's actions. Furthermore, "You shouldn't have done that!" is a judgmental statement, which is non-therapeutic. This is not an appropriate nursing response.*
2. *INCORRECT. This response is judgmental because it implies that the client did something wrong. It may also imply that he did it because he wants to die, and the nurse does not know the client's reason for his action. The nurse's response also puts the client on the defensive by requesting an explanation with a "why" question, which is a block to therapeutic communication.*
3. ***CORRECT. This response allows the client to tell the nurse how he feels about the tube and what it means to him. It promotes therapeutic communication and doesn't judge the client's actions. This response is therapeutic for the client.***
4. *INCORRECT. This response focuses on the doctor. It also expresses the opinion of the nurse, which is not important. The response is judgmental in that it implies that the client did something wrong. Therapeutic communication promotes the expression of the client's feelings. This option doesn't promote any communication and is not therapeutic.*

7. The nurse is caring for a client who is mourning a recent loss. The nurse understands that it is important to avoid saying that mourning:

1. Is a normal response to loss.
2. Functions to free the individual from an attachment to the lost object so that future relationships can be established.
3. Is accompanied by a growing realization that the loss has occurred.
4. Occurs only in humans.

1. *INCORRECT. The process of mourning or grieving is a normal response to a loss. This is a true statement, so it isn't the correct option in this question with a false response stem.*
2. *INCORRECT. The ultimate goal of mourning is to free the individual from too close an attachment to the lost object and permits the person to move on and establish new relationships. This is a true statement, so it isn't the correct option in this question with a false response stem.*
3. *INCORRECT. The initial phase of the grief process is usually shock and denial. This is followed by a growing realization that the loss has occurred. This is a true statement, so it isn't the correct opinion in this question with a false response stem.*
4. ***CORRECT. This option is NOT a true statement. Mourning occurs in animals other than humans, particularly those that form individual attachments, such as primates and household pets.***

> ***TEST-TAKING TIP:*** This question with a false response stem is designed to test your understanding of the grieving process.

8. The wife of an alcoholic client says to the nurse "I told my husband I would leave him if he did not get into treatment. Now that he is here, I feel differently. What can I do to help him?" The most therapeutic nursing response is:

1. "You should attend an Al-Anon meeting. The group can teach you how best to help him stay sober."
2. "You have already done a great deal by getting him to come into treatment. Now it is up to him to make the best use of his time here."
3. "Are you feeling some responsibility for his drinking?"
4. "Tell me more about the kind of help you feel you are able to provide at this time."

1. *INCORRECT. The nurse is giving advice which is not therapeutic. In addition, the nurse is inaccurately describing the Al-Anon program. Al-Anon provides information to family members on enabling behaviors and how to cope more effectively with the person who drinks, but the Al-Anon program emphasizes that the decision to stay sober rests with the alcoholic. Al-Anon members are encouraged to focus more closely on meeting their own needs and less on those of the alcoholic.*

> ***TEST-TAKING TIP:*** Any response that includes incorrect information or uses a communication block, like giving advice, cannot be the answer. Read all of the options before selecting the best!

2. *INCORRECT. This response is not therapeutic, because it implies that there is no further role for the wife, and overlooks the wife's need for help in dealing more effectively with her husband's behaviors. Alcoholism is identified as a "family disease," because each member is affected by the drinking behavior. Most programs include the family in aspects of the treatment process.*
3. *INCORRECT. This is not a therapeutic response. It asks for a "yes" or "no" answer, and it addresses an inappropriate issue. The wife did not present any information to indicate that she felt responsible for her husband's drinking. A therapeutic response would address the issue raised by the client.*
4. ***CORRECT. The wife is the client in this question. This response will help the wife clarify what assistance she can realistically provide without sacrificing her own needs in the process.***

TEST-TAKING TIP: The word "help" is used in both this option and the introductory statement. This is a clue that this MAY be the correct answer. Another clue is that it uses a therapeutic communication tool.

9. An elderly client asks the nurse to telephone her husband and ask him if he remembered to pick up his suit at the cleaners. The nurse knows that her husband died five years before. The best nursing response initially is:

1. "It may seem like your husband is still here, but he died five years ago."
2. "You miss your husband a lot, don't you? It must seem like he's almost here with you."
3. "You've forgotten that your husband is dead, haven't you?"
4. "Don't worry. Your husband will remember to pick up his cleaning."

1. INCORRECT. This response is an attempt to orient the client to reality, and it appears sympathetic, but it does not actually address the client's feelings or encourage further communication.

TEST-TAKING TIP: The key word in the stem is "initially," and communication theory identifies that the nurse should first address the client's feelings.

2. CORRECT. This nursing response validates the client's feelings and acknowledges her experience. This is the best option because the nurse is responding to the feelings underlying the client's comment, instead of the disordered content. This response uses the therapeutic communication tool of empathy.

3. INCORRECT. The nurse responds only to the content in the client's statement, and indicates no empathy for how the client is feeling.

TEST-TAKING TIP: The key word in the stem is "initially," and communication theory identifies that the nurse should first address the client's feelings.

4. INCORRECT. The nurse should not reinforce the client's belief that her husband is still alive.

10. The nurse enters a client's room. The client's son tells the nurse, "You people can't do anything right. Ever since my father was admitted to this hospital, it has been one mistake after another. I am taking him out of here before you kill him." The appropriate response to the son is:

1. "You feel that your father is not being well taken care of?"
2. "We have the best intentions for the clients."
3. "I'll get the supervisor for you."
4. "Your father hasn't complained about the care. What specifically is the problem?"

1. CORRECT. The son is the client in this question. This response uses the communication tool of restatement. It focuses on the client's issue and encourages him to express his concerns to the nurse. The nurse needs more information from the client before problem-solving can occur. This response also focuses therapeutically on the "here and now."

2. INCORRECT. This response is a defensive remark by the nurse, which is a communication block. This response implies that whatever is bothering the son cannot be valid, and this response may escalate the situation. A therapeutic response would encourage the son to tell the nurse why he feels upset concerning his father's care.

3. INCORRECT. This response puts the feelings of the son on hold by asking him to wait until the supervisor arrives. Therapeutic communication addresses the "here and now" and does not "pass the buck" to another person. Indeed, the supervisor may become involved, but the best response by the nurse is to address the client's immediate needs.

4. INCORRECT. This response focuses on the father, but the son is the one with the concerns—and the son is the client in this question. This response implies that the son's feelings cannot be valid since his father has not voiced any complaints. This is not a therapeutic nursing response. It contains the communication blocks of not addressing the client and devaluing his feelings.

11. A client has been told by the doctor that he has cancer and that it has advanced so far that treatment will not help. When the nurse comes to help him with his bath, he says to the nurse, "I'm not an invalid, you know! I can take care of myself. Get out and leave me alone." How should the nurse respond?

1. "I know that you are not an invalid. However, I was trying to help you."
2. "It sounds to me like you are angry about something. Did somebody do something wrong?"
3. "You are pretty upset. Let's talk about it."
4. "I'll just set up this equipment for you to bathe and come back later when you're not so angry."

1. INCORRECT. This response is defensive and focuses on the nurse, not on the client.

2. INCORRECT. This option assumes that the client is angry. By asking if "somebody" did something wrong, it focuses on "somebody" else instead of focusing on the client's feelings.

3. CORRECT. This option addresses the emotional state of the client by stating that he is upset. The communication tool of clarification is used to promote therapeutic communication, which focuses on the client's feelings.

4. INCORRECT. This option does not promote any communication with the client. It implies that his behavior is inappropriate and that the nurse is not willing to deal with it.

12. The nurse tells a client that the doctor has ordered an intravenous line to be started. The client appears to be upset but says nothing. What should the nurse say?

1. "Do you have any questions about the procedure?"
2. "The doctor wants you to have antibiotics, and this method eliminates getting frequent injections."
3. "What is there about this procedure that concerns you?"
4. "It only hurts a little bit. It'll be over before you know it."

1. *INCORRECT. This response focuses on the procedure but ignores the client's feelings.*
2. *INCORRECT. This response focuses on an inappropriate person (the doctor) and on an inappropriate issue (antibiotics by injection). This is a block to communication, since the client's feelings aren't addressed.*
3. ***CORRECT. This response uses the communication tool of clarification. The nurse inquires about the client's concerns in a way that indicates a willingness to talk with the client about both the procedure and the client's feelings.***
4. *INCORRECT. An intravenous puncture hurts more than a little bit. This communication block is identified as false reassurance.*

13. An elderly client is admitted to the hospital. His daughter, who takes care of him at home, says to the nurse, "I'm so glad he is here. You can take much better care of him than I can." What is the best nursing response to the daughter?

1. "We do have the equipment and people to take care of sick clients."
2. "It is not easy to care for the elderly. How do you manage?"
3. "Sir, your daughter takes good care of you at home, doesn't she?"
4. "Are you feeling guilty because your father has pneumonia?"

1. *INCORRECT. This response does not focus on the appropriate person (the daughter). This response also focuses on inappropriate issues concerning other people and hospital equipment. To be therapeutic, the nurse's response should focus on the daughter's feelings and concerns.*
2. ***CORRECT. This response uses the communication tools of showing empathy, and asks for clarification of the statement made to the nurse.***

> ***TEST-TAKING TIP:*** Be sure to correctly identify the client in communication questions! The daughter is the client in this question, and the nurse's response should address her concerns. Note that Options 1 & 3 focus on inappropriate issues, and Option 4 implies to the client that she may be to blame for her father's pneumonia.

3. *INCORRECT. The daughter is the client in this communication question, and this response is not directed to her. Even though the father is the person with the medical problem, the daughter has addressed a comment to the nurse, and the nurse's response should be addressed to the daughter.*
4. *INCORRECT. This response indirectly places blame on the daughter for her father's pneumonia. This type of response can put the client on the defensive, which is not therapeutic.*

14. A client is to have a nasogastric tube inserted. The nurse explains the procedure to him and is about to begin the insertion, when the client says, "No way! You are not putting that hose down my throat. Get away from me." Which is the most appropriate nursing response?

1. "You have the right to refuse treatment. Why don't you talk to your doctor about it."
2. "Something is upsetting you. Can you tell me what it is?"
3. "What do you feel about this hose?"
4. "I would just get it over with, because you won't get better without this tube."

1. *INCORRECT. The client does have the right to refuse treatment, but this is not the best response by the nurse. This response puts the client's feelings on hold, referring them to another person at a later time. This response blocks communication.*
2. ***CORRECT. This response addresses the client's feelings. This option uses the communication tool of clarification, which encourages communication by the client and helps the nurse assess the situation.***

> ***TEST-TAKING TIP:*** This response is more global than Option 3, which focuses on the client's feelings about the nasogastric tube.

3. *INCORRECT. This option is a good distractor. It asks for a response from the client concerning the hose. The nurse does not need information concerning the hose. The nurse needs information concerning the client's feelings about the whole situation.*
4. *INCORRECT. In this response, the nurse is blocking communication by giving advice.*

15. The nurse observes an elderly client trying to climb over the side rails of the bed. When the nurse begins to place a vest restraint on the client, the client's daughter says to the nurse, "My mother does not need to be tied down in bed. I've been caring for her for years, and she hasn't fallen out of bed yet." Which response is therapeutic for the daughter?

1. "I just saw your mother trying to climb over the side rails. Since I am concerned about her falling and hurting herself, I think this is best for her safety."
2. "Tell me how you managed to care for her at home."
3. "Hospital policy requires restraint vests on clients who are at risk for falling. I just saw your mother trying to climb over the rails. You don't want her to get hurt, do you?"
4. "The elderly may become confused in an unfamiliar place and do things they wouldn't do at home. It is difficult to see her restrained. While you are with her, the restraints can be off. Let me know when you are ready to leave."

1. *INCORRECT. The daughter is the client in this test question. The nurse should address the daughter's concerns about restraints being placed on her mother. This response by the nurse focuses only on safety and restraints. Note that, since the daughter and nurse are with the mother, she is not in immediate danger.*

2. *INCORRECT. This response does not focus on the specific issue in the question, which concerns the client's feelings about restraints being placed on her mother. This more general question about caring for the mother may be appropriate later in the conversation, but is not the best initial response.*
3. *INCORRECT. This response implies that the daughter is not interested in her mother's safety and makes her defensive. It also focuses on hospital policy and not the daughter's concerns.*
4. ***CORRECT. This option focuses on the daughter's concerns, provides information and rationale for the restraints, and uses the communication tool of empathy. It also provides for the mother's safety and offers a compromise to the daughter that addresses her concerns and gives her some control.***

16. The nurse is preparing to give an elderly client a bath. The client says to the nurse, "I don't think that I need a bath today. I just had one yesterday. My skin is going to get too dry. I bathe every other day at home." Which is the most appropriate nursing response?

1. "My head nurse wants all of the clients bathed daily. She believes that it decreases the number of germs on your skin that cause infection. Would you like to talk to her?"
2. "A bath can make you feel refreshed and make the day seem brighter. Don't you agree?"
3. "Would you like to compromise and just wash your face and hands today?"
4. "I heard you say that you don't want a bath today."

1. *INCORRECT. This option blocks communication by "passing the buck" to the head nurse and by referring to an inappropriate issue (the head nurse's wishes and beliefs). The nurse should address the client's concerns.*

> ***TEST-TAKING TIP:*** A response that uses a communication block cannot be correct.

2. *INCORRECT. This client is concerned about dry skin, and this cliché' does not address the client's concerns. It is an inappropriate response.*
3. ***CORRECT. Allowing the client to make a choice in her plan of care promotes a sense of independence and self-worth. The issue in this question is not a physiological need or a safety issue.***
4. *INCORRECT. Restatement is used to clarify and allow the client to express her feelings, but this client has already explained to the nurse why she doesn't want a bath. This communication tool is used inappropriately in this question.*

17. A visitor asks the nurse about the client in the next room, who cries out frequently. "That person must have a terrible disease. What is the matter with him?" The most appropriate response by the nurse is:

1. "That client has cancer and is quite uncomfortable."
2. "Mr. Jones is being kept as comfortable as possible."
3. "That person is quite uncomfortable. Does his crying out bother you?"
4. "I cannot reveal anything about his diagnosis. Why don't you ask his family when they visit. I'm sure they would appreciate your concern."

1. *INCORRECT. Identifying the client in the next room and revealing his diagnosis is an invasion of the client's privacy.*
2. *INCORRECT. Identifying the client in the next room by name is a breach of confidentiality.*
3. ***CORRECT. This option states the obvious and focuses on the client's feelings, rather than on confidential information concerning the uncomfortable person.***
4. *INCORRECT. This option does not address the immediate concern of the client, and it ignores the family's right to privacy.*

18. A young client has been admitted to the acute diseases unit. She has recently been diagnosed with AIDS. When the nurse enters her room, the nurse finds the client is crying. What is the most appropriate response demonstrated by the nurse?

1. Ignore the crying and proceed to take the client's vital signs.
2. Acknowledge her feelings and offer to help.
3. Consult with the charge nurse immediately.
4. Notify her physician and suggest an antidepressant medication.

1. *INCORRECT. This is disrespectful of the client's feelings and demonstrates a lack of caring by the nurse. The nurse should never ignore the client.*
2. ***CORRECT. This demonstrates acceptance of the client by the nurse. Acknowledging the client's feelings is the therapeutic communication tool of empathy. Offering to help is the therapeutic communication tool of offering self. This response is therapeutic for the client.***
3. *INCORRECT. This is not indicated at this time. The nurse should address the client's feelings.*
4. *INCORRECT. This is not an appropriate nursing response to this situation. The nurse must address the client's feelings and try to help her deal with them.*

> ***TEST-TAKING TIP:*** There is no physiological or safety need identified in the introductory statement. Look for a response that uses a therapeutic communication tool.

19. The nurse learns that an elderly client's sleeping problems began six months ago when his physician diagnosed prostatic cancer. Prior to that time, he had enjoyed good physical health. The nurse also knows that his wife of 50 years died one year ago. One day the client tells the nurse, "I'd be better off dead because I am totally worthless." The nurse's most therapeutic response is:

1. "I have seen some very valuable things about you."
2. "You feel worthless now because you are so depressed. You will feel different when your depression begins to improve."
3. "You really have a great deal to live for."
4. "You have been feeling very sad and alone for some time."

1. *INCORRECT. This may look like a positive and encouraging statement, but it is not therapeutic for the client because it does not address the client's feelings. The nurse should accept the client's perceptions without agreeing with any conclusions.*
2. *INCORRECT. This response does address the client's feelings of worthlessness, but in an incorrect manner. This client has suffered some serious losses, and the nurse should accept the client's feelings and help the client to explore them. Instead, this response blocks communication by using false reassurance because the nurse does not know how the client will feel in the future.*
3. *INCORRECT. This response is not therapeutic. It uses cliché and false reassurance. From the client's point of view, this statement is simply not true. The nurse should accept the client's feelings and encourage further exploration of them.*
4. ***CORRECT. Depressed persons have great difficulty expressing their feelings. This response by the nurse uses the communication tool of empathy and is a good way to begin to provide help and help the client become more aware and accepting of his feelings.***

20. A client who has just been diagnosed with cancer tells the nurse that he would rather be dead than go through the treatment for cancer. The most appropriate nursing response is:

1. "What is it about the cancer treatment that concerns you."
2. "If you don't receive the treatment, you will get your wish."
3. "Why don't you talk to your doctor about your feelings?"
4. "That wouldn't be fair to your family, would it?"

1. ***CORRECT. This response is therapeutic because it focuses on the client's feelings and concerns. This response encourages the client to further express his feelings about cancer treatments. The nurse may also be able to clarify any misinformation that the client may have concerning the treatments.***

> ***TEST TAKING TIP:*** Note that in addressing the client's concerns, this response uses the words "cancer" and "treatment" from the introductory statement. This is a clue that this may be the correct answer.

2. *INCORRECT. This response is inappropriate and unprofessional. It fails to respect the client's feelings and does not address the client's immediate concerns. This response blocks further communication, instead of encouraging the client to express his feelings concerning the treatments. The nurse must always be in a therapeutic role.*
3. *INCORRECT. With this response, the nurse avoids the discussion with the communication block of "putting the client's concern on hold." This response is not appropriate because it tells the client that the nurse does not want to hear about the client's feelings. The nurse must always be in a therapeutic role.*
4. *INCORRECT. This response uses the communication block of "referring to an inappropriate person." By addressing the needs of the family instead of the needs of the client, the nurse indicates that the needs of the family are more important. This statement also expresses disapproval by the nurse, which is not therapeutic.*

21. The client tells the nurse that he does not know how he is ever going to stay on the low cholesterol diet that his doctor ordered after his heart attack. The best response by the nurse is:

1. "If you don't follow the diet, you will probably have another heart attack, which could kill you."
2. "What is it about the low cholesterol diet that seems to be a problem for you?"
3. "I've been on that diet for the past five years, and I'm sure you will learn how to change you eating habits after a while."
4. "I will have the dietitian talk to you before you are discharged. She's the expert, and she can be really helpful."

1. *INCORRECT. A low cholesterol diet decreases the amount of fat in the diet. High fat content in the diet causes plaque to be deposited in the blood vessels, which results in narrowed blood vessels that can cause a heart attack. Telling the client that he may die if he doesn't follow the diet, however, is perceived as a threat and blocks therapeutic communication.*
2. ***CORRECT. This response uses the therapeutic communication tool of clarification. It lets the client know that his concerns are important to the nurse, and encourages him to tell the nurse more about his concerns. When you cannot identify a therapeutic response focusing on the client's feelings, look for a response that addresses the client's concerns and uses a therapeutic communication tool.***

> ***TEST TAKING TIP:*** Note that in seeking to clarify the client's concerns, this response uses the words "low cholesterol diet" from the introductory statement. This may be a clue that this is the correct answer.

3. *INCORRECT. The fact that the nurse has personal experience with this diet may be beneficial when teaching the client about the diet. As a response to the client's comment in the case scenario, however, this response is not therapeutic. It blocks communication by focusing on an inappropriate person—the nurse—instead of on the client's feelings and concerns. The nurse must always be in a therapeutic role.*
4. *INCORRECT. This response blocks communication by putting the client's concerns on hold. The nurse should address the client's concerns and should obtain more information from the client about the problem before deciding to ask the dietitian to talk with the client.*

22. A client has advanced cancer of the lung with metastasis. His wife says to the nurse, "I know my husband is in severe pain. I wish I could do something to make him feel better." Which of the following responses by the nurse would be most helpful to the wife?

1. "It must be very difficult for you to see your husband suffering."
2. "I wish there was more that I could do to relieve his pain, too."
3. "I'm sure he will begin to feel better after his next pain medication."
4. "Your husband tries hard not to show the pain when you are with him."

1. ***CORRECT. The wife is the client in this question. The nurse is responding to her feelings. Her response is therapeutic and illustrates the communication tool of empathy.***
2. *INCORRECT. This option focuses on the nurse rather than the client and is not therapeutic. It may also make the client feel more helpless.*
3. *INCORRECT. The wife is the client in this question. This response addresses the wife's concerns but not her feelings, and it illustrates the non-therapeutic communication block of false reassurance.*
4. *INCORRECT. The client in this question is the wife. The response in this option is incorrect because it focuses on the husband. It might also cause the wife to feel guilty and is non-therapeutic. Look for a response that addresses the wife's feelings and uses a therapeutic communication tool.*

23. A young male diabetic is admitted to the hospital for dialysis because of poor renal function. He says to the nurse, "I don't even know why I'm doing this. There is no cure." Which of the following is the most appropriate nursing response?

1. "There is always a chance that through research a cure will be found."
2. "Dialysis will help you live longer."
3. "You shouldn't complain! You are fortunate to be in this good a shape, considering the type of diabetes you have."
4. "It sounds as though you have given up on life."

1. *INCORRECT. This statement is an example of cliché and false reassurance. The client has expressed his feelings to the nurse. Instead of helping the client deal with his feelings in the here and now, however, the nurse focuses on the possibility of a cure.*
2. *INCORRECT. Although this statement is true, it does not address the client's feelings. To be therapeutic, the nurse's response should focus on the client's feelings.*
3. *INCORRECT. This statement expresses the nurse's disapproval of the client's feelings, and devalues his concerns about the future. This response blocks communication and is not appropriate in the nurse-client relationship.*
4. ***CORRECT. The nurse is using the communication tool of restatement to encourage the expression of feelings, which is therapeutic for the client. The nurse must maintain a nonjudgmental attitude so that the client will feel free to express his feelings. Note that Option 3 blocks communication by expressing the nurse's disapproval of the client's feelings.***

24. A couple is in the hospital because of a fetal death at 37 weeks' gestation. The husband is trying to comfort the wife, who is crying. The husband says to the nurse, "We wanted this baby so much." Which of the following is an appropriate response by the nurse?

1. "You are both young and you can have other children."
2. "It is God's will, and it must be accepted."
3. "It must be very difficult for you both. I will be available if you need anything."
4. "I think you should call your minister. He can help comfort you."

1. *INCORRECT. This statement may be true, but the nurse cannot know what will happen in the future. This response does not acknowledge the feelings of the clients and blocks communication. This is an example of cliché and false assurance.*
2. *INCORRECT. This is a cliché that expresses the nurse's beliefs and values. It is not empathetic and does not recognize the clients' feelings. This is a communication block.*
3. ***CORRECT. This statement acknowledges the clients' feelings. The nurse is showing empathy, and is also offering self by offering to assist them.***
4. *INCORRECT. This statement implies that the minister is needed for comforting and that the nurse is not available to discuss the clients' feelings. This response is also giving advice to the clients.*

25. A woman is crying continuously after the death of her husband. The son is distressed over his mother's crying and reports to the nurse that she has said that she wants to die. He asks the nurse to help "calm her down." The appropriate nursing response is:

1. "All right, I'll talk with her and see if I can comfort her."
2. "If you just sit quietly with her, I'm sure she will calm down when she gets these feelings out."
3. "It's hard to see her so upset, but she needs to let these feelings out; we can both stay with her for a while."
4. "This seems to bother you more than it does her."

1. *INCORRECT. This is not the best option because the nurse is ignoring the son's feelings of distress and is not basing her response on an understanding of the grief process.*
2. *INCORRECT. This option is partially correct in that the nurse recognizes his mother has a need to express her feelings through crying. However, this response does not recognize that the son is having difficulty with his feelings and his understanding of the grief process.*
3. ***CORRECT. The nurse's response acknowledges the son's feelings while also informing him of his mother's need to express her feelings through crying. The nurse is also offering self by offering to stay with both of them.***
4. *INCORRECT. This is not an accurate response. It appears judgmental and is not therapeutic for the son.*

26. A woman is distressed over the death of her husband. The son remarks to the nurse, "My father has been dead for six months now. I think my mother needs to get on with her life." What response from the nurse is appropriate?

1. "A death is usually a crisis for the whole family. How has your father's death affected you?"
2. "I agree. How can you help her find more pleasure in her life?"
3. "I think it would be helpful if you could give her more support."
4. "Perhaps she needs more time. Grieving often takes a year or more to complete."

1. *INCORRECT. This response does not address the son's concerns, so it is not the correct option. This might be an appropriate question for the nurse after she has responded to the son's concern.*
2. *INCORRECT. This response is not appropriate based on current information about the grief process.*
3. *INCORRECT. This response does not recognize the nature of the grief process. It also is not helpful to the son because the nurse does not explain what is meant by "support."*
4. ***CORRECT. This response communicates the correct information that acute grieving often takes one to two years to complete for the loss of a spouse or other loved one.***

27. The nurse observes an elderly depressed client in the day room. The client is shivering. Which response by the nurse would be most helpful to this client?

1. "Come with me to your room, and we will get a sweater for you."
2. "Why do you sit here without a sweater when you are cold?"
3. "What color sweater do you want me to get from your room for you?"
4. "When you are in the day room, you should dress so that you are not cold."

1. ***CORRECT. By volunteering to go with the client to get a sweater, the nurse is communicating therapeutically by offering self.***
2. *INCORRECT. This option uses a "why" question. This is an example of the communication block of requesting an explanation.*
3. *INCORRECT. It would be more therapeutic to assist the client in meeting her own need. Also, the color of the sweater is not significant and making decisions is often difficult for depressed clients.*
4. *INCORRECT. In this option, the nurse is giving advice. Giving advice is not therapeutic.*

28. Soon after being admitted to a rehabilitation unit, a chronic alcoholic says to the nurse, "I don't really need to be here. My wife and family make me drink! My wife spends all my money. My kid just had an accident with his car that will cost me a fortune in repairs!" The therapeutic nursing response is:

1. "Tell me more about how your wife is spending all of your money."
2. "Could you tell me more about why your child's car accident cost you money?"
3. "If sounds like you are having a great deal of financial difficulty."
4. "Tell me more about your feelings about being here in the hospital."

1. *INCORRECT. The client is a chronic alcoholic who is in denial. ("I don't really need to be here.") Before the client can accept help for his problem, he must examine his feelings and acknowledge that he is an alcoholic who needs help. This option focuses on his financial difficulties rather than his feelings.*

> ***TEST-TAKING TIP:*** Options 2 and 3 also focus on financial difficulties; these similar distracters can all be eliminated.

2. *INCORRECT. The client is a chronic alcoholic who is in denial. ("I don't really need to be here.") Before the client can accept help for his problem, he must examine his feelings and acknowledge that he is an alcoholic who needs help. This option focuses on his financial difficulties rather than his feelings.*

> ***TEST-TAKING TIP:*** Options 1, 2 and 3 all focus on financial difficulties; these similar distractors call all be eliminated.

3. *INCORRECT. The client is a chronic alcoholic who is in denial. ("I don't really need to be here.") Before the client can accept help for this problem, he must examine his feelings and acknowledge that he is an alcoholic who needs help. This option focuses on his financial difficulties rather than his feelings.*

> ***TEST-TAKING TIP:*** Options 1, 2 and 3 all focus on financial difficulties; these similar distractors call all be eliminated.

4. ***CORRECT. The client is a chronic alcoholic who is in denial ("I don't really need to be here.") Before the client can accept help for his problem, he must examine his feelings and acknowledge that he is an alcoholic who needs help. This option focuses on the client's feelings about being in the hospital.***

> ***TEST-TAKING TIP:*** Note that the other three options all focus on money and financial difficulties. Options that express the same idea can be eliminated.

29. An elderly client is admitted to the hospital for an exploratory laparotomy. The client's daughter says to the nurse, "I wish I could stay with my father, but I need to go home to see how my children are doing. I really hate to leave my father alone at this time." The most helpful response by the nurse to the daughter is:

1. "Your father needs opportunities to be independent. This will help him become self-sufficient."
2. "Your father is capable of taking care of himself. Try to allow him more independence."
3. "Stress is not good for your father at this time. Perhaps you could call your children."
4. "You are feeling concern for both your dad and your children. Let me know when you are leaving, and I'll stay with him."

1. *INCORRECT. This response is not focused on the client. The client in this question is the daughter, who has shared with the nurse her need to go home to see her children and her reluctance to leave her father. This response is focused on an inappropriate person.*

> ***TEST-TAKING TIP:*** Look for a client-centered option that uses a therapeutic communication tool.

2. *INCORRECT. The client in this question is the daughter who has shared with the nurse her need to go home to see her children and her reluctance to leave her father. This response is focused on the father, not the daughter. It also uses the communication block of giving advice.*

> ***TEST-TAKING TIP:*** Look for a client-centered option that uses a therapeutic communication tool.

3. *INCORRECT. This response is focused on an inappropriate person. The client in this question is the daughter and the issue is her need to go home to check on her children as well as care for her father. There is no data to indicate that the father would find it stressful if his daughter went home, or that his condition requires the daughter to remain constantly at the hospital, This response also uses the communication block of giving advice, and denies the daughter the opportunity to make her own decision and to meet her own needs.*

> ***TEST-TAKING TIP:*** Look for a client-centered option that uses a therapeutic communication tool.

4. ***CORRECT. This option illustrates the tools of showing empathy and offering self. The client in this question is the daughter. The issue is her need to go home to check on her children. This response recognizes her feelings about both her father and her children. In offering to stay with the father while she is away, the nurse if offering self.***

30. A 20-day-old infant is recovering from surgery for pyloric stenosis. The client's mother asked the nurse, "Now that my son has had this surgery, is it likely that pyloric stenosis will cause trouble later?" An appropriate nursing response to the mother would be:

1. "Why don't you talk to the doctor about your uncertainties regarding your son's future."
2. "He might develop obstructive symptoms later. If so, take him immediately to an emergency room."
3. "He will not have symptoms again in childhood, but may have digestive difficulties in his adult life."
4. "Recurrence of the obstruction or repetition of the surgical procedure would be unlikely."

1. *INCORRECT. This is a block that places the client's concerns on hold. An answer to the client's question is within the realm of nursing.*
2. *INCORRECT. This response provides incorrect information. A child who has had a surgical repair of pyloric stenosis is not likely to develop obstructive symptoms later. There is no need to evoke fear in the mother by responding in this way.*
3. *INCORRECT. The words "will not" make this an absolute statement, which is wrong. The primary symptom of pyloric stenosis, projectile vomiting, can be caused by a variety of factors. It is incorrect for the nurse to say that the client will not have this symptom again.*
4. ***CORRECT. This option is the correct answer because the nurse is addressing the client's concern and providing correct information. Following surgical repair of pyloric stenosis, recurrence of the obstruction or the surgical procedure is not expected.***

31. A chronic alcoholic has been hospitalized following a drinking binge. During a lengthy conversation with the nurse about his long history of alcoholism, the client becomes tense and uncomfortable. Which of the following is the initial response by the nurse?

1. "What did I say to make you feel so uncomfortable?"
2. "Drinking for a long time can make anyone feel uncomfortable."
3. "At what point did you begin to feel uncomfortable?"
4. "Talking about your drinking will help you to recover."

1. *INCORRECT. This response is an illustration of the non-therapeutic communication block of focusing on an inappropriate person. The response is focused on the nurse rather than on the client. The nurse is also accepting responsibility for the client's feelings.*
2. *INCORRECT. This response is an assumption by the nurse. The nurse should seek additional information (do an assessment) before stating the cause of the client's feelings.*
3. ***CORRECT. This response illustrates the therapeutic communication tool of clarification. The nurse needs to gather more information about the client's feelings (do an assessment).***
4. *CORRECT. This response illustrates the non-therapeutic communication block of giving advice. It also does not focus on the issue, which is the client's discomfort.*

32. A 62-year-old female has been diagnosed with breast cancer. She has become quiet and thoughtful and says to the nurse, "What do you think people will say about me when I'm gone?" Which response by the nurse is the most helpful to the client?

1. "You will be remembered as a very nice person."
2. "Do you feel that people will be talking about you after your death?"
3. "At this time, a positive attitude can influence your recovery."
4. "The thought of your breast cancer must seem hopeless."

1. *INCORRECT. This response uses the communication block of false reassurance. We have no data to indicate that the nurse would know what others might say about the client. More importantly, how-*

ever, this response is not therapeutic because it does not address the client's feelings of hopelessness.

2. *INCORRECT. This response does not focus on the appropriate issue. The nurse's response should address the client's feelings of hopelessness.*
3. *INCORRECT. This response blocks communication by giving advice. The nurse's response should encourage the client to explore her feelings.*
4. ***CORRECT. This response uses the tool of restatement to focus on the client's feelings of hopelessness. This response is therapeutic because it allows the client to talk about what she has been thinking since she has learned of her diagnosis.***

> ***TEST-TAKING TIP:*** The words "breast cancer" from the introductory statement are repeated in this option. This is a clue that this might be the correct option.

33. A woman is admitted to the ICU on a ventilator after attempting suicide. As the husband is talking with the nurse, he begins to cry. He says, "It's all my fault. I should have been home more often to keep an eye on her." Which response to the husband by the nurse would be most helpful initially?

1. "You seem to regret not being there for your wife. How can you feel that way when you have to earn a living?"
2. "At this time you need your privacy. I will return later, and we can talk then."
3. "This is an important issue that you need to bring up at your family therapy session."
4. "It must have been hard to be away when your wife was so sick."

1. *This response is partly correct, since it begins with the nurse showing empathy for the client. However, the second part of the nurse's response actually rejects the client's feelings and minimizes them, while appearing to show approval for his actions. This response is not therapeutic.*

> ***TEST-TAKING TIP:*** When part of an option is a communication block, the option is incorrect.

2. *INCORRECT. In this response, the nurse abandons the client when he needs to talk about his feelings, putting his feelings on hold. The client's feelings must be dealt with at this time. Remember, the client in this question is the husband.*
3. *INCORRECT. This response puts the client's feelings on hold. The nurse's response should address the client's feelings and encourage him to express them. Remember, the client in this question is the husband.*
4. ***CORRECT. This response shows empathy by showing that the nurse understands the husband's feelings. The husband is the client in this question. Communication theory identifies that the nurse must address his feelings first. Note that Options 1, 2, and 3 put the client's feelings on hold.***

34. A hospitalized client says to the nurse, "I'm a terrible person, and I should be dead." Which response by the nurse would be appropriate initially?

1. "That is why you are here. We are trying to help you with your bad feelings."
2. "Feeling that way must be awful. What makes you feel so terrible?"
3. "Feeling like a terrible person is part of your illness. As you get better, those feelings will lessen."
4. "You are not terrible. You are not a bad person."

1. *INCORRECT. The client did not ask why she is here, so this question addresses an inappropriate issue. More importantly, this response appears to support the client's feelings that she is a terrible person. In addition, the second part of the response also blocks therapeutic communication by focusing on inappropriate persons—the nurse and others who "are trying to help" the client. This response is not therapeutic.*
2. ***CORRECT. This response shows empathy, and then seeks clarification of the client's feelings. These two communication tools combine to make a therapeutic response that allows the client to talk about her feelings.***
3. *INCORRECT. This response does give the client information about her illness, but the client's feelings must be addressed before information is given. When a client is distressed and upset, giving an explanation is inappropriate.*

> ***TEST-TAKING TIP:*** Look for an option that addresses the client's feelings and uses a therapeutic communication tool.

4. *INCORRECT. In this response, the nurse is giving a personal opinion. The nurse's opinion is not important! This response blocks therapeutic communication by putting the nurse in the role of an authority figure, using false reassurance, and devaluing the client's feelings. The nurse's response should encourage the client to explore her feelings with the nurse.*

> ***TEST-TAKING TIP:*** Look for an option that addresses the client's feelings and uses a therapeutic communication tool.

35. An elderly client with Alzheimer's disease is admitted to the hospital. His daughter says to the nurse, "I really feel guilty about leaving my father, but I need to go home." The most helpful response by the nurse to the daughter is:

1. "Your father is well cared for here."
2. "Your worried feelings are normal."
3. "When you are getting ready to leave, tell me. I will sit with your father."
4. "Can I call another family member to stay with him?"

1. *INCORRECT. This response blocks therapeutic communication by using cliché and false reassurance. Remember, the client in this test question is the daughter! The nurse's response should address the feelings and concerns that the daughter has shared with the nurse.*
2. *INCORRECT. This is an example of the communication block of cliché and false reassurance, which*

devalues the client's feelings. Also, this response incorrectly identifies the client's feelings as "worry," and it does not address the client's concern about leaving her father.

3. ***CORRECT. The daughter is the client in this test question. The nurse addresses the daughter's concern about leaving her father by her offer to help the daughter by sitting with the father. The nurse is using the therapeutic communication tool of offering self.***
4. *INCORRECT. There is no information that the father's condition requires the daughter or other family member to remain with him at the hospital. It is very important to note that the daughter is the client in this question. The nurse's response must be therapeutic for the daughter. This response uses the communication block of referring to inappropriate persons—the "other family members." In addition, by suggesting getting someone else to sit with the father, the nurse may make the daughter feel all the more guilty about leaving. This response is not therapeutic for the client.*

NOTES

Chapter 13

REVIEW OF TEST-TAKING STRATEGIES FOR THE NCLEX

Section I: Preparing for the NCLEX

A. What You Should Know About the NCLEX-RN Exam
   1. General information
      a. The first integrated exam was given in July 1982
      b. The purpose of the exam is to determine that a candidate is prepared to practice nursing safely
      c. The exam is designed to test essential knowledge of nursing and a candidate's ability to apply that knowledge to clinical situations
      d. The purpose of the new test plan is to bring the exam in line with current nursing behaviors (the nursing process and decision making)
      e. Exam is "pass/fail," and no other score is given
   2. Computerized Adaptive Testing
      a. Computer program continuously scores answers and selects questions suitable for each candidate's competency level for a more precise measurement of competency
      b. A higher weight is assigned to difficult questions so a passing score can be obtained by answering a lot of easier questions-or a smaller number of more difficult questions
      c. Special screen design is used
      d. Use the mouse to move the cursor on the screen to the desired location. Double-click your mouse to select an option as your answer.
      e. A drop-down calculator also is featured. Double-click your mouse

on the calculator icon, and the drop-down calculator will appear.

3. Exam schedule
   a. Given year-round
   b. May only take a single exam in one day
   c. Retake policy: not more than once in a three month period, with a maximum of four times in one year
4. Number of questions and time allowed
   a. No minimum amount of time; however, a candidate must answer a minimum of 75 test questions
   b. Maximum time is five hours, with a maximum of 265 test questions
   c. About one out of three candidates completes the exam in less than two hours; one in three will use the complete five hours
   d. The computer will automatically stop as soon as one of the following occurs:
      1) Candidate's measure of competency is determined to be above or below the passing standard
      2) Candidate has answered all 265 test questions
      3) Maximum amount of time (five hours) has expired
5. A candidate will pass by either:
   a. Answering 75 to 265 questions above the passing standard (the required weighted score) for all questions answered, within the time allowed; or
   b. Answering at least 75 questions within the time allowed and achieving the passing standard for the last 60 questions answered

SCREEN DESIGN

On the psychiatric unit, a nurse observes a client standing near a window and touching the glass. The client also mutters from time to time. Which comment by the nurse indicates the best understanding of the client's behavior?

1. "Why are you standing by the window and touching the glass?"
2. "There you are. I came to see if you wanted to see the video we are showing on the unit?"
3. "What are you looking at through the window?"
4. "Are you hearing voices or seeing things?"

Case Scenario and Stem

Choices 1, 2, 3, and 4

6. Types of questions
   a. All questions are multiple choice
      1) Each question has four options
      2) The best option is the only correct answer
   b. Exam includes 15 unmarked experimental or "try-out" questions
7. Exam procedure:
   a. Look for the BEST answer to each question
   b. It is not possible to skip questions or return to previous questions
   c. Mandatory 10-minute break after first two hours and after another one-and-one-half hours
   d. Scratch paper provided for calculations must be returned at end of exam
8. Structure of the test plan *
   a. Safe, Effective Care Environment
      1) Coordinated of Care 7-13%
      2) Safety and Infection Control 5-11%
   b. Health Promotion and Maintenance
      1) Growth and Development Through the Lifespan 7-13%
      2) Prevention and Early Detection of Disease 5-11%
   c. Psychosocial Integrity
      1) Coping and Adaptation 5-11%
      2) Psychosocial Adaptation 5-11%
   d. Physiological Integrity
      1) Basic Care and Comfort 7-13%
      2) Pharmacological Therapies 5-11%
      3) Reduction of Risk Potential 12-18%
      4) Physiological Adaptation 12-18%

      **Information courtesy of the National Council of State Boards Nursing, Inc., Test Plan 2003.*

B. Schedule Your Study Time
   1. The minimum time for preparation is two hours a day for six to eight weeks
      a. Spend 1/3 of your time reviewing content
      b. Spend 2/3 of your time answering test questions
   2. For content review, use an NCLEX-RN exam review book such as this one, which outlines content
   3. Begin with areas that are most difficult for you, or the areas that are least familiar

4. For more detailed information on your difficult or less familiar areas, use a good nursing reference manual
5. Review medical-surgical, pediatric, women's health, and psychiatric nursing, as well as nursing management and alternate test item formats
6. Use a body systems approach for medical-surgical and pediatric nursing areas
7. When studying body systems and the associated diseases, remember to:
   a. Define the disease in terms of the pathophysiological process that is occurring
   b. Identify the client's early and late manifestations
   c. Identify the most important or life-threatening complications
   d. Define the medical treatment
   e. Identify and prioritize the nursing interventions associated with early and late manifestations
   f. Identify what the nurse teaches the client/family to prevent or adapt to disease
8. To schedule your study time:
   a. List the areas you need to review
   b. Count the number of days you have available to study
   c. Estimate the amount of time needed for each area
   d. On your calendar, write the area to review, the number of questions to answer, and the amount of time needed for each study day

C. Answer Many Questions
1. Answering questions will develop your test-taking skills
2. Use questions similar to those on the NCLEX exam
3. Answer a minimum of 3,000 test questions
4. Include answering test questions in your study plan. For example, answer 100 questions each day for a month.
5. If you are at high risk, answer 5,000 test questions
6. Use at least three different question-and-answer books, including MEDS Publishing's *Complete Q&A for the NCLEX-RN* with CD-ROM
7. Using a variety of books provides a more comprehensive preparation

D. Assess Your Progress
1. Each time you answer questions, check the number of questions you answered correctly
   a. If you answer less than 65% correctly, this is a warning signal! Spend lots of time reviewing content and answering more questions in this area of nursing.
   b. If you answer 65 to 75% correctly, your performance is average. Success in this area is uncertain. Continue working with this content

until your score is above 75%. Work on building your confidence by answering more questions in this area.

c. If you answer 75 to 85% correctly, your performance is very good. Only return to this area after you have at least 75% in all other areas. Feel confident.

d. If you answer 85 to 95% correctly, your performance is superior. Don't waste time on this. Feel very confident.

2. For each wrong answer, identify why you answered wrong
   a. You may have answered a question wrong because you did not know the facts or got confused about the information
      1) Identify this as a content weakness
      2) Review the content again
   b. You may have answered a question wrong because you misread the question, did not understand what it was asking, or did not know how to select the best answer
      1) Identify this as a test-taking deficiency
      2) For further assistance with test-taking deficiencies, we recommend MEDS test-taking book, *Test Question Logic for the NCLEX-RN Exam.*
3. Check the number of questions that you identified as difficult and went back to answer later. See how many of them you answered correctly.

Section II: Answering Questions

A. Identify the Critical Elements in the Question
   1. Identify the issue in the question
      a. The issue is the problem about which the question is asking
      b. The issue may be a:
         1) Drug: for example, digoxin (*Lanoxin*), furosemide (*Lasix*)
         2) Nursing problem: for example, alteration in comfort, potential for infection
         3) Behavior: for example, restlessness, agitation
         4) Disorder: for example, diabetes mellitus, ulcerative colitis
         5) Procedure: for example, glucose tolerance test, cardiac catheterization
   2. Identify the client in the question
      a. The client in the question is usually the person with the health problem
      b. The client in a test question may also be a relative or significant other or another member of the health care team with whom the nurse is interacting

   c. The correct answer to the question must relate to the client in the question
3. Look for the key words
   a. Key words focus attention on what is important
   b. Key words may appear in bold print
   c. Examples:
      1) During the early period, which of the following nursing procedures would be **best**?
      2) The nurse would expect to find which of the following characteristics in an **adult** diabetic?
      3) Which of the following nursing actions is **vital**?
      4) Which of the following nursing actions would be best **initially**?
4. Identify what the stem is asking and determine whether the question has a true response stem or false response stem
   a. Be clear about what the stem is asking before you look at the options
   b. If the question is not clear to you, rephrase it using your own words
   c. Determine whether the question has a true response stem or a false response stem
      1) True response stem
         a) Definition: A true response stem requires an answer that is a true statement
         b) Examples:
            (1) Which of these interpretations is most justifiable?
            (2) The nurse would demonstrate best judgment by taking which of the following actions?
            (3) The chief purpose of the drug is to:
            (4) The nurse should give immediate consideration to which of the following findings?
      2) False response stem
         a) Definition: A false response stem requires an answer that is a false statement
         b) Examples:
            (1) Which of the following nursing actions would be inappropriate?
            (2) Which of the following statements by the client would indicate a need for further instruction?
            (3) Which of the following describes incorrect placement of the hands during CPR?
            (4) Which of the following actions would place the client at risk?

B. Use a Selection Procedure to Eliminate Incorrect Options
   1. Most NCLEX questions have four options. The correct answer is the BEST answer. The other three options are "distractors."
   2. Distractors are options made to look like correct answers. They are intended to distract you from answering correctly.
   3. As you read each of the four options, make a decision about it.
      a. This option is true (+)
      b. This option is false (–)
      c. I am not sure about this option (?)
   4. If the stem is a true response stem:
      a. An option that is true (+) might be the correct answer
      b. An option that is false (–) is a distractor. Eliminate this option
      c. An option that you are not sure about (?) is possibly the correct answer
   5. If the stem is a false response stem:
      a. An option that is true (+) is a distractor. Eliminate this option.
      b. An option that is false (–) may be the correct answer
      c. An option that you are not sure about (?) is possibly the correct answer
   6. Do not return to options you have eliminated
   7. If you are left with one option, that is your answer
   8. If you are left with one (+) option and one (?) option, select the (+) option as your answer
   9. If you are left with two (+) options, use strategies to select the best answer

C. Use Test-Taking Strategies When You Are Unable to Select the Best Option
   1. The Global Response Strategy
      a. A global response is a general statement that may include ideas of other options within it
      b. Look for a global response when more than one option appears to be correct
      c. The global response option will probably be the correct answer
   2. The Similar Distractors Strategy
      a. Similar distractors say basically the same thing using different words
      b. Since there is only one correct answer in a question, similar distractors must be wrong
      c. Eliminate similar distractors. Select for your answer an option that is different.

3. The Similar Word or Phrase Strategy
   a. When more than one option appears to be correct, look for a similar word or phrase in the stem of the question and in one of the four options
   b. The option that contains the similar word or phrase may be the correct answer
   c. Use this strategy after you have tried to identify a global response option and eliminated similar distractors

D. Answering Communication Questions
1. The NCLEX exam includes many communication questions because the ability to communicate therapeutically is essential for safe practice
2. Identify the critical elements as in all questions. Pay particular attention to identification of the client in the question. Remember that the answer must relate to the client.
3. Learn to identify communication tools that enhance communication.
   a. Being silent: Nonverbal communication
   b. Offering self: "Let me sit with you."
   c. Showing empathy: "You are upset."
   d. Focusing: "You say that . . ."
   e. Restatement: "You feel anxious?"
   f. Validation/clarification: "What you are saying is . . .?"
   g. Giving information: "Your room is 423."
   h. Dealing with the here and now: "At this time, the problem is . . ."
4. Learn to identify non-therapeutic communication blocks.
   a. Giving advice: "If I were you, I would . . ."
   b. Showing approval/disapproval: "You did the right thing."
   c. Using clichés and false reassurances: "Don't worry. It will be all right."
   d. Requesting an explanation: "Why did you do that?"
   e. Devaluing client feelings: "Don't be concerned. It's not a problem."
   f. Being defensive: "Every nurse on this unit is exceptional."
   g. Focusing on inappropriate issues or persons: "Have I said something wrong?"
   h. Placing the client's issues "on hold": "Talk to your doctor about that."
5. When answering communication questions, select an option that illustrates a therapeutic communication tool. Eliminate options that illustrate non-therapeutic communication blocks.

E. Answering Questions that Focus on Setting Priorities
1. Priority-setting questions ask the test taker to identify either what comes first, is most important, or gets the highest priority

2. Examples:
   a. What is the nurse's initial response?
   b. The nurse should give immediate consideration to which of the following?
   c. Which nursing action receives the highest priority?
   d. What should the nurse do first?
3. Use guidelines to help you to answer priority setting questions
   a. Maslow's Hierarchy of Needs indicates that physiological needs come first
   b. Maslow's Hierarchy of Needs indicates that when no physiological need is identified, safety needs come first
   c. Nursing Process indicates that assessment comes first
   d. Communication Theory indicates focusing on feelings first
   e. Teaching/Learning Theory indicates focusing on motivation first

Section III: Preparing for Exam Time

A. Plan for Everything
   1. Assemble everything you will need for the exam the night before:
      a. Identification: two IDs with signatures, including one with recent photograph
      b. Watch
      c. Several sharpened pencils (with erasers) for calculations
   2. Plan to arrive at the test site early:
      a. Know the route to the exam site
      b. Know how long it will take to get there
      c. Know where you will park and if you will need coins for a parking meter
   3. Pay close attention to your own physiological needs:
      a. Dress in layers
      b. Get a good night's sleep the night before the exam
      c. Eat a good breakfast
      d. Avoid stimulants and depressants
      e. Use the bathroom just before the exam
   4. During the exam:
      a. Listen to the instructions
      b. Pace yourself; don't spend too long on any one question
      c. Don't let yourself become distracted. Focus your attention on answering the questions.

d. Go with your first choice. Use test-taking strategies only when you cannot decide between close options.
e. Keep your thoughts positive!

B. Manage Your Anxiety Level
1. Moderate levels of anxiety increase your effectiveness
2. Don't cram the night before the exam
3. Do something enjoyable and relaxing the night before the exam
4. Learn and practice measures to manage your anxiety level during the exam as needed
   a. Take a few deep breaths
   b. Tense and relax muscles
   c. Tell yourself positive affirmations
   d. Visualize a peaceful scene
   e. Visualize your success

C. Test-Taking Tips
1. Prepare comprehensively and be sure to be well rested for the exam
2. Read each question carefully, identifying the critical elements. Each question must be answered in sequence, and you may not skip or go back to change your answers to any questions.
3. Don't panic if the computer stops after a short time! It does not mean that you failed. The computer stops when the exam is able to determine with at least 95% certainty that you have demonstrated the ability, or inability, to practice safely at the minimal level of nursing competency.
4. It is helpful to know that most students pass by answering a maximum of all 265 questions.
5. If you are having difficulty choosing between the best two options, use the three test-taking strategies you learned in this review:
   a. Look for the global response option
   b. Eliminate similar distractors
   c. Look for similar words in the question and one of the options
6. You should anticipate that the test questions will increase in difficulty
7. Use your scratch paper wisely. Since you cannot review earlier questions to help recall previous facts, use the scratch paper provided for calculations to remember facts from previous questions. Sometimes, information from one question is helpful in answering another question.
8. Don't panic if someone finishes before you! The test adapts to each candidate's level of ability, and it means that you may take longer to prove that you are capable of practicing competently at the beginning level of nursing.
9. Keep a positive attitude! Remember that you have learned a great amount of nursing knowledge, and the exam is only designed to determine whether you are able to practice safely at the entry level.

Chapter 14

NCLEX ALTERNATE TEST ITEM FORMATS

Section I: Overview

A. NCLEX Item Types
   1. Standard Multiple Choice Question
      a. Traditionally, the format of NCLEX questions
      b. Still the most commonly seen type of question on the NCLEX
      c. Has four options, only one of which is correct ("one best option")
      d. Mastering this format is critical to your success on the NCLEX.
   2. As of April 2003, the NCLEX started including items other than standard multiple choice questions. These items are known as Alternate Test Item Formats.
      a. Fill-in-the-Blank
         1) Calculation
         2) Sequence
      b. Multiple Response
      c. Hot Spot
      d. Charts, Tables, Graphic Images
   3. The average standard question takes 60 to 70 seconds to answer.
   4. The average candidate will be administered only one or two of these alternate items.

POINTS TO REMEMBER:

You should allot a slightly longer time for alternate test items.

Section II: Fill-in-the-Blank

A. Overview
   1. Definition: Fill-in-the-blank items are a type of alternate item that will be primarily numerical. This type of question typically involves either solving a math problem or putting a list of options into the correct sequence.
   2. Method of Answer: To answer these questions, you will need to type a number into the answer box on the screen.

B. Types
   1. Calculation item
      a. This type of fill-in-the-blank question typically involves solving a math problem.
      b. Method of Answer: To answer these questions, you will need to type a number into the answer box on the screen.
      c. Read the question carefully. If you see the question is asking for the answer in a specific unit amount, it is not necessary to put units in your answer.

POINTS TO REMEMBER:

1. Write equation down on your scrap paper.
2. Be certain you are solving for the correct unit value!
3. Show all of your work.
4. Bring up drop-down calculator.
5. Double-check your work

GRAPHIC 14-1.
FILL-IN-THE-BLANK CALCULATION ITEM

There are 13 clients being seen in the emergency room and 5 clients in the waiting room. What is the total number of clients?

Type your answer in the box below.

18

2. Sequence item
   a. This type of fill-in-the-blank question requires you to put a list of options into the correct order.
   b. Method of Answer: To answer these questions, you will need to type a series of numbers into the answer box on the screen.
   c. Read the question carefully. Sequence items on the NCLEX may require you to put the options in the order that you would perform them, or in order of priority.
   d. It is not necessary to separate the numbers in any way, so do not insert spaces, dashes, commas, slashes or any other spacing device between the numbers.

POINTS TO REMEMBER:

Remember that there is only one correct sequence that preserves the client's safety at all stages during the procedure.

GRAPHIC 14-2.
FILL-IN-THE-BLANK SEQUENCE ITEM

Put the following words in alphabetical order.

1. Pizza
2. Apples
3. Onion
4. Bacon
5. Rice

Type your answer in the box below.

24315

Section III: Multiple Response

A. Overview
   1. Definition: Multiple response items are a type of alternate item that require you to choose more than one answer from up to six options. Any number of the options may be correct.
   2. Method of Answer: To answer these questions, you will need to click on all the answers that apply.
   3. On the NCLEX, you will receive credit only for completely correct answers; there is no "partial credit" given for these item types.

POINTS TO REMEMBER:

Consider each response as you would a true-false question; is that statement true about the question or false? Click on all that you determine are true.

GRAPHIC 14-3.
MULTIPLE RESPONSE ITEM

Which of the following are types of vegetables?

Select all that apply.

- [x] 1. Broccoli
- [x] 2. Cucumber
- [ ] 3. Peach
- [ ] 4. Orange
- [ ] 5. Grape

Section IV: Hot Spot

A. Overview

1. Definition: Hot spot items are a type of alternate item that will be a "point and click" exercise. Hot spot items will usually require you to identify an anatomical location on a figure.
2. Method of Answer: To answer these questions, you will need to point at an area on the screen with your cursor and click on the correct spot. As you move your mouse around the screen, you will see an arrow. Once you select a spot and click, the arrow will change into a circle with an "X" in it.
3. Read the question carefully, then analyze the image.
4. The NCLEX will allow you to reclick as many times as necessary.

POINTS TO REMEMBER:

It is very important to remember that the screen is NOT a mirror image! If you see that the question is asking for an answer on the right or left side of the body, make sure you are clicking on the correct side.

GRAPHIC 14-4.
HOT SPOT ITEM

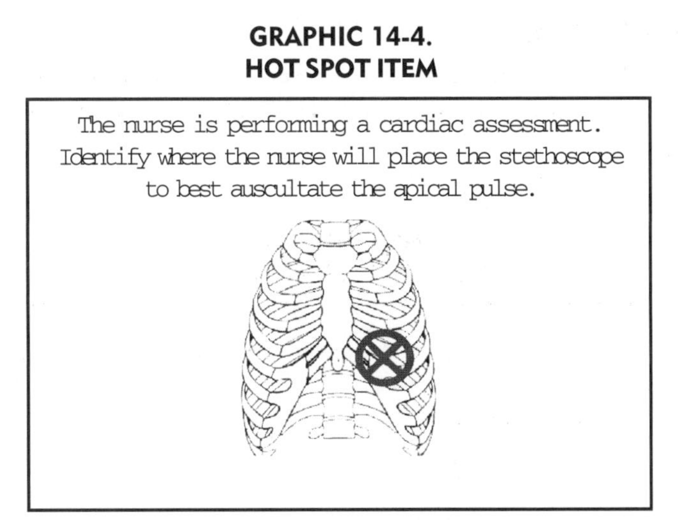

Section V: Charts, Tables, & Graphic Images

A. Overview
   1. Any of the NCLEX standard multiple choice or alternate items may also include charts, tables or other graphic images that you must analyze and understand in order to correctly answer the question.
   2. It is important that you read the question carefully first, then analyze the image.

GRAPHIC 14-5.
CHARTS, TABLES, GRAPHIC IMAGES ITEM

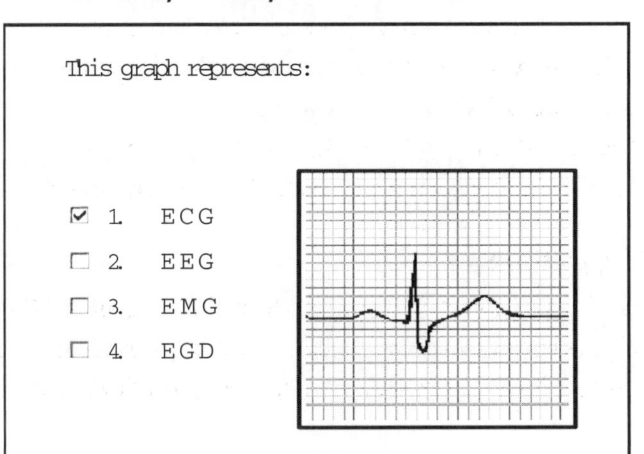